Endometriosis in Clinical Practice

Endometriosis in Clinical Practice

Edited by

David L. Olive
Chief of Reproductive Endocrinology
Department of Obstetrics and Gynecology
University of Wisconsin/Madison
Madison, WI, USA

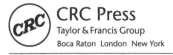

CRC Press
Taylor & Francis Group
Boca Raton London New York

CRC Press is an imprint of the
Taylor & Francis Group, an **informa** business

© 2005 Taylor & Francis, an imprint of the Taylor & Francis Group

First published in the United Kingdom in 2005
by Taylor & Francis, an imprint of the Taylor & Francis Group,
2 Park Square, Milton Park, Abingdon, Oxfordshire OX14 4RN

Tel.:   +44 (0) 1235 828600
Fax.:   +44 (0) 1235 829000
E-mail: info@dunitz.co.uk
Website: http://www.dunitz.co.uk

Although every effort has been made to ensure that all owners of
copyright material have been acknowledged in this publication, we would
be glad to acknowledge in subsequent reprints or editions any omissions
brought to our attention.

A CIP record for this book is available from the British Library.

Library of Congress Cataloging-in-Publication Data

Data available on application

ISBN 1 84214 343 1

Distributed in North and South America by
Taylor & Francis
2000 NW Corporate Blvd
Boca Raton, FL 33431, USA

Within Continental USA
Tel.: 800 272 7737; Fax.: 800 374 3401
Outside Continental USA
Tel.: 561 994 0555; Fax.: 561 361 6018
E-mail: orders@crcpress.com

Distributed in the rest of the world by
Thomson Publishing Services
Cheriton House
North Way
Andover, Hampshire SP10 5BE, UK
Tel.: +44 (0)1264 332424
E-mail: salesorder.tandf@thomsonpublishingservices.co.uk

Composition by EXPO Holdings, Malaysia

Printed and bound in Spain by Grafos SA

Contents

Contents

List of Contributors

Sanober Amin
Department of Obstetrics and Gynecology
Division of Reproductive Biology Research
Northwestern University
303 East Chicago Ave
Tarry 13-764
Chicago, Il 60611, USA

Aydin Arici M.D.
Department of Obstetrics and Gynecology
Yale University School of Medicine
333 Cedar Street
PO Box 208063
New Haven, CT 06520-8063, USA

Kaylon L. Bruner-Tran M.D.
Women's Reproductive Health Research Center,
Vanderbilt University, B-1100 MCN 2519
Nashville, TN 37232-2519, USA

John D. Buek M.D.
Dept of Obstetrics and Gynecology
Georgetown University Hospital
3800 Reservoir Road
Washington DC 20007, USA

Serdar E. Bulun M.D.
Chief, Division of Reproductive Biology Research
Department of Obstetrics and Gynecology
Feinberg School of Medicine
Northwestern University
333 E. Superior St., Suite 484
Chicago, IL 60611, USA

Daniel W. Cramer M.D., Sc.D.
Ob/Gyn Epidemiology Center
Department of Obstetrics, Gynecology and
Reproductive Biology
Brigham and Women's Hospital
221 Longwood Avenue
Boston, MA 02115, USA

Sanatu Deb M.D.
Department of Obstetrics and Gynecology
Division of Reproductive Biology Research
Northwestern University
303 East Chicago Ave
Tarry 13-764
Chicago, Il 60611, USA

Thomas D'Hooghe M.D., Ph.D.
Leuven University Fertility Center
Department of Obstetrics and Gynecology
University Hospital Gasthuisberg
3000 Leuven, Belgium
and
Institute of Primate Research
Department of Reproduction
Nairobi, Kenya

Henrik Falconer M.D.
Division of Obstetrics and Gynecology
Department of Women and Child Health
Karolinska Hospital
Stockholm, Sweden
and
Institute of Primate Research
Department of Reproduction
Nairobi, Kenya

Zongjuan Fang M.D.
Department of Obstetrics and Gynecology
University of Illinois at Chicago
820 Polk Street
Chicago, IL 60612, USA

Bilgin Gurates M.D.
Firat University
Department of Obstetrics and Gynecology
Division of Reproductive Endocrinology and
Infertility
Elazig, Turkey

Daniela Hornung M.D., Ph.D.
Department of Obstetrics and Gynecology
University of Schleswig-Holstein, Campus
Luebeck
Ratzburgerallee 160
23538 Luebeck, Germany

Gonca Imir M.D.
Department of Obstetrics and Gynecology
Division of Reproductive Biology Research
Northwestern University
303 East Chicago Ave
Tarry 13-764
Chicago, Il 60611, USA

Crispin Jenkinson D.Phil.
Health Services Research Unit
Department of Public Health and Primary
Care
University of Oxford
Old Road Campus
Headington
Oxford OX3 7LF, UK

Umit Kayisli Ph.D.
Department of Obstetrics and Gynecology
Yale University School of Medicine
333 Cedar Street
PO Box 208063
New Haven, CT 06520-8063, USA
and
Department of Histology and Embryology
Akdeniz University School of Medicine
07070 Antalya, Turkey

Stephen Kennedy M.D.
Nuffield Department of Obstetrics and
Gynecology
University of Oxford
John Radcliffe Hospital
Oxford OX3 9DU, UK

Pinar H. Kodaman M.D., Ph.D.
Department of Obstetrics, Gynecology and
Reproductive Sciences
Yale University School of Medicine
333 Cedar Street
PO Box 208063
New Haven, CT 06520-8063, USA

David Langoi M.D.
Department of Obstetrics and Gynecology
University of Illinois at Chicago
820 Polk Street
Chicago, IL 60612, USA

Steven R. Lindheim M.D.
Reproductive Endocrinology and Infertility
Department of Obstetrics and Gynecology
University of Wisconsin Medical School
H4-628 Clinical Science Center
600 Highland Ave
Madison, WI 53792-6188, USA

Timothy S. Loy M.D.
Department of Pathology and Anatomical Sciences
University of Missouri Health Center
One Hospital Drive
Columbia, MO 65212, USA

Neal G. Mahutte M.D.
Reproductive Endocrinology and Fertility
Dartmouth Medical School
One Medical Center Drive
Lebanon, NH 03756, USA

Enda McVeigh M.D.
Nuffield Department of Obstetrics and Gynecology
Level 3, Women's Centre
John Radcliffe Hospital
Oxford OX3 9DU, UK

Stacey A. Missmer Sc.D.
Ob/Gyn Epidemiology Center
Department of Obstetrics, Gynecology and
Reproductive Biology
Brigham and Women's Hospital
221 Longwood Avenue
Boston, MA 02115, USA

Jason M. Mwenda
Institute of Primate Research
Department of Reproduction
Nairobi, Kenya

David L. Olive M.D.
Chief of Reproductive Endocrinology
Department of Obstetrics and Gynecology
University of Wisconsin/Madison
CSC, H4/630
600 Highland Ave
Madison, WI 53792-6188, USA

Kevin G. Osteen Ph.D., H.C.L.D.
Women's Reproductive Health Research Center,
Vanderbilt University, B-1100 MCN 2519
Nashville, TN 37232-2519, USA

Elizabeth Pritts M.D.
Department of Obstetrics and Gynecology
University of Wisconsin Medical School
CSC, H4/628
600 Highland Avenue
Madison, WI 53792, USA

Lisa Story M.D.
Department of Obstetrics and Gynecology
John Radcliffe Hospital
Oxford OX3 9DU, UK

Eric S. Surrey M.D.
Colorado Center for Reproductive Medicine
799 East Hampden Avenue, Suite 300
Englewood, CO 80110, USA

Misutoshi Tamura M.D.
Tohoku University
Graduate School of Medicine
Department of Obstetrics and Gynecology
1-1 Seiryou-machi
Aboa-ku
Sendai 980-8574, Japan

Hugh S. Taylor M.D.
Division of Reproductive Endocrinology and
Infertility
Department of Obstetrics, Gynecology and
Reproductive Sciences
Yale University School of Medicine
333 Cedar Street, New Haven, CT 06520, USA

Nik Taylor D.Phil.
Department of Obstetrics and Gynecology
John Radcliffe Hospital
Oxford OX3 9DU, UK

Sijun Yang M.D.
Department of Obstetrics and Gynecology
Division of Reproductive Biology Research
Northwestern University
303 East Chicago Ave
Tarry 13-764
Chicago, Il 60611, USA

Bertan Yilmaz
Department of Obstetrics and Gynecology
Division of Reproductive Biology Research
Northwestern University
303 East Chicago Avenue
Tarry 13-764
Chicago, IL 60611, USA

Steven L. Young M.D., Ph.D.
Department of Obstetrics and Gynecology
University of North Carolina at Chapel Hill
Chapell Hill
NC 27599-7570, USA

Craig A. Winkel M.D.
Dept of Obstetrics and Gynecology
Georgetown University Hospital
3800 Reservoir Road
Washington DC 20007, USA

Craig A. Witz M.D.
Obstetrics and Gynecology
University of Texas Health Science Center at San
Antonio
7703 Floyd Curl Drive, MSC 7836
San Antonio, TX 78229, USA

Preface

As a medical student in 1977, working with Dr Robert Franklin in Houston, I was first introduced to a disease called endometriosis. It seemed an odd disorder at the time, for it was being blamed for a number of different symptoms in the women I saw: pain of all sorts, infertility, fatigue, gastrointestinal upset, even psychological disorders. The frequency with which I encountered endometriosis was astounding; the variety of effects it was associated with seemed perplexing.

In those early years of my career I asked many questions about endometriosis, but few good answers were forthcoming. I began performing simple retrospective investigations at that point in an attempt to better decipher the mysteries of this disorder, and I scoured the literature to learn what others had found. Unfortunately, I discovered that when it came to endometriosis, knowledge had taken a back seat to passion and belief. Although rigorous clinical and basic research principles were finding their way into investigation of many diseases, this was not the case with endometriosis where studies were poorly constructed, analysis was simplistic and incomplete, and conclusions were frequently unsupported by data.

Fortunately, times change. A quarter of a century later the amount of quality research involving endometriosis is orders of magnitude greater than in my youth. However, all too often these 'breakthroughs' are lost amid the high volume of publications in today's medical literature. Furthermore, updated knowledge often has difficulty displacing longstanding dogma in the minds of practicing clinicians. As an investigator, I had been of the opinion that providing scientific information was the key to altering practice patterns. What I have learned is that the modern researcher must do more than publish; he/she must also place the new information in context, revise existing mythologies, and publicize the new theoretical construct surrounding a disease.

This book is an attempt to do exactly that. I have tried to assemble a group of experts in their areas to provide the most current information available and to piece these bits of information together, when possible, into a coherent story. Clearly there are holes in our understanding, and surely we have on occasion drawn incorrect conclusions from available data, but overall the message is clear: we are making tremendous headway into understanding and treating this disease. Should we continue to make such progress, I believe that in short order endometriosis will be a disease that is well understood and easily treated. While that may put many of this book's authors out of business, it will represent a major victory for the health of women. It is to this hope that I offer *Endometriosis in Clinical Practice*.

David L. Olive

To my parents Jerald and Leah, who dedicated a piece of their lives to make me the person I am today.
To my wife Elizabeth, whose partnership and love for me keep me focused and grounded.
To my sons Zachary, Matthew, and Alexander, and their pursuit of happiness and success.
It is to each of you that I dedicate this book.

1. Normal Cycling Endometrium: Molecular, Cellular, and Histologic Perspectives

Steven L. Young and Timothy S. Loy

The primary functions of the human endometrium are to allow the implantation of a normal embryo and provide mechanisms for the clearance of tissue and hemostasis at menstruation. At the same time, the endometrium must also provide a defense against invasion by potential pathogens and prevent the implantation of an abnormal embryo. In order to achieve these functions, the endometrium undergoes profound changes in structure and function during each cycle that result in defined periods of proliferation, embryo receptivity, and menstruation. The cyclic structural changes are evident on every level of examination, from gross inspection to electron microscopy. Both structural and functional changes are the result of changes in the molecular components of each cell, whereas a lack of appropriate cyclic changes is thought to underlie many common disorders, including abnormal uterine bleeding, infertility, endometriosis, and endometrial cancer. Therefore, a thorough understanding of the molecular and cellular alterations of the endometrium across the cycle should provide new approaches to the prevention, diagnosis, and treatment of endometrial disorders.

Considering that implantation of the embryo is fundamental to the survival of every human being at the earliest stage of his or her existence as an individual, it is remarkable that our current understanding of the molecular and cellular biology of the endometrium remains modest. Clearly, ethical and moral issues present significant hurdles to scientific inquiries into human embryo implantation, but an understanding of molecular and cell biology of the menstrual and immune functions of the endometrium also remains surprisingly incomplete. This chapter will provide an overview of the tissue, cellular, and molecular architecture of the endometrium, with an emphasis on changes across the cycle.

ENDOMETRIAL STRUCTURE – CELL TYPES

The endometrium is composed of multiple cell types, including epithelium, stroma, resident bone-marrow-derived immunocompetent cells, and blood vessel endothelium (Figure 1.1).

EPITHELIUM

The endometrial epithelium, embryonically derived from müllerian duct epithelium, forms a continuous layer, some of which is in direct contact with the uterine lumen (luminal) and some of which lines thin, glandular invaginations of the lumen (glandular). The luminal epithelium consists of both ciliated and non-ciliated cells, whose relative number and morphology change over the cycle.

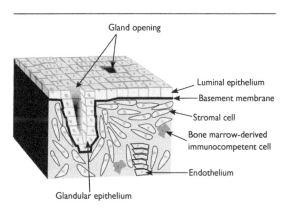

Figure 1.1 Structural organization of human endometrium.

The luminal epithelium is the first endometrial cell type to encounter an implanting embryo and the first cell type to encounter ascending foreign cells, including sperm and microbes. Thus, luminal epithelial cells must be immunologically unresponsive to foreign sperm, allow invasion by a normal embryo, and prevent invasion by abnormal embryos and foreign microbes. The luminal barrier to invasion is multifaceted and includes tight junctions between epithelial cells as well as specific apical membrane proteins and glycocalyx. During the embryo-receptive phase, the luminal epithelium undergoes a loss of apical–basal polarity, alterations in tight junction and cytoskeletal architecture, and thinning of the basal lamina. These structural changes are probably responsible, in part for increased trophoblast adhesion and the ability of trophoblasts to invade.[1–4]

Although the epithelial barrier to invasion is an important facet of endometrial defense, the barrier is probably weakened during implantation and certainly by menstruation. Also, the endometrium, like other mucosal surfaces, must detect potentially pathogenic microorganisms as early as possible to allow appropriate innate and adaptive responses. The immunologic problem of tolerating the presence of foreign sperm and invasion by a semi-foreign embryo while protecting against invasion by microbes and abnormal embryos was first recognized by the transplant immunologist Medawar over 50 years ago.[5] To date, however, the mechanisms by which the endometrium accomplishes this immunologic feat remain an active subject of investigation.

The glandular epithelial cells, as the name implies, line a secretory gland, which during the secretory phase produces specific products thought to be important to the implanting trophoblast.[6] These products include proteins and glycoproteins (e.g. prolactin and uteroglobin) as well as sialoglycoproteins (mucins). Changes in secretory glands are a major determining feature of endometrial differentiation, and many of the characteristic changes in the microscopic anatomy of the endometrium involve changes in the glands (see below).

STROMA

Endometrial stromal cells are derived from differentiated urogenital ridge mesenchymal cells immediately surrounding the müllerian duct, and the stroma is probably induced by the developing epithelium. The stroma cells are surrounded by a complex extracellular matrix[7] produced, in large part, by the stromal cells themselves. Intermixed with the stromal cells are blood vessels and a variety of bone marrow-derived immunocompetent cells (see below). Perhaps the most distinctive change apparent in stromal structure across the cycle is decidualization. Decidualization involves enlargement and differentiation of the stromal cells, beginning with the perivascular stroma in the mid-secretory phase and continuing toward the stromal cells adjacent to the luminal and glandular epithelium. Decidualization is maintained during pregnancy.

BONE-MARROW DERIVED IMMUNOCOMPETENT CELLS

Lymphocytes (including natural killer (NK) cells) account for about 40% of the endometrial cells in early pregnancy, but little is known about their physiologic role. By far the most prevalent endometrial leukocyte in the secretory phase and early pregnancy is a specialized NK cell with granular morphology known as a large granular lymphocyte or uterine NK (uNK) cell. uNK cells have distinct differences from peripheral NK cells. uNK cells have cytolytic potential, which is low in the early proliferative phase but comparable to that of peripheral blood NK cells in the secretory phase and pregnancy.[8] Furthermore, whereas 85–90% of peripheral NK cells display a CD16+ CD56dim immunophenotype, >90% of endometrial NK cells display a CD16- CD56bright immunophenotype.[9,10] The proportion of CD16- CD56bright uNK cells rises from about 30–50% of total endometrial leukocytes in the proliferative phase to about 50–70% in the mid and late secretory phases, whereas CD16+ CD56dim NK cells remain at about 5–10% throughout the cycle.[9,11] The recruitment of this rare subset of NK cells probably arises from expression of the CXCL12 chemokine by decidual cells and its receptor CXCR4 by peripheral CD16− NK cells.[12]

The other major type of leukocyte in the endometrium is the T lymphocyte. These cells make up approximately 5% of the total uterine cell population. Whether the numbers of T lymphocytes change during the cycle is unclear, although increased proliferation is seen in the secretory phase.[13,14] Furthermore, the distribution and activity of T cells may undergo significant changes.[9,11]

Although macrophages and B-lymphocytes are found in the endometrium, they represent less than 10% and 5%, respectively, of endometrial leukocytes. Interestingly, lymphoid aggregates containing a B-cell core surrounded by CD8+ T cells and a halo of macrophages have been observed in the endometrium, and the size of these aggregates increases in the secretory phase.[11,14,15] In addition, prominent infiltrates of neutrophils are seen on histologic sections taken from the very late secretory phase.

ENDOTHELIUM

Radial arteries penetrate the myometrium and split into basal and spiral arteries. The basal arteries form a rich network of anastomoses, supplying the relatively stable endometrial basalis and, like the basalis, undergo little cyclic change. In contrast, the spiral arteries do not anastomose and change markedly over the cycle, to supply the first proliferating and then differentiating endometrial functionalis.

ENDOMETRIAL STRUCTURE: HISTOLOGY

It has been almost 100 years since Hitschmann and Adler first reported cyclic changes in the microscopic architecture of endometrial functionalis, and more than 50 years since Noyes et al. established the basic histologic criteria currently used by pathologists for the assessment of endometrial differentiation on endometrial biopsies stained with hematoxylin and eosin.[16–18] A careful reassessment of the classic histologic dating criteria using fertile subjects, modern cycle-monitoring techniques, and modified analytic methods has confirmed that the histologic changes described in 1950 represent a good description of the usual cyclic changes in endometrial structure and composition, but has also suggested that classic histologic evaluation of the endometrium is insufficiently precise to be used for clinical evaluation of endometrial function.[19]

Most authors describe cyclic changes in endometrial histology using an idealized 28-day cycle, with menses on day 1, lutenizing hormone (LH) surge on day 13 (d13), ovulation on d14, followed by 14 more days of secretory phase. Typical cyclic changes in endometrial morphology, demonstrated in Figure 1.2, have been extensively described and will only be outlined here.[17,18,20,21]

The proliferative phase follows the menses and thus is initially characterized by re-epithelialization, which begins as early as d2 of the cycle.[22] By the early proliferative phase (d5–7; Figure 1.2A), the endometrial epithelium covers the surface, and straight glands with a small circular cross-section are evident. The luminal and glandular epithelial cells are short, with basal nuclei, whereas the stroma is composed of oval cells with little cytoplasm. In early proliferative endometrium, mitotic figures are rare in both epithelium and stroma. Under the influence of increasing levels of estrogen, the midproliferative endometrium, (d8–10; Figure 1.2B) is characterized by increased epithelial and stromal mitosis, more columnar epithelium with pseudostratified nuclei, slightly coiled glands, and stromal edema. Estrogen continues to rise markedly in the late proliferative phase (d11–14; Figure 1.2C), causing continued glandular mitoses and increased stromal mitoses. The glands become more tightly coiled, with a wide lumen, and the glandular epithelium shows maximal pseudostratification, whereas the stromal edema lessens.

The high, sustained levels of estradiol trigger the LH surge, which in turn triggers ovulation about 34–36 hours after the onset of the surge.

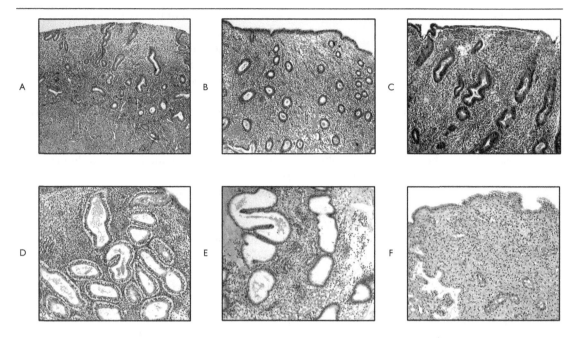

Figure 1.2 Light micrographs of endometrium across the cycle. A, menstrual; B, midproliferative; C, late proliferative; D, early secretory; E, midsecretory; F, late secretory.

The day of ovulation is defined as day 14 of the idealized 28-day cycle, and secretory days are often referred to as post-ovulatory days (POD) 1–14, instead of cycle days 15–28. After follicular rupture, the resulting corpus luteum begins producing estradiol and progesterone, resulting in secretory transformation of the endometrial glands. Interestingly, electron microscopy reveals continued secretion of products into the glandular lumen throughout the cycle, although in the 'secretory' phase their character changes. During the second half of the secretory phase, three zones of endometrium can be distinguished. In order from lumen to myometrium, these zones are called the zona compacta, the zona spongiosum, and the basalis. The functionalis layer, which is shed during menses, is composed of both compacta and spongiosum, and the endometrium regenerates from the basalis layer. The basalis is largely unchanged over the cycle.

In the early secretory phase (d15–18, POD 1–4, Figure 1.2D), progesterone levels are low and the endometrium continues to show mitoses; however, by d16, the first progestational effects are seen as secretory vacuoles appear beneath the glandular nuclei. Large glycogen deposits can be appreciated by electron microscopy beneath the glandular nuclei just before ovulation, at least 2 days before subnuclear vacuoles appear. As these appear at the same time as giant mitochondria, it is thought that the glycogen store may be required as an energy source in the secretory phase. The secretory vacuoles move toward the apical aspect of the glandular epithelial cell, passing the nucleus on d18. Also by d18, mitoses have virtually disappeared.

In the midsecretory phase (d19–23, POD 5–9; Figure 1.2E), the endometrial glands begin to secrete increasing amounts of material into the lumen, and maximal secretory material in the glands is seen on d20 (POD 6). Stromal edema is also prominent in this phase, with maximal edema seen on d22 (POD 8). The arterioles become more spiral in appearance by d23 (POD 9). Apoptosis has been described in the epithelial cells of the midsecretory phase, although this is not apparent on routine histologic sections.

Embryo implantation usually occurs between d20 and d24, termed, 'the window of implantation'. The window of implantation is characterized by ultrastructural changes including decreased density of tight junctions,[23] alterations in basal lamina architecture,[4] and the appearance of pinopods on the luminal surface.[24] The emergence of pinopods correlates with uterine receptivity to implantation and represents a marked alteration in the apical cytoskeleton. An example of the appearance of pinopods is given in Figure 1.3. The pinopod-like structures persist through the implantation window and then appear to deflate in the late secretory phase.[25]

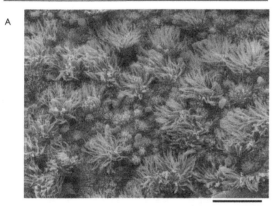

10μm 2070X

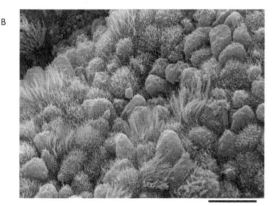

10μm 2020X

Figure 1.3 Scanning electron micrographs of endometrial lumen. A, 2–3 days after LH surge; B, 9–10 days after LH surge.

In the absence of embryo implantation, the late secretory phase ensues (d24–28; Figure 1.2F) characterized by falling levels of E and P, glandular involution, and predecidual changes in the stroma. On day 24, thick 'cuffs' of decidualizing stroma are seen around the arterioles and glandular epithelium begins to regress, showing diminished height, indistinct cytoplasmic borders, and a serrated appearance. Predecidual change is seen in the stroma cells immediately adjacent to the epithelium by d25. By d26, solid sheets of predecidua are seen between the subepithelial and perivascular stroma. Marked infiltration by specialized uterine NK cells and neutrophils occurs by d27 (POD 13). Finally, focal necrosis and hemorrhage are observed on d28 (POD 28), presaging the onset of menstrual bleeding (d1–4).

MOLECULAR AND CELLULAR BIOLOGY OF CYCLIC ENDOMETRIAL CHANGES

STEROID HORMONES AND RECEPTORS

Cyclic changes in endometrial structure and function are almost entirely due to the effects of cyclic changes in estradiol (E) and progesterone (P). The effects of E and P are best illustrated by studies of women with non-functioning ovaries, whose endometrium is atrophic and inactive. In women without ovarian function, treatment with estrogen and progesterone in a manner closely approximating the normal cycle results in changes in endometrial structure and function very similar to those seen normally.[26–30] Since E and P largely determine endometrial function, a deep understanding of the mechanisms of their action would greatly advance our knowledge of the mechanisms determining fertility, endometrial proliferation control, and menstruation. Because E and P act primarily at the level of gene expression and have different effects on different cell types, a deeper knowledge of their action on the endometrium requires investigation at the cellular and molecular levels.

In the most basic sense, E and P act through specific, high-affinity receptors to alter levels of gene expression. Classic models suggested that estrogen and progesterone each acted by binding a single cognate receptor (ER or PR), which, upon occupation by hormone, could bind to specific DNA target sequences in the promoter regions of specific genes to increase or decrease transcription. However, evidence accumulated over the last 15 years demonstrates that the classic model is vastly oversimplified and inadequate to explain the marked differences of effects of the same steroid on different genes and different cell types, as well as the effects of selective progesterone and estrogen receptor-modulating drugs.

The modern concept of estrogen and progesterone action is based on the following findings. There are at least two estrogen receptor types, encoded by two separate genes (ERα and Erβ, with a third form described in fish) and at least two progesterone receptor types, encoded by the same gene as alternate splice variants (PRA and PRB). Each of the receptor types can have distinct effects in cells, and the expression of each may be regulated in a cell-type-specific and cycle-specific pattern. Since the ER and PR bind DNA as a dimer, each may act as a homodimer and/or heterodimer. Furthermore, the action of each receptor dimer is determined partly by coregulators (coactivators and corepressors) which serve as an intermediary between the receptor and the transcriptional complex.[31,32] The expression of these co-regulators is also cell-type specific and cycle regulated.[33,34] The actions of receptors and co-regulators can be further modified by dynamic post-transcriptional alterations such as phosphorylation. ER and PR may also act via pathways not involving DNA binding, including binding to other transcription factors as well as activating second messenger pathways used by cell-surface receptors. At the tissue level, cells may communicate with one another by secreting paracrine factors or by altering extracellular matrix in response to E and/or P. The intercellular communication may result in hormone effects on nearby cells lacking a particular receptor. Finally, the endometrium can express enzymes responsible

for hormone synthesis (e.g. aromatase) and degradation (e.g. 17β-hydroxysteroid dehydrogenase), thereby allowing endometrial cells to alter their own endocrine environment. Thus, E and P act by complex and modifiable mechanisms that vary over the cycle.

As shown in Figure 1.4, ER and PR expression by endometrial stroma and epithelium varies markedly over the cycle. In endometrial stroma and epithelium, ERβ expression appears to parallel ERα expression.[35,36] Interestingly, the loss of endometrial epithelial PR during the period of uterine receptivity (midsecretory phase) is seen in most, if not all, placental mammals, suggesting a conserved function in early pregnancy.[37] The loss of PR seen in the mid-secretory phase glan-

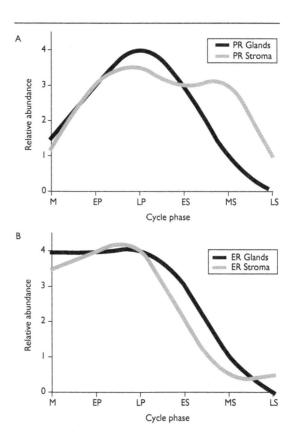

Figure 1.4 Abundance of ER and PR through the menstrual cycle. M, menstrual; EP, early proliferative; LP, late proliferative; ES, early secretory; MS, mid secretory; LS, late secretory.

dular endometrium is predominantly a loss of PRB, although PRA is maintained.[38-40] In the mouse model, PRA appears to be involved in decidualization and PRB in implantation-specific events, suggesting that progesterone-dependent actions on endometrial epithelium at the time of embryo implantation may be largely mediated via paracrine factors (progestomedins) stimulated by stromal PRB.[41] Studies in human tissues have suggested that progesterone may act both indirectly, through stromal production of progestomedins, and directly, through epithelial PRA.[42] Although the identity of progesterone-induced stromal factors acting on the epithelium (progestomedins) is unclear, growth factors and cytokines are likely candidates for progestomedins and other paracrine regulators of endometrial function. Thus the modes of action of E and P are complex, cell-type specific, and dependent on multiple endocrine, paracrine, and autocrine factors.

GROWTH FACTORS AND CYTOKINES

The first two growth factors to be discovered were epidermal growth factor (EGF) and insulin-like growth factor 1 (IGF-1).[43,44] Although growth factors were first described as regulators of cellular growth and replication, the same factors have been shown to serve many other functions as paracrine communicators between cells. Interestingly, both EGF and IGF families are thought to be important paracrine regulators of endometrial function. Heparin-binding EGF-like growth factor (HB-EGF) is thought to function as a progestomedin as well as in maternal-fetal communication in the early stages of implantation.[45,46] IGF-1, produced by stroma during decidualization, is thought to be a key regulator of decidualization and placental invasion.[47,48] The expression of both these factors is cyclic and can be regulated by E and P.[45,47] The potential roles of many other growth factors and their receptors have been described in several review articles.[49,50]

In addition to growth factors, cytokines are the other class of paracrine factor known to be involved in endometrial intercellular communication. Cytokines, including the chemotactic cytokines or chemokines, were originally identified as immunoregulatory factors produced by and acting on leukocytes. However, further work has demonstrated that many cytokines share structural and functional features with both growth factors and neurotransmitters. Thus, cytokines, growth factors, and neurotransmitters can be regarded as overlapping subclasses of factors that serve most of the body's paracrine, juxtacrine, autocrine, and intracrine regulatory functions. Cytokines are now recognized to play important roles in the essential functions of endometrium, including host immunity, embryo implantation, pregnancy maintenance, and menstruation. Furthermore, all endometrial cell types can express one or more cytokine species, with epithelial expression being particularly pronounced.[51] Cytokines produced by endometrial epithelium and stroma can act in a paracrine fashion on receptors expressed by the blastocyst, invading embryo, endometrial epithelium and stroma, resident leukocytes, and endothelium.

The regulatory importance of cytokines in endometrial function has been best illustrated by studies exploring the roles of leukemia inhibitory factor (LIF) and interferon-τ (IFN-τ) during early pregnancy. In mice, endometrial production of LIF, is essential for embryo implantation.[52,53] Interestingly, human and rhesus (monkey) endometrium also produce LIF at the time of embryo implantation, and a role in the rhesus has been demonstrated experimentally.[54-56] In the sheep, embryonic production of a unique type 1I interferon, IFN-τ, is required for early pregnancy survival.[57-59] No homolog of the IFN-τ gene is present in rodents or primates, but endometrial and embryonic expression of other type 1 interferons is known. Furthermore, endometrial expression of many interferon-stimulated genes is increased during the period of embryo receptivity, and at least one interferon-stimulated gene can be induced by the blastocyst.

Cytokines are also thought to play important roles in pregnancy maintenance versus loss, menstrual function, and the establishment and growth of endometriosis.[56,60–62] Given the importance of cytokines in endometrial function, it is not surprising that the expression of many endometrial cytokines is cyclic.[51] In addition, the expression and function of some cytokines are directly regulated by E and P.[63,64] Other potential regulators of endometrial cytokine expression are human chronionic gonatotropin (hCG), prolactin, other cytokines, and a recently-discovered class of receptors termed Toll-like receptors (TLR), whose endometrial expression has been recently demonstrated.[65] Cytokines and growth factors, are therefore, important molecules involved in paracrine regulation of endometrial function.

ADHESION MOLECULES AND EXTRACELLULAR MATRIX

Both growth factors and cytokines can bind specifically to the extracellular matrix (ECM), with effects on factor targeting and half-life. Thus, the composition and location of ECM can markedly alter paracrine signaling. Furthermore, the type of ECM to which a cell is bound via its adhesion molecules can alter its gene expression pattern as well as its responses to endocrine and paracrine factors. Finally, adhesion molecules on the apical surfaces of endometrial epithelium, stroma, and trophoblast have been implicated as regulators of implantation. Thus, the content of the ECM and the adhesion molecules that bind it are important regulators of endometrial function. A review of the composition and function of endometrial ECM has recently been published and the information summarized here is taken from that source.[7]

The interstitial ECM and the epithelial and endothelial basal laminae are initially laid down during the regeneration of endometrial functionalis after the initiation of menses. The interstitial ECM, whose components include collagens (types I, III, IV, VI, and XIII), fibrillin, fibronectin, tenascin C, thrombospondin I, and decorin, is thought to provide structural support for the tissue and may also be involved in cellular regulation via ECM receptors, such as integrins, on the cell surface. A continuous basement membrane exists between the epithelium and the stroma, as well as between the endothelium and the stroma. In addition, the decidualized stromal cells are surrounded by basement membrane. The endometrial basement membrane components include multiple laminin subunits as well as type IV collagen, heparin sulfate proteoglycan, and BM-40. These components are recognized by epithelial and endothelial integrin receptors potentially altering cellular function and allowing the differentiation of basal and apical membrane regions. Both interstitial ECM and basement membrane components change over the menstrual cycle, probably reflecting changing structural and functional needs.

The endometrium is remarkable in that some integrin receptors are present on the apical side of the epithelium. Because apical integrins have no ECM with which to interact, it has been suggested that these receptors are involved in the initial interaction between the embryo and the endometrium.[66,67] One particular integrin, $\alpha v\beta 3$, appears to be temporally correlated with embryo implantation and is absent in many forms of infertility.[68] Interestingly, a gene regulatory protein, HOXA-10, whose absence prevents implantation in mice, has been shown to regulate both $\alpha v\beta 3$ expression and (in the mouse) pinipod formation.[69,70] The demonstrated connections between $\alpha v\beta 3$, HOXA-10, and pinopods are among the first findings that allow synthesis between molecular, structural, and functional lines of research.

If taken further, the investigation of interacting factors at multiple levels of analysis will allow a much deeper understanding of endometrial function and dysfunction. However, the identification of sets of molecules important to endometrial function has been hampered by techniques that allow the detection of changes in only one (or a few) specific molecule: polymerase chain reaction, Northern blot, and in situ hybridization for RNA and ELISA, Western blot, and immunohistochemistry, and phosphoprotein analyses for protein. In order to understand the overall function of endometrial cells in health and disease, it will be necessary to investigate the interactions among many proteins and genes and their effects on structure and function. Genomic and proteomic tools developed in the last few years are now beginning to allow simultaneous analysis of changes in hundreds to tens of thousands of endometrial genes and proteins.

FURTHER APPLICATION OF CELLULAR AND MOLECULAR ANALYSES

The genomic technique of microarray hybridization of whole human endometrium has recently been applied to the study of endometrial gene expression, resulting in the identification of genes heretofore not known to be expressed.[71-75] This work is further bolstered by similar studies in other animal species.[76-78] These studies are somewhat hampered by the use of whole endometrial specimens as an RNA source, which may be influenced by alterations in the relative proportion of each cell type in the endometrium. The difference between changes in gene expression by particular cells and a change in the number of cells expressing the particular gene is important, as many of the gene products, such as cytokines, growth factors, receptors, and intracellular proteins, have local, concentration-dependent effects.

A handful of investigators have also studied the global gene profiles of individual cell types, including endometrial stroma before and after in vitro decidualization,[79-81] or before and after progesterone treatment,[81,82] uterine NK cells compared to peripheral NK cells,[83] and 'receptive' versus 'non-receptive' endometrial epithelial cell lines.[84]

As genomic and proteomic approaches identify candidate molecules involved in specific cellular functions, a large amount of work will need to be done to verify the findings as well as assess functional relevance. Thus, proteomic and genomic approaches generate many answers and many more questions.

CONCLUSIONS

Our current understanding of the molecular and cell biology of the endometrium is limited but growing. Increased knowledge of normal endometrial structure and function will allow identification of the causes and treatments of endometriosis and other disorders involving the endometrium.

REFERENCES

1. Murphy CR, Swift JG, Need JA, Mukherjee TM, Rogers AW., A freeze-fracture electron microscopic study of tight junctions of epithelial cells in the human uterus. Anat Embryol (Berl) 1982;163:367–70.
2. Murphy CR, Rogers PA, Hosie MJ, Leeton J, Beaton L. Tight junctions of human uterine epithelial cells change during the menstrual cycle: a morphometric study. Acta Anat (Basel) 1992;144:36–8
3. Denker HW. Implantation: a cell biological paradox. J Exp Zool 1993;266:541–58.
4. Dockery P, Khalid J, Sarani SA, et al. Changes in basement membrane thickness in the human endometrium during the luteal phase of the menstrual cycle. Hum Reprod Update 1998;4:486–95.
5. Medawar P. Some immunological and endocrinological problems raised by the evolution of viviparity in vertebrates. Symp Soc ExpBiol.1953;44:320–8.
6. Aplin JD. Cellular biochemistry of the endometrium. In: Wynn RM, Jollie WP, eds. Biology of the Uterus, 2nd ed. New York: Plenum Medical, 1989;89–119.
7. Aplin JD. Endometrial extracellular matrix. In: Glasser S, Aplin J, Giudice L, Tabibzadeh S, eds. The Endometrium. London: Taylor & Francis, 2002;294–307.
8. Jones RK, Bulmer JN, Searle RF. Cytotoxic activity of endometrial granulated lymphocytes during the menstrual cycle in humans. Biol Reprod 1997;57:1217–22.
9. Kodama T, Hara T, Okamoto E, Kusunoki Y, Ohama K. Characteristic changes of large granular lymphocytes that strongly express CD56 in endometrium during the menstrual cycle and early pregnancy. Hum Reprod 1998;13:1036–43.
10. Bulmer JN, Morrison L, Longfellow M, Ritson A, Pace D. Granulated lymphocytes in human endometrium: histochemical and immunohistochemical studies. Hum Reprod 1991;6:791–8.
11. Wira CW, Fahey JV, White HD, et al. The mucosal immune system in the human female reproductive tract: influence of stage of the menstrual cycle and menopause on mucosal immunity in the uterus. In: Glasser S, Aplin J, Giudice L, Tabibzadeh S, eds. The Endometrium. London: Taylor & Francis, 2002;294–307.
12. Hanna J, Wald O, Goldman-Wohl D, et al. CXCL12 expression by invasive trophoblasts induces the specific migration of CD16- human natural killer cells. Blood 2003;102:1569–77.
13. Booker SS, Jayanetti C, Karalak S, Hsiu JG, Archer DF. The effect of progesterone on the accumulation of leukocytes in the human endometrium. Am J Obstet Gynecol 1994;171:139–42.

14. Tabizbadeh S. Proliferative activity of lymphoid cells in human endometrium throughout the menstrual cycle. J Clin Endocrinol Metab 1990;70:437–43.

15. Yeaman GR, Guyre PM, Fanger MW, et al. Unique CD8+ T cell-rich lymphoid aggregates in human uterine endometrium. J Leukoc Biol 1997;61:427–35.

16. Hitschmann F, Adler L. Der Bau der Uterusschleimhaut des Geschlechtsreifen Weibes mit besonderer Beruckssichtigung der Menstruation. Geburtsh Gynaekol 1908;27:1–82.

17. Wynn RM. The human endometrium: cyclic and gestational changes. In: Wynn RM, Jollie WP, eds. Biology of the Uterus, 2nd edn. New York; Plenum Medical, 1989;289–329.

18. Noyes R, Heritg A, Rock J. Dating the endometrial biopsy. Fertil Steril 1950;1:3–25.

19. Murray M, Meyer W, Zaino R, et al. A critical reanalysis of the accuracy, reproducibility, and clinical utility of histologic endometrial dating: a systematic study of the secretory phase in normally cycling, fertile women, Fertil Steril 2004;81:1333–43.

20. Dockery P. The fine structure of the human endometrium., In: Glasser S, Aplin J, Giudice L, Tabizbadeh S, eds. The Endometrium. London: Taylor & Francis, 2002;21–37.

21. Dinh TV. Syllabus of Gynecologic Pathology. Austin, TX: University of Texas Press, 1990.

22. Ludwig H, Metzger H. The Human Female Reproductive Tract: a Scanning Electron Microscopic Atlas. New York: Springer- Verlag, 1976.

23. Rogers PA, Murphy CR. Morphometric and freeze fracture studies of human endometrium during the peri-implantation period. Reprod Fertil Dev 1992;4:265–9.

24. Johannisson E, Nilsson L. Scanning electron microscopic study of the human endometrium. Fertil Steril 1972;23:613–25.

25. Usadi RS, Murray MJ, Bagnell RC, et al. Temporal and morphologic characteristics of pinopod expression across the secretory phase of the endometrial cycle in normally cycling women with proven fertility. Fertil Steril 2003;79:970–4.

26. Lessey BA. Embryo quality and endometrial receptivity: lessons learned from the ART experience. J Assist Reprod Genet 1998;15:173–6.

27. Tanos V, Friedler S, Zajicek G, et al. The impact of endometrial preparation on implantation following cryopreserved–thawed-embryo transfer. Gynecol Obstet Invest 1996;41:227–31.

28. Davis OK, Rosenwaks Z. Preparation of the endometrium for oocyte donation. J Assist Reprod Genet 1993;10:457–9.

29. Li TC, Warren MA, Dockery P, Cooke ID. Human endometrial morphology around the time of implantation in natural and artificial cycles. J Reprod Fertil 1991;92:543–54.

30. Navot D, Bergh P. Preparation of the human endometrium for implantation. Ann N Y Acad Sci 1991;622:212–19.

31. Fernandes I, White JH. Agonist-bound nuclear receptors: not just targets of coactivators. J Mol Endocrinol 2003;31:1–7.

32. Edwards DP, Wardell SE, Boonyaratanakornkit V. Progesterone receptor interacting coregulatory proteins and cross talk with cell signaling pathways. J Steroid Biochem Mol Biol 2002;83:173–86.

33. Gregory CW, Wilson EM, Apparao KB, et al. Steroid receptor coactivator expression throughout the menstrual cycle in normal and abnormal endometrium. J Clin Endocrinol Metab 2002;87:2960–6.

34. Shiozawa T, Shih HC, Miyamoto T, et al. Cyclic changes in the expression of steroid receptor coactivators and corepressors in the normal human endometrium. J Clin Endocrinol Metab 2003;88:871–8.

35. Lecce G, Meduri G, Ancelin M, Bergeron C, Perrot-Applanat M. Presence of estrogen receptor beta in the human endometrium through the cycle: expression in glandular, stromal, and vascular cells. J Clin Endocrinol Metab 2001;86:1379–86.

36. Matsuzaki S, Fukaya T, Suzuki T, et al. Oestrogen receptor alpha and beta mRNA expression in human endometrium throughout the menstrual cycle. Mol Hum Reprod 1999;5:559–64.

37. Spencer TE, Bazer FW. Biology of progesterone action during pregnancy recognition and maintenance of pregnancy. Front Biosci 2002;7:d1879–98.

38. Mote PA, Balleine RL, McGowan EM, Clarke CL. Colocalization of progesterone receptors A and B by dual immunofluorescent histochemistry in human endometrium during the menstrual cycle. J Clin Endocrinol Metab 1999;84:2963–71.

39. Mote PA, Balleine RL, McGowan EM, Clarke CL. Heterogeneity of progesterone receptors A and B expression in human endometrial glands and stroma. Hum Reprod 2000;15 (Suppl 3):48–56.

40. Wang H, Critchley HO, Kelly RW, Shen D, Baird DT. Progesterone receptor subtype B is differentially regulated in human endometrial stroma. Mol Hum Reprod 1998;4:407–12.

41. Conneely OM, Mulac-Jericevic B, DeMayo F, Lydon JP, O'Malley BW. Reproductive functions of progesterone receptors., Recent Prog Horm Res 2002;57:339–55.

42. Lessey BA. Two pathways of progesterone action in the human endometrium: implications for implantation and contraception. Steroids 2003;68:809–15.

43. van Wyk JJ, Hall K, Weaver RP. Partial purification of sulphation factor and thymidine factor from plasma. Biochim Biophys Acta 1969;192:560–2.

44. Cohen S. The stimulation of epidermal proliferation by a specific protein EGF. Dev Biol 1965;12:394–407.

45. Lessey BA, Gui Y, Apparao KB, Young SL, Mulholland J. Regulated expression of heparin-binding EGF-like growth factor HB-EGF in the human endometrium: a potential paracrine role during implantation. Mol Reprod Dev 2002;62:446–55.

46. Stavreus-Evers A, Aghajanova L, Brismar H, et al. Co-existence of heparin-binding epidermal growth factor-like growth factor and pinopods in human endometrium at the time of implantation. Mol Hum Reprod 2002;8:765–9.

47. Irwin JC, de las Fuentes L, Giudice LC. Growth factors and decidualization in vitro. Ann N-Y Acad Sci 1994;734:7–18.

48. Nayak NR, Giudice LC. Comparative biology of the IGF system in endometrium, decidua, and placenta, and clinical implications for foetal growth and implantation disorders. Placenta 2003;24:281–96.

49. Giudice LC. Growth factors and growth modulators in human uterine endometrium: their potential relevance to reproductive medicine. Fertil Steril 1994;61:1–17.

50. Tazuke SI, Giudice LC. Growth factors and cytokines in endometrium, embryonic development, and maternal: embryonic interactions. Semin Reprod Endocrinol 1996;14:231–45.

51. Robertson SA, Hudson SN. Cytokines: pivotal regulators of endometrial immunobiology. In: Glasser S, Aplin J, Giudice L, Tabizbadeh S, eds. The Endometrium. London: Taylor & Francis, 2002;416–30.

52. Stewart CL, Kaspar P, Brunet LJ, et al. Blastocyst implantation depends on maternal expression of leukaemia inhibitory factor. Nature 1992;359:76–9.

53. Chen JR, Cheng JG, Shatzer T, et al. Leukemia inhibitory factor can substitute for nidatory estrogen and is essential to inducing a receptive uterus for implantation but is not essential for subsequent embryogenesis. Endocrinology 2000;141:4365–72.

54. Delage G, Moreau JF, Taupin JL, et al. In-vitro endometrial secretion of human interleukin for DA cells/leukaemia inhibitory factor by explant cultures from fertile and infertile women. Hum Reprod 1995;10:2483–8.

55. Laird SM, Tuckerman EM, Dalton CF, et al. The production of leukaemia inhibitory factor by human endometrium: presence in uterine flushings and production by cells in culture. Hum Reprod 1997;12:569–74.

56. Piccinni MP, Beloni L, Livi C, et al. Defective production of both leukemia inhibitory factor and type 2 T-helper cytokines by decidual T cells in unexplained recurrent abortions. Nature Med 1998;4:1020–4.

57. Roberts RM. Conceptus interferons and maternal recognition of pregnancy. Biol Reprod 1989;40:449–52.

58. Pontzer CH, Torres BA, Vallet JL, Bazer FW, Johnson HM. Antiviral activity of the pregnancy recognition hormone ovine trophoblast protein-1. Biochem Biophys Res Commun 1988;152:801–7.

59. Hansen TR, Imakawa K, Polites HG, et al. Interferon RNA of embryonic origin is expressed transiently during early pregnancy in the ewe. J Biol Chem 1988;263:12801–4.

60. Yue ZP, Yang ZM, Wei P, et al. Leukemia inhibitory factor, leukemia inhibitory factor receptor, and glycoprotein 130 in rhesus monkey uterus during menstrual cycle and early pregnancy. Biol Reprod 2000;63:508–12.

61. Seli E, Berkkanoglu M, Arici A. Pathogenesis of endometriosis. Obstet Gynecol Clin North Am 2003;30:41–61.

62. Lebovic DI, Shifren JL, Ryan IP, et al. Ovarian steroid and cytokine modulation of human endometrial angiogenesis., Hum Reprod 2000;15 (Suppl 3):67–77.

63. Seli E, Arici A. Modulation of the immune system by sex steroids. Infertil Reprod Med Clin North Am 2002;13:19–48.

64. Kelly RW, King AE, Critchley HO. Cytokine control in human endometrium. Reproduction 2001;121:3–19.

65. Young SL, Lyddon TD, Jorgenson RL, Misfeldt ML. Expression of Toll-like receptors in human endometrial epithelial cells and cell lines. Am J Reprod Immunology 2004;52:67–73.

66. Lessey BA, Ilesanmi AO, Lessey MA, et al. Luminal and glandular endometrial epithelium express integrins differentially throughout the menstrual cycle: implications for implantation, contraception, and infertility. Am J Reprod Immunol 1996;35:195–204.

67. Aplin JD. The cell biology of human implantation. Placenta 1996;17:269–/75.

68. Lessey BA. Adhesion molecules and implantation. J Reprod Immunol 2002;55:101–12.

69. Bagot CN, Kliman HJ, Taylor HS. Maternal Hoxa10 is required for pinopod formation in the development of mouse uterine receptivity to embryo implantation. Dev Dyn 2001;222:538–44.

70. Daftary GS, Troy PJ, Bagot CN, Young SL, Taylor HS. Direct regulation of beta3-integrin subunit gene expression by HOXA10 in endometrial cells. Mol Endocrinol 2002;16:571–9.

71. Riesewijk A, Martin J, van Os R, et al. Gene expression profiling of human endometrial receptivity on days LH+2 versus LH+7 by microarray technology. Mol Hum Reprod 2003;9:253–64.

72. Carson DD, Lagow E, Thathiah A, et al. Changes in gene expression during the early to mid-luteal receptive phase; transition in human endometrium detected by high-density microarray screening. Mol Hum Reprod 2002;8:871–9.

73. Kao LC, Tulac S, Lobo S, et al. Global gene profiling in human endometrium during the window of implantation. Endocrinology 2002;143:2119–38.

74. Chen HW, Chen JJ, Tzeng CR, et al. Global analysis of differentially expressed genes in early gestational decidua and chorionic villi using a 9600 human cDNA microarray. Mol Hum Reprod 2002;8:475–84.

75. Eyster KM, Boles AL, Brannian JD, Hansen KA. DNA microarray analysis of gene expression markers of endometriosis. Fertil Steril 2002;77:38–42.

76. Kim S, Choi Y, Bazer FW, Spencer TE. Identification of genes in the ovine endometrium regulated by interferon tau independent of signal transducer and activator of transcription 1. Endocrinology 2003;144:5203–14.

77. Ishiwata H, Katsuma S, Kizaki K, et al. Characterization of gene expression profiles in early bovine pregnancy using a custom cDNA microarray. Mol Reprod Dev 2003;65:9–18.

78. Reese J, Das SK, Paria BC, et al. Global gene expression analysis to identify molecular markers of uterine receptivity and embryo implantation. J Biol Chem 2001;276:44137–45.

79. Tierney EP, Tulac S, Huang ST, Giudice LC. Activation of the protein kinase A pathway in human endometrial stromal cells reveals sequential categorical gene regulation. Physiol Genomics 2003;16:47–66.

80. Brar AK, Handwerger S, Kessler CA, Aronow BJ. Gene induction and categorical reprogramming during in vitro human endometrial fibroblast decidualization. Physiol Genomics 2001;7:135–48.

81. Popovici RM, Kao LC, Giudice LC. Discovery of new inducible genes in in vitro decidualized human endometrial stromal cells using microarray technology. Endocrinology 2000;141:3510–13.

82. Okada H, Nakajima T, Yoshimura T, Yasuda K, Kanzaki H. Microarray analysis of genes controlled by progesterone in human endometrial stromal cells in vitro. Gynecol Endocrinol 2003;17:271–80.

83. Koopman LA, Kopcow HD, Rybalov B, et al. Human decidual natural killer cells are a unique NK cell subset with immunomodulatory potential. J Exp Med 2003;198:1201–12.

84. Martin J, Dominguez F, Avila S, et al. Human endometrial receptivity: gene regulation. J Reprod Immunol 2002;55:131–9.

2. Endometriosis and Implantation

Pinar H. Kodaman and Hugh S. Taylor

INTRODUCTION

Approximately 60% of women with endometriosis are subfertile, that is, their cumulative pregnancy rates are lower than those of controls.[1] Although not yet completely understood, it appears that the detrimental effects of endometriosis on fertility are pleiotropic in nature and include distortion of the pelvic anatomy by the formation of adhesions and biochemical alterations, resulting in a microenvironment that negatively affects folliculogenesis,[2-4] fertilization,[5] embryogenesis,[6] and implantation.[7-9] This chapter will address (a) the process of implantation and its frequency in natural and assisted reproductive technology (ART) cycles; (b) the molecular basis for implantation; (c) the effects of endometriosis on implantation; and (d) the potential treatment of implantation defects associated with endometriosis.

IMPLANTATION AND ENDOMETRIAL RECEPTIVITY

Implantation is a complex process that requires synchronization between the developing embryo and the progesterone-primed endometrium. After fertilization, the zygote migrates down the fallopian tube until it reaches the uterine cavity at the morula stage on day 18 of an ideal 28-day cycle.[10,11] On day 19 the blastocyst forms, sheds its zona pellucida, and superficially apposes and then adheres to the endometrium.[12] This is followed by trophoblast invasion through the endometrial epithelium and underlying stroma, which ultimately results in placentation.[13] Implantation occurs only during the 'window of implantation', which in humans corresponds to postovulatory days 6–10.[14] In fact, the endometrium is one of the few tissues in which implantation

cannot take place except during this restricted, narrow time period.[14]

Implicit in implantation is the concept of endometrial receptivity, which has been defined as 'the temporally and spatially unique set of circumstances that allow for successful implantation of the embryo'.[15] Traditionally, endometrial receptivity has been indirectly assessed by luteal-phase endometrial biopsy, with which a histological determination is made regarding whether the degree of differentiation of the endometrial sample corresponds to the cycle day on which the biopsy was performed.[16] The luteal-phase defect – that is, a greater than 2–3-day lag in endometrial maturation – implies a lack of endometrial receptivity, yet endometrial biopsies are often performed late in the luteal phase and thus may not directly reflect the window of implantation.[15] Furthermore, histological endometrial maturation does not necessarily correlate with a functionally mature endometrium.[17] Recent studies have suggested that there are two types of luteal-phase defect that may compromise endometrial receptivity; in the classic or type I defect histological endometrial maturation is delayed, whereas in the type II defect endometrial histology is within normal limits; however, the expression of biochemical markers of maturation is delayed.[18] The latter will be discussed in detail below, as many of these molecular markers of endometrial receptivity are affected by endometriosis and probably contribute to the decreased implantation rates seen with the disease.

IMPLANTATION RATES IN NATURAL CYCLES AND ART

In natural cycles the implantation rate is difficult to determine because although ovulation can be confirmed, knowledge about successful fertilization and transport of the embryo to the uterine cavity is limited. The estimated rate of implantation in natural cycles, assuming the formation of only one embryo, is 15–30%,[19] making the efficiency of human implantation quite low compared to that of other species.[20] The implantation rate decreases with age in a non-linear fashion until age 35, at which point there is an approximately 3% decrease per year.[21] As mentioned above, with endometriosis, pregnancy rates in natural cycles are lower than normal.[22] Thus, ART is often utilized in the treatment of endometriosis-related infertility. In fact, endometriosis represents the third most common indication for ART after tubal and male factors.[23]

In ART, and specifically in in vitro fertilization–embryo transfer (IVF-ET), implantation rates can be more accurately assessed. It has been estimated that, on average, the implantation rate – that is, the number of gestational sacs produced per number of healthy zygotes transferred into the uterine cavity – is only 10–15%.[24,25] Efforts to improve this rate have included allowing embryos to develop further until the blastocyst stage (day 5 versus day 3 embryos); using coculture techniques, in which tubal, granulosa, endometrial, or other cell lines are incubated with the embryos; and the implementation of sequential media changes for different stages of embryo development.[26] It is believed that blastocyst culture allows for self-selection of viable embryos and improves the synchronicity between endometrial and embryo development.[27] Although a recent meta-analysis found no difference in the pregnancy or livebirth rate between blastocyst and early cleavage (days 2–3) embryo transfer, it did show a significant improvement in implantation rates in the subgroup of studies in which blastocyst culture was performed in conjunction with sequential media changes.[27]

CELLULAR/MOLECULAR MARKERS AND MECHANISMS UNDERLYING IMPLANTATION

As described earlier, implantation is a complex process that requires synchronization between the developing embryo and the differentiating endometrium. Numerous studies have investigated potential markers of endometrial receptivity as predictors of successful implantation, and in so doing have helped to define the cellular and molecular mechanisms by which implantation occurs (Figure 2.1). These markers include pinopods, cell adhesion molecules, matrix metalloproteinases and their inhibitors, cytokines, homeobox genes, and growth factors. As will be discussed later, many of these markers are altered in the setting of endometriosis. This section will allude to the various markers of endometrial receptivity as they pertain to implantation, focusing on those that are mundane to endometriosis.

PINOPODS

With the onset of the secretory phase of the menstrual cycle, microvilli on the apical surface of the luminal endometrial epithelium fuse to form structures known as pinopods (Figure 2.2).[28] The appearance of these progesterone-dependent structures, which are involved in endocytosis, pinocytosis, and possibly blastocyst adhesion, occurs during the window of implantation.[29] Pinopods last for only 1–2 days – usually d20–21 in an ideal cycle, though there is up to 4 days' variation in the timing of their appearance.[28] Furthermore, their numbers correlate with implantation.[29,30] Interestingly, pinopods form earlier in gonadotropin-stimulated cycles (d19–20)[31] and later in artificial, hormone replacement cycles for donor recipients (d21–22),[32] resulting in a loss of synchronization between the developing embryo and the endometrium. Addressing this issue may represent a means of improving implantation rates in ART cycles. For example, it would be beneficial to postpone the window of implantation in women undergoing controlled ovarian hyperstimulation for IVF so that embryo maturation could catch up prior to embryo transfer.[28] Such a delay in endometrial development has been accomplished in the rat using the antiprogestin RU-486 after ovulation.[33]

INTEGRINS

Numerous cell adhesion molecules (CAM), including mucins[34,35] and trophinin,[36] have been

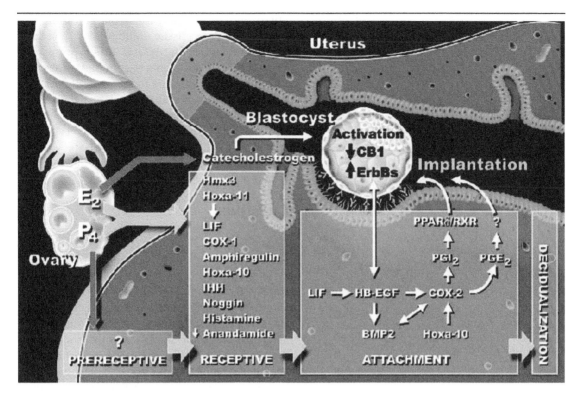

Figure 2.1 Molecular signaling during implantation. The follicular-phase endometrium is unreceptive to the blastocyst. After estradiol-induced proliferation, progesterone differentiates the endometrium into a receptive state. Multiple uterine factors mediate this process. Whereas sex steroid levels are unaltered in endometriosis, multiple intrauterine molecules involved in the implantation process are affected. (From Paria BC et al. Science 2002;296:2185–7)

implicated in the attachment phase of implantation, during which they serve to tether the blastocyst to the endometrium, as described by the receptor-mediated model of implantation.[37] Perhaps the best studied of the CAM have been the integrins, which are heterodimeric glycoproteins consisting of non-covalently associated α and β subunits.[38] At least 20 types of integrin heterodimer have been defined, which form from 14 α and 9 β subunits.[39] Integrins are unusual cell surface receptors in that they bind with low affinity and are present in large numbers, allowing for ligand motility without loss of attachment.

Endometrial epithelial cells constitutively express certain integrins, whereas others are cycle dependent.[40] Among the latter is αvβ3, which is present on the apical surface of both luminal endometrial cells and human embryos.[41]

Osteopontin (OPN), one of the ligands for αvβ3, is a glycoprotein secreted by the endometrium and probably serves as a bridging molecule between the embryo and the endometrium.[38,42] Interestingly, immunostaining for both αvβ3 and OPN corresponds to the endometrial pinopods that form during the window of implantation.[43]

During the secretory phase of the menstrual cycle, elevated progesterone levels increase OPN secretion[44] and result in a downregulation of endometrial progesterone receptors.[45] The latter is associated with an increase in αvβ3 expression, signaling the onset of endometrial receptivity.[46] The significance of αvβ3 is highlighted by the finding that in infertile women with type I luteal phase defects the loss of PR is delayed, as is the expression of αvβ3.[46,47] Furthermore, there is evidence that treatment of the condition

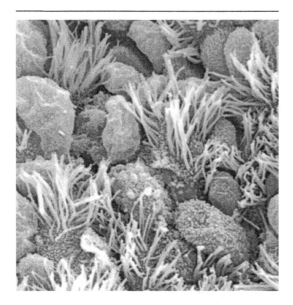

Figure 2.2 Scanning electron micrograph of endometrial epithelium on day 21 of a natural cycle. Most secretory cells bear fully developed pinopods, whereas the non-secretory cells are ciliated. (From Nikas G et al. Ann NY Acad Sci 2003;997:120–3)

underlying the luteal phase defect or progesterone supplementation restores PR downregulation and αvβ3 expression.[18,40] Although antibodies blocking αvβ3, or the use of ligands that compete with OPN, compromise implantation in rabbits,[48] gene knockout studies have demonstrated that β3-deficient mice are still fertile, implying that although αvβ3 has a role in implantation, there is redundancy within this process.[49]

PROTEASES AND PROTEASE INHIBITORS

In addition to acting as a receptor for the embryo, αvβ3 also activates matrix metalloproteinases (MMP), such as MMP-2,[50] which degrade extracellular matrix proteins and thereby facilitate the invasive phase of implantation.[51] Other MMP, including MMP-7 and MMP-11, are expressed in the endometrium during menses and the proliferative phase, but are downregulated by progesterone during the secretory phase.[52] Protease

activity, and consequently trophoblast invasion, is also regulated by tissue inhibitors of matrix metalloproteases (TIMP) and other protease inhibitors, such as α_2-macroglobulin.[15] Among the TIMP, TIMP-3 appears to be especially pertinent to implantation as it is expressed by murine decidua just adjacent to the sites of embryo implantation.[53] Furthermore, TIMP-3 is also expressed by human cytotrophoblasts[54] and decidualizing stromal cells, where it is upregulated by progesterone.[55]

CYTOKINES

As with the CAM, numerous cytokines have been implicated in implantation. Colony-stimulating factor (CSF-1), for example, is expressed by human endometrium during the midproliferative and midsecretory phases,[56] and mice with a null mutation in this gene have decreased implantation rates, which are improved with exogenous CSF-1 administration.[57] It has been postulated that CSF-1 facilitates blastocyst attachment;[15] similarly, the interleukins may be involved in the cross-talk between the embryo and the endometrium. Interleukin-1α (IL-1α), interleukin-1β (IL-1β), and the interleukin-1 receptor antagonist (IL-1RA), for instance, are expressed by human endometrium,[58] and levels of their receptor interleukin-1 receptor type 1 (IL-1R T1) are maximal during the secretory phase.[59] Interestingly, a recent study showed that that IL-1RA inhibits implantation by downregulating the integrin subunits α4, αv, and β3.[60] Still, as with the integrins, there is redundancy with respect to the role the IL-1 system plays in implantation, as null mutations in the IL-1α and IL-1β genes have no appreciable effects on fertility.[61]

Leukemia inhibiting factor, a member of the interleukin-6 family, is a well-substantiated marker of implantation. This glycoprotein is expressed by human endometrium and decidua,[62] where it is regulated by other cytokines and steroid hormones, such as estrogen.[63] There is very little LIF expression in proliferative endometrium, but levels increase during the secretory phase, reaching a maximum between days 19 and 25, which coincides with the implantation window.[62] The effects of LIF on cellular proliferation and differentiation are mediated by its receptors LIF-R and glycoprotein 130 (gp130), both of which are expressed constitutively by proliferative and secretory endometrium as well as by trophoblasts.[64] LIF stimulates trophoblasts to increase fibronectin production, which facilitates anchoring[65] and also differentiates these cells into an invasive phenotype.[66] Blastocysts cannot implant in mice lacking the LIF gene.[67] On the other hand, blastocysts from LIF-deficient mice can implant into wildtype, pseudopregnant mice, showing conclusively that implantation requires maternal LIF expression.[68]

That LIF is involved in human implantation is suggested by the findings that conditioned media from endometrial explants of women with unexplained infertility have decreased levels of LIF compared to those of fertile women,[69] and some infertile women have mutations in the coding region of the LIF gene.[70] Furthermore, antiprogestin treatment results in reduced LIF expression,[71] and women with unexplained infertility are more likely to have undetectable levels of LIF in their uterine flushings than are fertile women.[72]

HOMEOBOX GENES

Another group of markers that are clearly integral to implantation are the homeobox (HOX) genes, which encode a class of transcription factors. There are at least 39 Hox (mouse)/HOX (human) genes, all of which have a similar 183 base pair DNA sequence – the homeobox – that encodes a highly conserved 61-amino acid domain known as the homeodomain.[73] Many of these transcription factors mediate embryonic development by determining regional body patterning along the anterior–posterior body axis, including that of the reproductive tract.[74] Specifically, *Hoxa-9* is expressed in the developing oviduct, *Hoxa-10* in the uterus, *Hoxa-11* in the lower uterine segment and cervix, and *Hoxa-13* in the upper vagina (Figure 2.3).[75]

Unlike most Hox genes, which are expressed only during the embryonic period, those specific

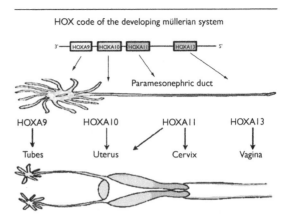

Figure 2.3 The HOX code of the developing müllerian tract. The HOX genes are arranged on the chromosome in the same order as they are expressed in the paramesonephric duct. Expression of a distinct HOX gene in the duct leads to the development of adult structures. The anterior boundary of expression of each gene forms the limit of each tissue

to the female reproductive tract continue to play a role in the adult.[75] For example, *HOXA-10* and *HOXA-11* are expressed by endometrial glands and stroma throughout the menstrual cycle,[76,77] and their levels increase maximally during the midsecretory phase at the time of implantation.[75] Both *HOXA-10* and *HOXA-11* are upregulated by 17β-estradiol and progesterone,[76] and the effects of these steroids are a direct result of their receptors (ER or PR) binding to the regulatory regions of the *Hoxa-10* or *Hoxa-11* genes.[77,78] The continued expression of Hox/HOX genes in the female reproductive tract facilitates the growth and differentiation of the endometrium, and thereby allows for the retention of developmental plasticity, which is important for successful implantation.

Although there are no known human mutations in *HOXA-10* or *HOXA-11*, women with decreased expression of these two genes during the secretory phase have lower implantation rates.[79] Targeted disruption of the *Hoxa-10* gene in mice results in a transformation of the upper uterine segment into an oviduct-like structure and inhibits implantation, even when embryos are transferred to the grossly unaffected lower uterine segment.[80,81] Similarly, mice with a homozygous mutation in the *Hoxa-11* gene are infertile owing to implantation defects,[82] and also have reduced expression of LIF.[83] Both *Hoxa-10* and *Hoxa-11* null mice produce normal numbers of embryos that are able to implant in wildtype surrogate mice, but wildtype embryos from the surrogate mice cannot implant in the *Hoxa-10* and *Hoxa-11*-deficient mice.[80–82] Thus, as with LIF, maternal expression of *Hoxa-10* and *Hoxa-11* by the endometrium is essential for implantation.

One downstream target of *HOXA-10* is *EMX2* (human)/*Emx2* (mouse).[84] *Emx2* is expressed in the developing brain and urogenital tract,[85] and mice lacking this gene have severe urogenital malformations that result in death shortly after birth.[86] During the midluteal phase, when *HOXA-10* levels are maximal, *EMX2* expression declines, and this downregulation occurs as a result of *HOXA-10* binding to the regulatory region of the *EMX2* gene.[84] Although the functional significance of *EMX2* downregulation is unclear, further elucidation of the HOX system should help to define the role of *EMX2* in endometrial development. Interestingly, *HOXA-10* also binds to the β3-integrin gene and upregulates its expression in endometrial cells, demonstrating that *HOXA-10* mediates integrin involvement in early embryo–endometrial interactions.[87]

GROWTH FACTORS

Growth factors are proteins that bind to specific receptors and thereby result in cellular differentiation and/or proliferation. Among the growth factors relevant to implantation are heparin-binding epidermal growth factor (HB-EGF)[88,89] and amphiregulin.[90] In the mouse, HB-EGF expression is limited spatially and temporally to the site of blastocyst implantation,[91] and is therefore thought to play a role in blastocyst attachment. In women, HB-EGF is also expressed during the window of implantation,[88,89] and this growth factor stimulates the growth and development of both human[92] and mouse[91] blastocysts in vitro. Interestingly, it appears that HB-EGF also regulates endometrial αvβ3 expression.[93] Although a role for amphiregulin in human implantation has not yet been defined, in the mouse this growth factor, which is

another member of the EGF family, is expressed during the period of maximal endometrial receptivity, initially throughout the uterine epithelium and then specifically at the sites of blastocyst implantation.[90]

Other growth factors, such as transforming growth factor-β (TGF-β), act as 'maternal restraints' during implantation, in that they limit trophoblast invasion.[94] TGF-β1 expression by endometrial glands and stroma increases during the secretory phase, and it inhibits proliferation of cytotrophoblasts, stimulates them to differentiate into a non-invasive phenotype, and induces protease inhibitors, such as plasminogen activator inhibitor (PAI) and TIMP-1, that counteract extracellular matrix degradation by trophoblast-derived proteases.[95]

Another apparent restraint on trophoblast invasion is insulin-like growth factor binding protein-1 (IGFBP-1), which is secreted by the secretory endometrium and decidua[96,97] and binds insulin-like growth factors I and II (IGF-I, IGF-II), thereby blocking their actions. The latter growth factor is expressed in large amounts by cytotrophoblasts,[97] and IGFBP-1 blocks the invasion of these cells into decidualized endometrial stromal cells in vitro.[98] The role of IGFBP-1 is not yet fully understood, as it has also been found to stimulate trophoblast invasion in other in vitro systems.[99,100] Furthermore, IGFBP-1 has been implicated in embryo recognition and the events associated with early implantation, as it directly interacts with integrins, such as α5β1, expressed by cytotrophoblasts.[98,99]

A relatively new addition to the TGF-β family of growth factors is endometrial bleeding associated factor (ebaf). This protein is a marker of uterine non-receptivity, as its expression is maximal immediately before and during menstrual bleeding, and it is also associated with abnormal uterine bleeding.[101] Endometrial expression of ebaf is limited to the stroma, where it is downregulated during the implantation window.[102]

PROSTAGLANDINS

In addition to apposition, attachment, and invasion, successful implantation requires increased endometrial vascular permeability followed by angiogenesis, the generation of new blood vessels from pre-existing ones. The process of angiogenesis in the peri-implantational endometrium is not completely understood; however, it is likely that, as in other tissues, angiogenic factors such as vascular endothelial growth factor (VEGF)[103] and the angiopoietins[104] are involved. Better characterized are the prostaglandins, which are arachidonic acid metabolites that mediate a wide array of biological processes, including angiogenesis, cellular proliferation, and differentiation. These compounds, which are generated by the cyclooxygenases (COX-1 and COX-2), facilitate increased vascular permeability in the endometrium during implantation.[105] Mice with null mutations in the inducible isoform of cyclooxygenase, COX-2, have multifactorial reproductive failure, including impaired ovulation, fertilization, implantation, and decidualization, whereas mice deficient in the constitutive enzyme COX-1 are not affected in this respect.[106] More recent studies investigating the role of COX-2 in implantation revealed that wildtype embryos are able to successfully implant in COX-2-deficient mice, although there is a delay in decidualization following implantation.[107] Thus, although COX-2-generated prostaglandins have a role in implantation, there again appears to be redundancy within this process.

EFFECTS OF ENDOMETRIOSIS ON IMPLANTATION

The clinical data consist of conflicting results with respect to the effect of endometriosis on implantation. Whereas some studies found significantly decreased implantation rates in patients with endometriosis,[7–9] others have found no difference at all.[6,108] Among the former group is the retrospective study by Simon et al[8] of approximately 200 IVF cycles in which half the patients had endometriosis and the other half had tubal factor. The two groups had pregnancy rates of 13 and 34% per cycle, respectively. The adverse effect of endometriosis on implantation was also demonstrated by Arici et al,[9] who retro-spectively analyzed almost 300 IVF cycles in women with endometriosis, tubal factor, and unexplained infertility, and found implantation rates of 3.9%, 8.1%, and 7.2%, respectively. Notably, there were no differences in the number and quality of oocytes or fertilization rates between the three groups. More recently, a large-scale meta-analysis of ART studies demonstrated that women with endometriosis have half the pregnancy rate of women with infertility due to tubal factor.[7] In addition, this comprehensive study showed that the detrimental effects of endometriosis on IVF are multifactorial and include diminished peak estradiol concentrations, fewer retrieved oocytes, and impaired fertilization and implantation rates.[7]

In contrast, another large, retrospective study, again comparing ART cycles for endometriosis versus tubal factor-related infertility, showed no significant differences in pregnancy rates, even when the endometriosis group was subdivided into stage of disease.[108] It has been argued that it is not endometrial receptivity, but rather oocyte quality, that is affected by endometriosis, thereby affecting fertilization and embryogenesis. For instance, a Swedish study found that although the fertilization rate was lower in patients with endometriosis, implantation rates among successfully fertilized oocytes were comparable.[5]

The study that directly addressed the controversy between oocyte quality and endometrial receptivity compared women with endometriosis undergoing IVF who used their own oocytes versus those who received donor oocytes from women without endometriosis.[6] Implantation rates were lower among women with endometriosis using their own oocytes for IVF; however, when donor oocytes were utilized, implantation rates were similar in patients with and without endometriosis. Conversely, when the donor oocytes were obtained from women with endometriosis, implantation rates were lower among all of the groups analyzed, including those with infertility secondary to endometriosis, tubal factor, male factor, and ovulation disorders.[6]

Although the above-mentioned study appeared to settle the debate between oocyte quality and endometrial receptivity defects as the etiology for implantation failure in endometriosis, it was limited, as most studies are, by the use of GnRH analogs and exogenous steroid hormones during the IVF cycles. Suppression of endogenous GnRH secretion for IVF simultaneously treats endometriosis; in fact, it has long been known that treatment of endometriosis patients with GnRH analogs significantly improves pregnancy rates in IVF.[109] Furthermore, controlled ovarian hyperstimulation and hormone treatment for IVF, as discussed earlier, also alter endometrial receptivity.[32] Thus, whether the findings described above hold true in natural cycles remains to be determined.

Despite the controversy in the clinical literature, the detrimental effect of endometriosis on implantation was clearly demonstrated by Hahn et al,[110] using a well-established rabbit model in which eutopic endometrial tissue is excised and then sutured into the peritoneal cavity. In this study, animals were artificially inseminated 11 weeks after surgery and then sacrificed at various time points. Whereas the number of corpora lutea and fertilized ova were comparable to those of the sham-operated controls, there was an almost 50% reduction in the implantation rate in the rabbits with endometriosis.

EFFECTS OF ENDOMETRIOSIS ON OOCYTE QUALITY

Successful implantation requires a receptive endometrium and a healthy embryo, and endometriosis affects both of these. The decreased fertilization rate in patients with endometriosis is probably a reflection of the quality of the oocytes obtained, as folliculogenesis is affected by endometriosis (Table 2.1). Aromatase activity and progesterone production, for example, are decreased in granulosa cells obtained from patients with mild endometriosis undergoing IVF compared to patients with tubal factor or unexplained infertility.[2] Conversely, granulosa cells from these patients produce higher levels of cytokines, such as tumor necrosis factor-α[111] and interleukin-6,[3] VEGF is decreased,[3] and they have

Table 2.1 Genes and gene products aberrantly expressed in follicles of women with endometriosis
Aromatase
Progesterone
TNF-α
IL-6
VEGF

increased rates of apoptosis.[4] As successful folliculogenesis relies on angiogenesis for the delivery of gonadotropins, steroid precursors, and other nutrients, VEGF levels correlate with follicular health.[112]

Some studies have suggested that the altered immune and endocrine environment in the follicles of patients with endometriosis may not be predictive of oocyte or embryo quality, yet natural cycle fertilization rates are clearly lower in these patients.[22] With respect to ART cycles, again there is controversy in the clinical literature. Whereas some studies have reported decreased fertilization rates,[5,113] others have not.[6,9] Recently, a retrospective study looking at ART outcomes based on stage of endometriosis found that increasing stage of disease does correlate negatively with fertilization rate.[114] With respect to the events after fertilization, Pellicer et al[6] demonstrated a significant decrease in the number of blastomeres at 72 hours post fertilization and an increase in the percentage of arrested embryos in women with endometriosis compared to those with tubal infertility.

EFFECT OF ENDOMETRIOSIS ON ENDOMETRIAL RECEPTIVITY

Many of the markers of endometrial receptivity are altered in the setting ofendometriosis and probably affect implantation (Table 2.2). Although a prospective study assessing pinopod formation found no difference between women with and without endometriosis,[115] the study subjects were receiving estrogen/progestin treatment for oocyte donation. It has been well docu-

Table 2.2 Markers of endometrial receptivity and other genes and gene products that are altered in endometriosis

Markers of endometrial receptivity altered in endometriosis	Other endometrial genes and gene products aberrantly expressed in endometriosis	
HOXA-10	COX-2	IL-15
HOXA-11	HGF	C4BP
LIF	IL-6	B61
αvβ3	MMP-7	Dickkopf-1
	MMP-11	Glycodelin
	suPA-R	GlcNAc6ST
	CA-125	G0S2 protein
	HSP-27	Purine nucleoside phosphorylase
	HSP-70	Semaphorin E
	Aromatase	Neuronal olfactomedin
	Estrogen receptors	SALP
		Neuronal pentraxin II

mented that the window of implantation and, concomitantly, pinopod formation are altered in the setting of exogenous gonadotropins and hormones.[31,32]

As described above, the integrin αvβ3 localizes to pinopods during the implantation window.[43] Aberrant expression of αvβ3 is associated with infertility related not only to endometriosis,[116] but also to luteal-phase defects,[46] hydrosalpinges,[117] and unexplained infertility.[18] In women with endometriosis the endometrium appears histologically normal and PR receptors are appropriately downregulated; however, there is a lack of β3-subunit expression.[116] These findings, which are consistent with a type II luteal-phase defect, are more pronounced with progressive stages of endometriosis.[116]

The injection of mice with peritoneal fluid from endometriosis patients decreases αvβ3 and LIF expression in the mouse and impairs implantation rates.[118] Similar studies on rabbits[110] and hamsters[119] have also shown reduced implantation. Although it is unknown whether the peritoneal fluid of endometriosis patients affects their eutopic endometrium, the animal studies suggest that peritoneal fluid contains factor(s) that affect implantation by directly altering the endometrial milieu.[110,118,119] Candidates for these

transferable factors include cytokines, such as RANTES,[120] monocyte chemoattractant protein-1 (MCP-1)[121] and CSF-1,[122] VEGF,[123] prostaglandins,[124] and activated macrophages,[121] all of which are increased in the peritoneal fluid of endometriosis patients.

The midluteal rise in HOXA-10 and HOXA-11 expression does not occur consistently in women with endometriosis (Figure 2.4).[79] Concomitantly, EMX2 expression in these patients is abnormally high during the peri-implantation period.[125] Ebaf expression is persistently elevated during the window of implantation in infertile women with endometriosis,[102] also indicating a lack of endometrial receptivity. There is decreased cyclic variation in COX-2 expression by eutopic endometrium in endometriosis patients, and levels of this enzyme are abnormally increased in both the proliferative and the secretory phase.[126] The significance of upregulated COX-2 during the implantation window is unclear, given that animal studies show impaired implantation[106] and decidualization[107] with deficient COX-2 expression; however, as prostaglandins mediate a host of biological functions, overexpression of COX-2 may have negative, as yet uncharacterized, effects on endometrial receptivity.

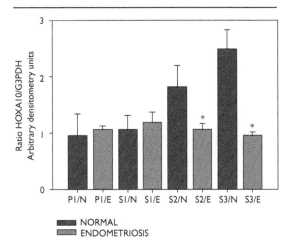

Figure 2.4 *HOXA-10* expression in the endometrium of women with and without endometriosis. Normal fertile women, shown in black, demonstrate a significant increase in endometrial *HOXA-10* expression in the mid and late secretory phases (S2 and S3, respectively) compared to the proliferative and early secratory phases (P1 and S1, respectively). This increase in *HOXA-10* expression at the time of implantation does not occur in women with endometriosis (grey). (After Taylor HS et al. Hum Reprod 1999;14: 1328–31.[79] European Society of Human Reproduction and Embryology. Reproduced by permission of Oxford University Press/Human Reproduction.)

Numerous other endometrial genes and gene products are altered in the setting of endometriosis and may also aberrantly affect implantation (see Table 2.2). For example, endometrial stromal cells from women with endometriosis secrete increased amounts of hepatocyte growth factor (HGF).[127] This has angiogenic properties and also stimulates endometrial epithelial cells to proliferate and differentiate in vitro;[127] thus, elevated HGF levels may lead to vascular and glandular abnormalities in the endometrium.[128] The HGF gene is transcriptionally activated by IL-6,[129] a cytokine that is also abnormally elevated in the eutopic endometrium of endometriosis patients.[130]

Cytokines have additionally been implicated in the dysregulation of MMP in patients with endometriosis. Both MMP-7 and MMP-11 are persistently expressed by the endometrium and fail to undergo downregulation by progesterone.[52] Soluble urokinase plasminogen activator receptor (suPA-R) is also overexpressed in endometrial cells from endometriosis patients, suggesting increased proteolytic potential.[131] Disruption of the balance between endometrial proteases and protease inhibitors could compromise implantation.

The upregulation of cytokines, proteases, and other proteins, such as CA-125,[132] in the endometrium reflects the inflammation associated with endometriosis, which probably has a negative impact on endometrial receptivity. This is further highlighted by the elevation of heat-shock protein-27 (HSP-27) and HSP-70 in eutopic endometrium from patients with endometriosis.[133] Heat-shock proteins are induced in response to a variety of stimuli, including inflammation, and they act as molecular chaperones in the folding of newly synthesized proteins.[134] Furthermore, heat-shock proteins may play a role in the immune system, as they appear to be involved in antigen processing, antigen presentation, or peptide binding.[135] HSP-70, for example, is recognized as a ligand by $\gamma\delta$ T cells,[135] a subset of T cells that are abnormally increased in the endometrial stroma of women with endometriosis.[136]

Aromatase, which catalyzes the conversion of androstenedione and testosterone to estrone and estradiol, respectively, is also aberrantly expressed in the endometrium of endometriosis patients.[137] At the same time, estrogen receptor (ER) mRNA expression, which normally decreases after ovulation, remains elevated,[138] demonstrating a loss of negative feedback regulation. Increased local concentrations of estrogen, specifically estradiol, have been implicated in the pathogenesis of endometriosis,[128,139] and may also have detrimental effects on implantation. Estradiol stimulates the production of prostaglandins, which in turn further stimulate aromatase activity.[140] Interestingly, the use of GnRH analogs to treat endometriosis decreases aromatase expression in eutopic endometrium by promoting a hypoestrogenic state[141] and simultaneously improves pregnancy rates in ART, as described above.[109]

Recently, a broader approach in the form of microarray analysis has been utilized to compare endometrium from women with and without endometriosis to identify potential differences associated with implantation failure.[142] Of the almost 13 000 genes analyzed, three groups of genes were found to be altered in endometriosis: group I consists of eight genes (IL-15, complement 4 binding protein, B61, Dickkopf-1, glycodelin, GlcNAc6ST, G0S2 protein, and purine nucleoside phosphorylase) that are upregulated during the normal window of implantation but significantly decreased in women with endometriosis; group II consists of three genes (semaphorin E, neuronal olfactomedin, and Sam68-like phosphotyrosine protein-α (SALP)) that are normally downregulated but which are significantly upregulated with endometriosis; and group III consists of one gene (neuronal pentraxin II) that is normally downregulated but which is further decreased with endometriosis.[142]

Although specific roles for many of the above-mentioned genes in endometriosis-related implantation failure remain to be characterized, some have been postulated based on known molecular functions in other systems.[142] For example, downregulation of *GlcNAc6ST*, which encodes an enzyme that glycosylates surface molecules, may impair embryo attachment by decreasing the glycosylation of mucins and other heavily glycosylated molecules involved in embryo–endometrial interactions.[142] Complement 4 binding protein, another group I gene, is thought to play a role in the endometrial immune defense system.[143]

Downregulation of IL-15, a cytokine that is normally upregulated during the implantation window[144] and which stimulates natural killer (NK) cell-mediated effects on decidualization,[145] may similarly alter endometrial receptivity. In fact, deficient NK activity resulting in impaired immune surveillance has been implicated in the pathogenesis of endometriosis.[146,147] Whereas IL-15 activates NK cells, glycodelin, a glycoprotein predominantly expressed by endometrium during the secretory phase, suppresses the actions of these cells.[148] Glycodelin thus helps to provide an immunosuppressive environment for the implanting embryo.[148] Although downregulation of glycodelin in endometriosis may counteract the effect of downregulated IL-15 on NK cells, a disruption of the potentially delicate balance between NK activation and suppression may lead to an unreceptive endometrial milieu.

Similarly, abnormal downregulation of neuronal pentraxin II, a group III gene, may also contribute to an inhospitable endometrial environment, as pentraxin proteins mediate the uptake of bacteria and other cell debris, including apoptotic cell remnants.[149] The latter may be integral in preventing an inflammatory or autoimmune response that could compromise implantation.[142]

Among the group II genes, semaphorin E encodes a secretory protein that has been implicated in angiogenesis;[150] thus, upregulation of this gene in endometriosis may result in an aberrantly vascularized endometrium. In contrast, increased expression of another group II gene, SALP, which acts as a negative regulator of cell growth,[151] may inhibit appropriate endometrial development.[142]

Although this genome-wide approach has led to the discovery of novel genes that may be crucial to our understanding of implantation failure in endometriosis, the challenge will be to specifically define the roles these genes play. Furthermore, microarray analysis is limited by the selection criteria utilized, as gene identification is based on degree of up- or downregulation. In the study described above[142] the algorithm used initially selected genes with twofold changes in expression, and then further limited the selection to those genes with 100-fold changes in expression. Notably, this approach failed to identify certain genes, including *HOXA-10*, LIF, and β3-integrin, which have well-established roles in implantation failure associated with endometriosis. Small differences in RNA expression that fall below a certain preset limit may still be of importance, and furthermore, may translate into significant functional differences at the protein level. Specifically, minimal changes in transcription factor levels can lead to amplification and increased expression of other genes.

TREATMENT OF IMPLANTATION DEFECTS SECONDARY TO ENDOMETRIOSIS

As the above discussion illustrates, the defects in implantation associated with endometriosis are still not fully understood. Treatments aimed at improving implantation rates include medical and surgical approaches, but they are inherently limited by the heterogeneous nature of the disease. Whereas two meta-analyses have argued against a benefit of medical therapy,[152,153] numerous other studies have demonstrated that prolonged treatment with GnRH analogs improves the outcome of both ovulation induction/artificial insemination and IVF cycles in patients with endometriosis.[109,154–156] Again, whether prolonged suppression of endometriosis improves oocyte quality or endometrial receptivity or both still remains to be clarified, but the increased pregnancy rates are self-evident. More recently, a preliminary study suggested that supplemental LIF via subcutaneous injection also increases implantation rates in patients with endometriosis.[157] As discussed earlier, maternal expression of LIF is critical to implantation in mice,[68] and peritoneal fluid from endometriosis patients decreases LIF expression and implantation in animal models.[110,118,119] Further studies are warranted to delineate the mechanism by which subcutaneous LIF injection increases pregnancy rates in women with endometriosis.

Surgical treatment of endometriosis is controversial as well. Although the two meta-analyses described above also found no clear benefit of surgical therapy,[152,153] others have shown a significant improvement in pregnancy rates following surgical ablation of minimal and mild endometriosis.[158,159] The discrepancies in the literature may be partly due to the fact that surgical treatment of endometriosis-associated adhesive disease is likely to be without impact when potential tubal compromise is bypassed with IVF. With respect to endometriomas, although there are no prospective randomized controlled trials addressing surgical treatment versus conservative management prior to ovarian stimulation, several retrospective studies indicate that the latter approach is preferable, at least in the setting of in vitro fertilization.[160–162]

A novel approach in the treatment of endometriosis-associated implantation impairment may involve the use of gene therapy. In mice, selective alteration of endometrial *Hoxa-10* expression, through the use of liposome-mediated gene transfection, dramatically altered implantation, and again demonstrated the importance of maternal *Hoxa-10* expression for endometrial receptivity.[163] In this study, the uteri of adult wildtype mice were transfected on postcoital day 2 with a *Hoxa-10* antisense oligodeoxyribonucleotide designed to prevent *Hoxa-10* expression. Indeed, *Hoxa-10* protein levels decreased, as did the number of implanted embryos and the size of the resulting litters. In contrast, when the mice were transfected with *Hoxa-10* complementary DNA (cDNA), the number of implanted embryos significantly increased, as did litter size.

Although similar studies have not yet been performed in higher animal models or in humans, transfection of a human endometrial adenocarcinoma cell line (Ishikawa cells) with a *Hoxa-10* antisense oligodeoxyribonucleotide also resulted in decreased *HOXA-10* expression.[163] Furthermore, efficient transfection and expression of an *Escherichia lacZ* reporter gene has been accomplished in intact human uteri ex vivo, showing that gene transfer to the intact female reproductive tract is feasible.[164,165] Thus, a gene therapy approach could potentially have a role in the enhancement of endometrial receptivity and implantation in patients with endometriosis.

SUMMARY

Endometriosis is a prevalent and heterogeneous gynecological disorder that often compromises fertility. Many aspects of fertility are altered in the setting of endometriosis, including oocyte/embryo development and endometrial receptivity, which can lead to decreased pregnancy rates in natural cycles. Although there is some controversy regarding the effect of endometriosis on implantation rates in ART cycles, the majority of the evidence clearly demonstrates that endometriosis aberrantly affects markers of endometrial receptivity in the eutopic endometrium, and thus probably has a detrimental impact on implantation. Further characterization of these markers of endometrial receptivity, and the discovery of others, will facilitate our understanding of the complex process of implantation. In this way, selective treatments for specific implantation defects in the setting of endometriosis and other disease entities could be implemented in addition to the medical and surgical approaches already available.

REFERENCES

1. Haney AF. Endometriosis-associated infertility. Reprod Med Rev 1997;6:145–61.
2. Harlow CR, Cahill CJ, Maile LA. Reduced preovulatory granulosa cell steroidogenesis in women with endometriosis. J Clin Endocrinol Metab 1996;81:426–9.
3. Pellicer A, Albert C, Mercader A. The follicular and endocrine environment in women with endometriosis: local and systemic cytokine production. Fertil Steril 1998;70:425–31.
4. Toya M, Saito H, Ohta N. Moderate and severe endometriosis is associated with alterations in the cell cycle of granulosa cells in patients undergoing in vitro fertilization and embryo transfer. Fertil Steril 2000;73:344–50.
5. Bergandal A, Naffah S, Nagy C. Outcome of IVF in patients with endometriosis in comparison with tubal-factor infertility. J Assist Reprod Genet 1998;15:530–4.
6. Pellicer A, Navarro J, Bosch E et al. Endometrial quality in infertile women with endometriosis. Ann NY Acad Sci 2001;943:122–30.
7. Barnhart KT, Dunsmoor R, Coutifaris C. The effect of endometriosis on IVF outcome. Fertil Steril 2000;74:576–84.
8. Simon C, Gutierrez A, Vidal A. Outcome of patients with endometriosis in assisted reproduction: results from in vitro fertilization and oocyte donation. Hum Reprod 1994;9:725–9.
9. Arici A, Oral E, Bukulmez O et al. The effect of endometriosis on implantation. Results from the Yale University in vitro fertilization and embryo transfer program. Fertil Steril 1996;65:603–7.
10. Hertig AT, Rock J, Adams EC. A description of 34 human ova within the first 17 days of development. Am J Anat 1956;98:435–91.
11. Croxatto HB, Diaz S, Fuentealba BA et al. Studies on the duration of egg transport in the human oviduct: The time interval between ovulation and egg recovery from the uterus in normal women. Fertil Steril 1972;23:447–58.
12. Enders AC, Schlafke S. Cytological aspects of trophoblast–uterine interactions in early implantation. Am J Anat 1969;125:1–30.
13. Cross JC, Werb Z, Fisher SJ. Implantation and the placenta: key pieces of the development puzzle. Science 1994;266:1508–18.
14. Fawcett DW. The development of mouse ova under the capsule of the kidney. Anat Rec 1950;108:71–91.
15. Giudice LC. Potential biochemical markers of uterine receptivity. Hum Reprod 1999;14(Suppl 2):3–16.
16. Noyes RW, Hertig AT, Rock J. Dating and the endometrial biopsy. Fertil Steril 1950;1:3.
17. Swiersz L, Giudice LC. Unexplained infertility and the role of uterine receptivity. Infertil Clin North Am 1997;8:523–43.
18. Lessey BA, Castlebaum AJ, Sawin SJ. Integrins as markers of uterine receptivity in women with primary unexplained infertility. Fertil Steril 1995;63:535–42.
19. Miller JF, Williamson E, Glue J et al. Fetal losses after implantation. Lancet 1980;2:554–6.
20. Valbuena D, Jasper M, Remohi J, Pellicer A, Simon C. Ovarian stimulation and endometrial receptivity. Hum Reprod 1999;14(Suppl. 2.):107–111.
21. Spandorfer SD, Chung PH, Kligman I et al. An analysis of the effect of age on implantation rates. J Assist Reprod Genet 2000;17:303–6.
22. Cahill DJ, Wardle PG, Maile LA. Ovarian dysfunction in endometriosis-associated and unexplained infertility. J Assist Reprod Genet 1997;14:554–7.
23. Assisted reproductive technology success rates: national summary and fertility clinic reports. In: National Center for Chronic Disease Prevention and Health Promotion, Division of Reproductive Health; 1998; Atlanta, GA: Centers for Disease Control and Prevention, 1998.
24. Paulson RJ, Sauer MV, Lobo RA. Embryo implantation after human in vitro fertilization: importance of endometrial receptivity. Fertil Steril 1990;53:870–4.
25. Lopata A. Implantation of the human embryo. Hum Reprod 1996(Suppl 1):175–84.
26. Menezo Y, Veiga A, Benkhalifa M. Improved methods for blastocyst formation and culture. Hum Reprod 1998;13(Suppl 4):256–65.
27. Blake D, Proctor M, Johnson N, Olive D. Cleavage state versus blastocyst stage embryo transfer in assisted conception. Cochrane Database of Systematic Reviews 2002;2:CD002118.
28. Nikas G. Endometrial receptivity: changes in cell-surface morphology. Semin Reprod Med 2000:229–36.
29. Nikas G. Cell surface morphological events relevant to human implantation. Hum Reprod 1999;14(Suppl. 2):37–44.
30. Nikas G. Pinopodes as markers of endometrial receptivity in clinical practice. Hum Reprod 1999;14(Suppl 2):99–106.
31. Nikas G, Develioglu OH, Toner JP, Jones HW. Endometrial pinopods indicate a shift in the window of receptivity in IVF cycles. Hum Reprod 1999;14:787–92.
32. Develioglu OH, Hsiu JG, Nikas G et al. Endometrial estrogen and progesterone receptor and pinopod expression in stimulated cycles in oocyte donation. Fertil Steril 1999;71:1040–7.
33. Sarantis L, Roche D, Psychoyos A. Displacement of receptivity for nidation in the rat by the progesterone antagonist RU 486: a scanning electron microscopy study. Hum Reprod 1988;3:251–5.
34. Carson DD, Rohde LH, Surveyor G. Cell surface glycoconjugates as modulators of embryo attachment to uterine epithelial cells. Int J Biochem 1994;26:1269–77.
35. Feinberg RF, Kliman HJ. MAG (mouse ascites Golgi) mucin in the endometrium: a potential marker of endometrial receptivity to implantation. In: Diamond MP, Osteen KG, eds. Endometrium and Endometriosis. Maldon, MA: Blackwell Science, 1997; 131–9.
36. Fukuda MN, Sato T, Nakayama J et al. Trophinin and tastin: a novel adhesion molecule complex with potential involvement in embryo implantation. Genes Dev 1995;9:1199–210.
37. Yoshinaga K. Receptor concept in implantation research. In: Yoshinaga K, Mori T, eds. Development of Preimplantation Embryos and their Environment. New York: Alan Liss, 1989; 379–87.
38. Lessey BA, Castlebaum AJ. Integrins and implantation in the human. Rev Endocrin Metab Disord 2002;3:107–17.

39. Lindhard A, Bentin-Ley U, Ravn V et al. Biochemical evaluation of endometrial function at the time of implantation. Fertil Steril 2002;78:221–33.

40. Lessey BA, Damjanovich L, Coutifaris C et al. Integrin adhesion molecules in the human endometrium. Correlation with the normal and abnormal menstrual cycle. J Clin Invest 1992;90:180–95.

41. Campbell S, Swann HR, Seif MW, Kimber SJ, Aplin JD. Cell adhesion molecules on the oocyte and preimplantation human embryo. Hum Reprod 1995;10:1571–8.

42. Apparao KBC, Zhang J, Truong P, Lessey BA. Osteopontin expression during the menstrual cycle in women: regulation and binding to the endometrial αvβ3 integrin. J Clin Endocrinol Metab 2001;86:4991–5000.

43. Apparo KB, Murray MJ, Fritz MA. Osteopontin and its receptor alphavbeta(3) integrin are coexpressed in the human endometrium during the menstrual cycle but regulated differentially. J Clin Endocrinol Metab 2001; 86: 4991–5000.

44. Young MF, Kerr JM, Termine JD et al. cDNA cloning, mRNA distribution and heterogeneity, chromosomal location and RFLP analysis of human osteopontin (OPN). Genomics 1990;7:491–502.

45. Slayden OD, Zelinski-Wooten MB, Chwalisz K, Stouffer RL, Brenner RM. Chronic treatment of cycling rhesus monkeys with low doses of the antiprogestin ZK 137316: morphometric assessment of the uterus and oviduct. Hum Reprod 1998;13:269–77.

46. Lessey BA, Yeh I, Castelbaum AJ et al. Endometrial progesterone receptors and markers of uterine receptivity in the window of implantation. Fertil Steril 1996;65:477–83.

47. Creus M, Balasch J, Ordi J et al. Integrin expression in normal and out-of-phase endometria. Hum Reprod 1998;13:3460–8.

48. Illera MJ, Lorenzo PL, Gui L-T et al. The role of αvβ3 integrin during implantation in the rabbit. Biol Reprod 2000; 62: 1285–90.

49. Hodivala-Dilke KM, Kairbaan M, McHugh KP. β3 integrin deficient mice are a model for Glanzmann thrombasthenia showing placental defects and reduced survival. J Clin Invest 1999;103:229–38.

50. Brooks PC, Stromblad S, Sanders LC et al. Localization of matrix metalloproteinase MMP-2 to the surface of invasive cells by interaction with integrin alpha v beta 3. Cell 1996;85:683–93.

51. Turpeenniemi-Hujanen T, Feinberg RF, Kauppila A, Puistola U. Extracellular matrix interactions in early human embryos: Implications for normal implantation events. Fertil Steril 1995;64:132–8.

52. Osteen KG, Keller NR, Feltus FA, Meiner MH. Paracrine regulation of matrix metalloproteinase expression in normal human endometrium. Gynecol Obstet Invest 1999;48(Suppl. 1):2–13.

53. Harvey MB, Leco KJ, Arcellana-Panlilio MY et al. Proteinase expression in early mouse embryos is regulated by leukemia inhibitory factor and epidermal growth factor. Development 1995;121:1005–14.

54. Bass KE, Li H, Hawkes SP et al. Tissue inhibitor of metalloproteinase-3 expression is upregulated during human cytotrophoblast invasion in vitro. Dev Genet 1997;21:61–7.

55. Higuchi T, Kanzaki H, Nakayama H et al. Induction of tissue inhibitor of metalloproteinase 3 gene during in vitro decidualization of human endometrial stromal cells. Endocrinology 1995;136:4973–81.

56. Bartocci A, Pollard JW, Stanley ER. Regulation of CSF-1 during pregnancy. J Exp Med 1986;164:956–61.

57. Wiktor-Jedrzejczak W, Urbanowska E, Aukerman SL. Correction by CSF-1 of defects in the osteopetrotic op/op mouse suggests

58. Simon C, Frances A, Pellicer A. Cytokines in implantation. Semin Reprod Endocrinol 1995;13:142–51.

59. Simon C, Piquette GN, Frances A. Localization of interluekin-1 type 1 receptor and interleukin-1 beta in human endometrium throughout the menstrual cycle. J Clin Endocrinol Metab 1993;77:549–55.

60. Simon C, Valbuena D, Krussel J et al. Interleukin-1 receptor antagonist prevents embryonic implantation by a direct effect on the endometrial epithelium. Fertil Steril 1998;70:896–906.

61. Yamada H, Mizumd S, Horai R. Protective role of interleukin-1 in mycobacterial infection in IL-1 alpha/beta double-knockout mice. US Can Acad Pathol 2000;80:759–67.

62. Charnock-Jones DS, Sharkey AM, Fenwick P, Smith SK. Leukemia inhibitory factor mRNA concentration peaks in human endometrium at the time of implantation and the blastocyst contains mRNA for the receptor at this time. J Reprod Fertil 1994;101:421–6.

63. Arici A, Engin O, Attar E, Olive DL. Modulation of leukemia inhibitory factor gene expression and protein synthesis in human endometrium. J Clin Endocrinol Metab 1995;80:1908–15.

64. Cullinan EB, Abbondanzo SJ, Anderson PS et al. Leukemia inhibitory factor (LIF) and LIF receptor expression in human endometrium suggests a potential autocrine/paracrine function in regulating embryo implantation. Proc Natl Acad Sci USA 1996;93:3115–200.

65. Natchtigall MJ, Kliman HJ, Feinberg RF et al. The effect of leukemia inhibitory factor on trophoblast differentiation: a potential role in human implantation. J Clin Endocrinol Metab 1996;81:801–6.

66. Bischof P, Haenggeli L, Campana A. Effect of leukemia inhibitory factor on human cytotrophoblast differentiation along the invasive pathway. Am J Reprod Immunol 1995;34:225–30.

67. Stewart CL, Kaspar P, Brunet LJ et al. Blastocyst implantation depends on maternal expression of leukemia inhibitory factor. Nature 1992;359:76–9.

68. Stewart CL. Leukemia inhibitory factor and the regulation of pre-implantation development of the mammalian embryo. Mol Reprod Dev 1994;39:233–8.

69. Hambartsoumian E. Endometrial leukemia inhibitory factor (LIF) as a possible cause of unexplained infertility and multiple failures of implantation. Am J Reprod Immunol 1998;39:137–43.

70. Giess R, Tanasescu I, Steck T, Sendtner M. Leukemia inhibitory factor gene mutations in infertile women. Mol Hum Reprod 1999;5:581–6.

71. Danielsson KG, Swahn ML, Bygdeman M. The effect of various doses of mifepristone on endometrial leukemia inhibitory factor expression in the midluteal phase – an immunohistochemical study. Hum Reprod 1997;12:1293–7.

72. Laird SM, Tuckerman EM, Dalton CF et al. The production of leukaemia inhibitory factor by human endometrium: presence in uterine flushings and production by cells in culture. Hum Reprod 1997;12:569–74.

73. McGinnis W, Krumlauf R. Homeobox genes and axial patterning. Cell 1992;68:283–302.

74. Taylor HS. The role of HOX genes in the development and function of the female reproductive tract. Semin Reprod Med 2000;18; 311–20.

75. Taylor HS, Vanden Heuvel GB, Igarahi P. A conserved Hox axis in the mouse and human female reproductive system: late establish-

ment and persistent adult expression of the Hoxa cluster genes. Biol Reprod 1997;57:1338–45.

76. Taylor HS, Arici A, Olive D, Igarashi P. Hoxa10 is expressed in response to sex steroids at the time of implantation. J Clin Invest 1998;101:1379–82.

77. Taylor HS, Igarashi P, Olive D, Arici A. Sex steroids mediate HOXA11 expression in human peri-implantation endometrium. J Clin Endocrinol Metab 1999;84:1129–35.

78. Ma L, Lim H, Dey SK, Maas RL. Abdominal B (AbdB) Hoxa genes: regulation in the adult uterus by estrogen and progesterone and repression in the mullerian duct by the synthetic estrogen diethylstilbestrol. Dev Biol 1998;197:141–54.

79. Taylor HS, Bagot C, Kardana A, Olive D, Arici A. Hox gene expression is altered in the endometrium of women with endometriosis. Hum Reprod 1999;14:1328–31.

80. Benson GV, Lim H, Parai BC. Mechanisms of reduced fertility in Hoxa-10 mutant mice: uterine homeosis and loss of maternal Hoxa-10 expression. Development 1996;58:337–47.

81. Satokata I, Benson G, Maas R. Sexually dimorphic sterility phenotypes in Hoxa-10 deficient mice. Nature 1995;374:460–3.

82. Hsieh-Li HM, Witte DP, Weinstein M. Hoxa11 structure, extensive antisense transcription, and function in male and female infertility. Development 1995;121:373–85.

83. Gendron RL, Paradis H, Hsieh-Li HM et al. Abnormal uterine stromal and glandular function associated with maternal reproductive defects in Hoxa-11 null mice. Biol Reprod 1997;56:1097–105.

84. Troy P, Daftary G, Bagot C, Taylor HS. Transcriptional repression of peri-implantation EMX2 expression in mammalian reproduction by HOXA10. Mol Cell Biol 2003;23:1–13.

85. Simeone A, Acampora D, Gulisand M. Nested expression domains of four homeobox genes in developing rostral brain. Nature 1992;358:687–90.

86. Pellegrini M, Mansouri A, Simeone A, Bocinelli E, Gruss P. Dentate gyrus formation requires Emx2. Development 1996;2:335–45.

87. Daftary G, Troy P, Bagot C, Young SL, Taylor HS. Direct regulation of beta3-integrin subunit gene expression by HOXA10 in endometrial cells. Mol Endocrinol 2002;16:571–9.

88. Yoo HJ, Barlow DH, Mardon HJ. Temporal and spatial regulation of expression of heparin-binding epidermal growth factor-like growth factor in the human endometrium: a possible role in blastocyst implantation. Dev Genet 1997;21:102–8.

89. Birdsall MA, Hopkisson JF, Grant KE, Barlow DH, Mardon HJ. Expression of heparin-binding epidermal growth factor messenger RNA in the human endometrium. Mol Hum Reprod 1996;2:31–4.

90. Das SK, Chakraborty I, Paria BC et al. Amphiregulin is an implantation-specific and progesterone regulated gene in the mouse uterus. Mol Endocrinol 1995;9:691–705.

91. Das SK, Wang XN, Paria BC et al. Heparin biding EGF-like growth factor gene is induced in the mouse uterus temporally by the blastocyst solely at the site of its apposition: a possible ligand for interaction with blastocyst EGF-receptor in implantation. Development 1994;120:1071–83.

92. Martin KL, Barlow DH, Sargent IL. Heparin-binding epidermal growth factor significantly improves human blastocyst development and hatching in serum-free medium. Hum Reprod 1998;13:1645–52.

93. Lessey BA, Gui Y, Apparao KB, Young SL, Mulholland J. Regulated expression of heparin-binding EGF-like growth factor (HB-EGF) in the human endometrium: a potential paracrine role during implantation. Mol Reprod Dev 2002;62:446–55.

94. Graham CH, McCrae KR, Lala PK. Molecular mechanisms of controlling trophoblast invasion of the uterus. Trophoblast Res 1993;7:237–50.

95. Graham CH, Lysiak JJ, McCrae KR, Lala PK. Localization of transforming growth factor beta at the human fetal–maternal interface: role in trophoblast growth and differentiation. Biol Reprod 1992;46:561–72.

96. Zhou J, Bondy C. Insulin-like growth factor II and its binding proteins in placental development. Endocrinology 1992;131:1230–40.

97. Han VK, Bassett N, Walton J, Challis JR. The expression of insulin-like growth factor (IGF) and IGF binding protein genes in the human placenta and membranes: evidence for IGF:IGFBP interactions at the feto-maternal interface. J Clin Endocrinol Metab 1996;81:2680–93.

98. Irwin JC, Giudice LC. IGFBP-1 binds to the $\alpha5\beta1$ integrin in human cytotrophoblasts and inhibits their invasion into decidualized endometrial stromal cells in vitro. GH & IGF Res 1998;8:21–31.

99. Irving JA, Lala PK. Functional role of cell surface integrins on human trophoblast cell migration: regulation by TGF-beta, IGF-II, and IGFBP-1. Exp Cell Res 1995;217:419–27.

100. Hamilton GS, Lysiak JJ, Han VKM, Lala PK. Autocrine–paracrine regulation of human trophoblast invasiveness by IGF-II and IGFBP-1. Exp Cell Res 1998;244:147–56.

101. Kothapalli R, Buyuksal I, Wu S-Q, Chegini N, Tabibzadeh S. Detection of ebaf, a novel human gene of the transforming growth factor beta superfamily: association of gene expression with endometrial bleeding. J Clin Invest 1997;99:2342–50.

102. Tabibzadeh S, Mason JM, Shea W et al. Dysregulated expression of ebaf, a novel molecular defect in the endometri of patients with infertility. J Clin Endocrinol Metab 2000;85:2526–36.

103. Ma W, Tan J, Matsumoto H et al. Adult tissue angiogenesis: evidence for negative regulation by estrogen in the uterus. Mol Endocrinol 2001;15:1983–92.

104. Maisonpierre PC, Suri C, Jones PF et al. Angiopoietin-2, a natural antagonist for Tie2 that disrupts in vivo angiogenesis. Science 1997;277:55–60.

105. Chakraborty I, Das SK, Wang J, Dey SK. Developmental expression of the cyclo-oxygenase 1 and cyclo-oxygenase 2 genes in the peri-implantational mouse uterus and their differential regulation by the blastocyst and ovarian steroids. J Mol Endocrinol 1996;16:107–22.

106. Lim H, Paria BC, Das SK et al. Multiple female reproductive failures in cyclooxygenase-2 deficient mice. Cell 1997;91:297–308.

107. Cheng J-G, Stewart CL. Loss of cyclooxygenase-2 retards decidual growth but does not inhibit embryo implantation or development to term. Biol Reprod 2002;68:401–4.

108. Olivennes F, Feldberg D, Liu HC, Cohen J, Moy F, Rosenwaks Z. Endometriosis: a stage by stage analysis – the role of in vitro fertilization. Fertil Steril 1995;64:392–8.

109. Marcus SF, Edwards RG. High rates of pregnancy after long-term down-regulation of women with severe endometriosis. Am J Obstet Gynecol 1994;171:812–17.

110. Hahn DW, Carraher RP, Foldesy RG, McGuire JL. Experimental evidence for failure to implant as a mechanism of infertility associated with endometriosis. Am J Obstet Gynecol 1986;155:1109–13.

111. Carlber M, Nejaty J, Froysa B. Elevated expression of tumor necrosis factor alpha in cultured granulosa cells from women with endometriosis. Hum Reprod 2000;15:1250–5.

112. Van Blerkom J, Antczak M, Schrader R. The developmental potential of the human oocyte is related to the dissolved oxygen

content of follicular fluid: association with vascular endothelial growth factor levels and perifollicular blood flow characteristics. Hum Reprod 1997;12:1047–55.

113. Wardle PG, Mitchell JD, McLaughlin EA et al. Endometriosis and ovulatory disorder: reduced fertilization in vitro compared with tubal and unexplained infertility. Lancet 1985;2:236–9.

114. Pal L, Shifren JL, Isaacson KB. Impact of varying stages of endometriosis on the outocme of in vitro fertilization–embryo transfer. J Assist Reprod Genet 1998;15:27–31.

115. Garcia-Velasco JA, Nikas G, Remohi J, Pellicer A, Simon C. Endometrial receptivity in terms of pinopode expression is not impaired in women with endometriosis in artificially prepared cycles. Fertil Steril 2001;75:1231–3.

116. Lessey BA, Castelbaum AJ, Sawin SW et al. Aberrant integrin expression in the endometrium of women with endometriosis. J Clin Endocrinol Metab 1994;79:643–9.

117. Meyer WR, Castelbaum AJ, Somkuti S et al. Hydrosalpinges adversely affect markers of endometrial receptivity. Hum Reprod 1997;12:1393–8.

118. Ilera MJ, Yuan L, Stewart CL, Lessey BA. Effect of peritoneal fluid from women with endometriosis on implantation in the mouse model. Fertil Steril 2000;74:41–8.

119. Steinleitner A, Lambert H, Kazensky C, Danks P. Peritoneal fluid from endometriosis patients affects reproductive outcome in an in vivo model. Fertil Steril 1990;53:926–9.

120. Khorram O, Taylor RN, Ryan IP, Schall TJ, Landers DV. Peritoneal fluid concentrations of the cytokine RANTES correlate with the severity of endometriosis. Am J Obstet Gynecol 1993;169:1545–9.

121. Akoum A, Lemay A, McColl S, Turcot-Lemay L, Maheux R. Elevated concentration and biologic activity of monocyte chemotactic protein-1 in the peritoneal fluid of patients with endometriosis. Fertil Steril 1996;66:17–23.

122. Fukaya T, Sugarawa J, Yoshida H, Yajima A. The role of macrophage colony stimulating factor in the peritoneal fluid in infertile patients with endometriosis. Tohoku J Exp Med 1994;172:221–6.

123. Shifren JL, Tseng JF, Zaloudek CJ et al. Ovarian steroid regulation of vascular endothelial growth factor in the human endometrium: implications for angiogenesis during the menstrual cycle and in the pathogenesis of endometriosis. J Clin Endocrinol Metab 1996;81:3112–18.

124. Drake TS, O'Brien WF, Ramwell PW, Metz SA. Peritoneal fluid thromboxane B2 and 6-keto-prostaglandin F1 alpha in endometriosis. Am J Obstet Gynecol 1981;140:401–4.

125. Daftary G, Taylor HS. EMX2 gene expression in the female reproductive tract and aberrant expression in the endometrium of patients with endometriosis. J Clin Endocrinol Metab 2004;89:2390–6.

126. Ota H, Igarashi S, Sasaki M, Tanaka T. Distribution of cyclooxygenase-2 in eutopic and ectopic endometrium in endometriosis and adenomyosis. Hum Reprod 2001;16:561–6.

127. Sugawara JT, Fukaya T, Murakami T, Yoshida H, Yajima A. Increased secretion of hepatocyte growth factor by eutopic endometrial stromal cells in women with endometriosis. Fertil Steril 1997;68:468–72.

128. Giuduce LC, Telles TL, Lobo S, Kao L. The molecular basis for implantation failure in endometriosis: On the road to discovery. Ann NY Acad Sci 2002;955:252–64.

129. Matsumoto K, Okazaki H, Nakamura T. Up-regulation of hepatocyte growth factor gene expression by interleukin-1 in human skin fibroblasts. Biochem Biophys Res Commun 1992;188:235–43.

130. Tseng JF, Ryan IP, Milam TD et al. Interleukin-6 secretion in vitro is up-regulated in ectopic and eutopic endometrial stromal cells from women with endometriosis. J Clin Endocrinol Metab 1996;81:1118–22.

131. Sillem M, Prifti S, Monga B et al. Soluble urokinase-type plasminogen activator receptor is over-expressed in uterine endometrium from women with endometriosis. Mol Hum Reprod 1997;3:1101–5.

132. McBean JH, Brumsted JR. In vitro CA-125 secretion by endometrium from women with advanced endometriosis. Fertil Steril 1993;59:89–92.

133. Ota H, Igarashi S, Hatazawa J, Tanaka T. Distribution of heat shock proteins in eutopic and ectopic endometrium in endometriosis and adenomyosis. Fertil Steril 1997;68:23–8.

134. Jacquier-Sarlin MR, Fuller K, Dinh-Xuan AT, Richard M-J, Polla BS. Protective effects of hsp70 in inflammation. Experientia 1994;50:1031–8.

135. Beagley KW, Fujihashi K, Black CA. The *Mycobacterium tuberculosis* 71-kDa heat shock protein induces proliferation and cytokine secretion by murine gut epithelial lymphocytes. Eur J Immunol 1993;23:2049–52.

136. Ota H, Igarashi S, Tanaka T. Expression of gamma delta T cells and adhesion molecules in endometriotic tissue in patients with endometriosis and adenomyosis. Am J Reprod Immunol 1996;35:477–82.

137. Noble LS, SImpson ER, Johns A, Bulun SE. Aromatase expression in endometriosis. J Clin Endocrinol Metab 1996;81:174–9.

138. Fujimoto J, Ichigo S, Hirose R, Sakaguchi H, Tamaya T. Expression of estrogen receptor wild type and exon 5 splicing variant mRNAs in normal and endometriotic endometria during the menstrual cycle. Gynecol Endocrinol 1997;11:11–16.

139. Zeitoun KM, Takayama K, Sasano H et al. Deficient 17-b hydroxysteroid dehydrogenase type 2 expression in endometriosis: failure to metabolize 17 b estradiol. J Clin Endocrinol Metab 1998;83:4474–80.

140. Noble LS et al. Prostaglandin E2 stimulates aromatase expression in endometriosis-derived stromal cells. J Clin Endocrinol Metab 1997;82:600–6.

141. Ishihara H, Kitawaki J, Kado N et al. Gonadtropin-releasing hormone agonist and danazol normalize aromatase cytochrome P450 expression in eutopic endometrium from women with endometriosis, adenomyosis, or leiomyomas. Fertil Steril 2003;79(Suppl 1):735–42.

142. Kao LC, Germeyer A, Tulac S et al. Expression profiling of endometrium from women with endometriosis reveals candidate genes for disease-based implantation failure and infertility. Endocrinology 2003;144:2870–81.

143. Bartosik D, Damjanov I, Viscarello RR, Riley JA. Immunoproteins in the endometrium: clinical correlates of the presence of complement fractions C3 and C4. Am J Obstet Gynecol 1987;156:11–15.

144. Carson DD, Lagow E, Thathiah A et al. Changes in gene expression during the early to mid-luteal (receptive) phase transition in human endometrium detected by high-density microarray screening. Mol Hum Reprod 2002;8:871–9.

145. Dunn CL, Critchley HO, Kelley RW. IL-15 regulation in human endometrial stromal cells. J Clin Endocrinol Metab 2002;87:1898–901.

146. Oosterlynck DJ, Meuleman C, Waer M, Vandeputte M, Koninckx PR. The natural killer activity of peritoneal fluid lymphocytes is decreased in women with endometriosis. Fertil Steril 1992;58:290–5.

147. Wu MY, Yang JH, Chao KH et al. Increase in the expression of killer cell inhibitory receptors on peritoneal natural killer cells in women with endometriosis. Fertil Steril 2000;74:1187–91.

148. Okamoto N, Uchida A, Takakura K et al. Suppression by human placental protein 14 of natural killer cell activity. Am J Reprod Immunol 1991;26:137–42.

149. Rovere P, Peri G, Fazzini F et al. The long pentraxin PTX3 binds to apoptotic cells and regulates their clearance by antigen-presenting dendritic cells. Blood 2000;96:4300–6.

150. Soker S, Miao HQ, Nomi M, Takashima S, Klagsburn M. VEGF165 mediates formation of complexes containing VEGFR-2 and neurophilin-1 that enhance VEGF165-receptor binding. J Cell Biochem 2002;85:357–68.

151. Lee J, Burr JG. SALPa and SALPb, growth arresting homologs of Sam68. Gene 1999;240:133–47.

152. Hughes EG, Fedorkow DM, Collins JA. A quantitative overview of controlled trials in endometriosis-associated infertility. Fertil Steril 1993;59:963–70.

153. Adamson GD, Pasta DJ. Surgical treatment of endometriosis-associated infertility: meta-analysis compared with survival analysis. Am J Obstet Gynecol 1994;171:1488–505.

154. Nakamura K, Oosawa M, Kondou I et al. Menotropin stimulation after prolonged gonadotropin releasing hormone agonist pretreatment for in vitro fertilization in patients with endometriosis. J Assist Reprod Genet 1992;9:113–17.

155. Dicker D, Goldman JA, Levy T, Feldberg D, Ashkenazi J. The impact of long-term gonadotropin-releasing hormone analogue treatment on preclinical abortions in patients with severe endometriosis undergoing in vitro fertilization–embryo transfer. Fertil Steril 1992;57:597–600.

156. Kim CH, Cho YK, Mok JE. Simplified ultralong protocol of gonadotrophin-releasing hormone agonist for ovulation induction with intrauterine insemination in patients with endometriosis. Hum Reprod 1996;11:398–402.

157. Brinsden PR, Ndukwe G, Engrand P et al. Does recombinant human leukemia inhibitory factor improve implantation in women with recurrent failure of assisted reproduction treatment? Hum Reprod 2003;18(Suppl):Abstract 050.

158. Nowroozi K, Chase JS, Check JH, Wu CH. The importance of laparoscopic coagulation of mild endometriosis in infertile women. Int J Fertil 1987;32:442–4.

159. Marcoux S, Maheux R, Berube S. Laparoscopic surgery in infertile women with minimal or mild endometriosis. N Engl J Med 1997;337:217–22.

160. Tinkanen H, Kujansuu E. In vitro fertilization in patients with ovarian endometriomas. Acta Obstet Gynecol Scand 2000;79:119–22.

161. Pagidas K, Falcone T, Hemmings R, Miron P. Comparison of reoperation for moderate (stage III) and severe (stage IV) endometriosis-associated infertility with in vitro fertilization–embryo transfer. Fertil Steril 1996;65:791–5.

162. Isaacs JD, Hines RS, Sopelak VM, Cowan BD. Ovarian endometriomas do not adversely affect pregnancy success following treatment with in vitro fertilization. J Assist Reprod Genet 1997;14:551–3.

163. Bagot C, Troy PJ, Taylor HS. Alteration of maternal Hoxa10 expression by in vivo gene transfection affects implantation. Gene Ther 2000;7:1378–84.

164. Daftary G, Taylor HS. Efficient liposome-mediated gene transfection and expression in the intact human uterus. Hum Gene Ther 2001;12:2121–27.

165. Daftary GS, Taylor HS. Reproductive tract gene transfer. Fertil Steril 2003;80:475–84

3. The Endometrium and Angiogenesis

Elizabeth Pritts

Angiogenesis is the process by which new blood vessels develop from existing vessels. They accomplish this through a variety of methods, including sprouting,[1] intussusception, and vessel elongation. There may also be a role in angiogenesis for circulating endothelial progenitor cells[2] (Figure 3.1). Sprouting, also known as classic angiogenesis, begins with the activation of endothelial cells. Through the release of proteases, the basement membranes underlying the mature vessels are degraded, and activated endothelial cells migrate through that breach towards an angiogenic attractant. Through proliferation and intercellular communication, the active endothelial cells then organize to form tubules. During intussusception, the lumen of a mature vessel is partitioned into two separate vessels when activated endothelial cells are induced to separate from their mature vessel walls. The inward migration of the activated endothelial cells ultimately creates a system of interlocking or parallel vessels. Angiogenesis through vessel elongation occurs with the remodeling of existing vessels under the influence of metabolic demands.

Angiogenesis, and ultimately blood vessel development, depends upon intricate interactions between the endometrial glands and stroma, the basement membranes of the vessels, and the vessels themselves. These interactions are orchestrated through the secretion of a variety of growth factors. Although the ovarian steroid hormones are the major regulators of the growth factors, the factors themselves have both paracrine (secretion by one cell with effects on cells in close proximity) and autocrine (secretion by a cell with effects upon itself) functions in the tissues in which they reside.

Angiogenesis is found throughout the human body during embryogenesis; however, it occurs uncommonly in adult tissues and organs. In adults, it has been linked to disease states such as rheumatoid arthritis, psoriasis, chronic inflammatory disorders, and malignancies. In non-diseased states, angiogenesis occurs in the female adult reproductive tract on a monthly basis. Both the corpus luteum and the endometrium undergo blood vessel regrowth during the normal menstrual cycle.

Angiogenesis is different from vasculogenesis which, although it is a continuation of angiogenesis, is a different entity. Angiogenesis is the outgrowth of vessels from those already in existence, whereas vasculogenesis is the formation of vascular networks de novo.

During vasculogenesis, angioblasts, or endothelial progenitor cells, form a primitive vascular network. This process occurs predominantly during embryogenesis and fetal development, but has also been seen in adults in response to ischemic injury.[3,4] Vasculogenesis occurs in a stepwise fashion, with (1) the induction of hemangioblasts and angioblasts by stimulation from fibroblast growth factor (FGF); (2) the assembly of primordial vessels mediated through vascular endothelial growth factor (VEGF) and VEGF receptor complex; and (3) the transition from vasculogenesis to angiogenesis.

This chapter begins with a brief review of angiogenesis, followed by a profile of the

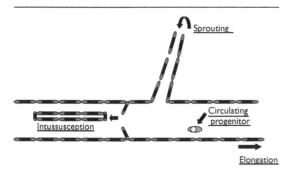

Figure 3.1 Types of angiogenesis. (Adapted from Gargett and Rogers. Reproduction 2001;121:181–6[141] with permission from Elsevier.)

morphogenesis of the uterus, a histologic review of the endometrium, and a review of cellular and vascular morphology and function during the menstrual cycle. The known endometrial angiogenic and antiangiogenic factors and their receptors will then be introduced, with a brief review of the cofactors involved as well. Each factor, cofactor, and receptor will then be localized temporally to the phase of the menstrual cycle and spatially to each cellular subtype in which they are found.

the uterus begins to regress in both size and cellular activity. This leads to a uterine cervix which in young girls is larger than the corpus.

In young girls the uterus remains quiescent until about age 7, at which time the total uterine volume, as well as the corpus to cervix ratio, begins to increase.[8,9] Under the influence of ovarian hormones the endometrium will begin the growth and regression of the glands and stroma that will continue for the next 40 years or so of a woman's life.

MORPHOGENESIS OF THE UTERUS

The uterus arises from the fusion of the paramesonephric ducts. These ducts, also known as müllerian ducts, arise from the longitudinal invaginations of the coelomic epithelium of the mesonephros. This fusion begins at around week 6 of gestation by dates for a normal female fetus.[5] This appears to be regulated by a set of homeobox (HOX) genes that control the transcriptions of growth modulation factors. These gene products, HOX 9-13, when dysregulated, can result in abnormalities in both the structure and the function of adult reproductive tissues. In particular, HOX-a 10 and 11 seem to be expressed in the paramesonephric duct during uterine embryogenesis.[6]

These fused ducts subsequently undergo a 'canalization' phase, during which the uterine septum resorbs, leaving a primordial uterus with a single cavity. The septum is actually made up of the lateral fused walls of the paramesonephric ducts. These ducts eventually give rise to the epithelium and glands of the uterus. The stromal component of the uterus, as well as the muscular covering, or myometrium, are derived from a different embryonic layer, the mesenchyme, which lies adjacent to the müllerian ducts.[7]

By week 22 of gestation the uterus is complete in its development. By week 32, glandular secretory activity, as evidenced by glycogen accumulation and stromal edema, are found. Throughout the rest of gestation the fetal uterus is still under control of maternal hormones. Just after delivery,

STRUCTURE OF THE ENDOMETRIUM

The endometrium can be divided into two major layers (Figure 3.2). The layer nearest the luminal surface is called the functionalis, which is further broken down into the compact and spongy zones. The functionalis zone undergoes dramatic changes throughout the menstrual cycle, and it is this zone that is sloughed each 28 days in a non-pregnant uterus.

The functionalis itself is then further subdivided histologically. The most superficial layer consists of the epithelial or glandular cells. These overlie a complex stromal compartment consisting of mesenchymal fibroblasts, such as vascular smooth muscle cells, stromal cells, and immunologic cells.

The second zone of the endometrium is the basal zone. This contains the fundi (basal portion) of the glands as well as the supporting vasculature. This zone undergoes much less change during the menstrual cycle, and is thought to be primarily responsible for the regeneration of the endometrium as early as the second day of menstrual bleeding.

The vessels of the endometrium are fed from the uterine artery in the basal layer of the endometrium. This artery feeds the spiral arteries located in the spongy and compact zones of the functionalis layer of the endometrium. Ultimately, the spiral arteries will give rise to and feed the subcapillary plexus, which is located in the compact zone. This subcapillary plexus, along with a segment of the spiral artery, will be lost to

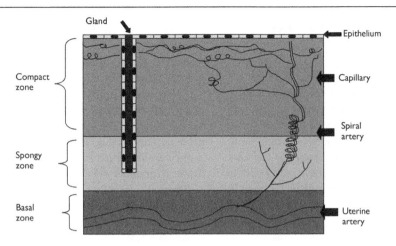

Figure 3.2 The endometrial architecture.

menstruation, only to be restored the next month in anticipation of implantation.

THE MENSTRUAL CYCLE

It has been shown that the growth of the endometrium during the menstrual cycle is intimately associated with the growth and maturity of the vasculature. In certain studies,[10] by blocking angiogenesis, the proliferation of the endometrium has been curtailed.

THE PROLIFERATIVE PHASE

Immediately post menstruation in the proliferative phase angiogenesis begins, with the repair of ruptured vessels. Elongation of the existing vessels is thought to be the major form of angiogenesis at this time. This was shown in an elegant study during which the investigators measured vessel length over a given area and compared it against vessel branching over that same area. When a segment elongates, it is more likely to be associated with angiogenesis by elongation. When the branching areas increase, they are more likely to be associated with intussusception. In this study, vessel elongation predominated during

the early proliferative phase.[11] The vessels form a loose capillary network which permeates the overlying and newly forming functionalis zone.[12] This process continues until the late proliferative phase.

The epithelium, which can measure as little as 2 mm in the early part of the proliferative phase, begins its regeneration from the nidus of the enduring basalis layer cells still present in the cornual regions and the lower uterine segment of the uterus. The mitotic activity of both the epithelial and the stromal cells begins its acceleration at this time. By day 5 of the menstrual cycle the epithelium has regenerated and forms a contiguous structure overlying the functionalis.

The angiogenesis that occurs during the mid-proliferative phase of the menstrual cycle does so under the influence of estradiol. It occurs in the spongy zone through the elongation of the spiral arteries, and in the compact zone through the elongation of the subluminal capillary plexus.[13]

It is during this time that the endometrium undergoes its most rapid growth phase, quadrupling in size. The endometrium increases its height as a result of hyperplasia of the glands and an increase in extracellular matrix. Ultrasound studies have shown at least a tripling of endometrial thickness during this period.[14,15]

THE TRANSITION FROM PROLIFERATIVE TO SECRETORY PHASE

In the transition from the proliferative to the secretory phase of the menstrual cycle, two angiogenic mechanisms have been suggested: sprouting and intussusception. Sprouting is not thought to be involved in endometrial angiogenesis,[13] but there are data to support intussusception as being the primary mode of angiogenesis. In a single study[16] sprouting angiogenesis was recognized in the endometrium, but unfortunately this finding has not so far been corroborated. In fact, when other investigators have examined endometrial tissue they have not found evidence of sprouting angiogenesis. Instead, they have found proliferating endothelial vessels within existing vessels, pointing to intussusception as the mode of angiogenesis in the endometrium.[13] Further evidence of intussusceptive angiogenesis exists as well. $\alpha v\beta 3$ Integrin is a marker for new endothelial growth. This marker has only been localized to the lumina of pre-existing vessels.[17] Endothelial cells undergo cytoplasmic growth during the secretory phase, and that growth seems to be inward towards the lumen. Some cells enlarge to fill the capillary lumen, a description that is again consistent with intussusceptive growth.[18]

THE SECRETORY PHASE

Initially in the secretory phase, a portion of the arterioles in the endometrium coil and thicken to form a spiral conformation. This phenomenon occurs because of the rather constant growth of both the spongy and the compact zones of the cellular endometrium, compared with the relatively increased proliferation of the spiral arteries.[13]

In the midsecretory phase, vessel length remains stable but there is an increase in vessel junction numbers. This is consistent with a switch from vessel elongation as the primary mode of angiogenesis to intussusception. By the late secretory phase, vascular length density is already beginning to decrease to early proliferative levels, possibly suggesting even vascular

regression.[11] This is also the time in the menstrual cycle during which increased vascular permeability is noted. This is evidenced by stromal edema, increased blood flow, and transudation of plasma proteins by the late secretory phase.[13,19-22]

After ovulation, the mitotic activity of the glandular and stromal cells decreases and the major activity is secretion, with only limited growth. This is due in part to the secretion of progesterone, which inhibits mitogenesis at least in the stromal as well as the glandular cells.

There is currently controversy as to the rate of angiogenesis in the different zones during the different phases of the menstrual cycle. Common sense suggests that the proliferation of the endothelium would increase throughout the menstrual cycle, and would do so in the functional zone of the endometrium rather than the basal zone. Limited data from the late 1970s appeared to corroborate this theory. In these early studies, proliferation rates in the basalis seemed lower than that found in the functionalis.[23] Other investigators confirmed that endothelial proliferation during the menstrual cycle increased as the cycle progressed.[17,24] It was thought that the basalis vessels were only the progenitor vessels, with most of the proliferation occurring in the functionalis layer of the endometrium.

Recent studies, however, have challenged this finding.[11,25] In these studies there was no difference in vessel segment length between the subepithelial capillary plexus, the functionalis, and the basalis during matched times in the menstrual cycle. If vessel growth were occurring at an increased rate in the functionalis zone, the vessels' segment lengths should be increased, but this is not the case. The rate of increase in the density of vessels was also similar between the basalis and functionalis. If, during intussusceptive growth, the functionalis zone had an increased rate of growth, the density of this endometrial layer should be increased. Again this is not the case. All other investigators, save one group, have found similar vessel length and density in each endometrial zone.[13,26,27] In a single study in which the mitogenic activity of the endothelial cells was directly examined, no peak growth rates were exhibited during the menstrual cycle.[26] At any rate, it is clear that angiogenesis must be accelerated in order to nourish the growth of the cellular and extracellular layers of the endometrium as they develop during the cycle.

THE MENSTRUAL PHASE

If implantation does not occur, then the decline of progesterone and estrogen leads to vasoconstriction of the arterioles and spiral arteries. As the vessels relax, an ischemic–reperfusion injury ensues.

The spiral arterioles are thought to play a major role in the control of menstrual bleeding, and are the major site of blood loss.[28,29] These vessels differ from other arterioles in two ways: their lack of elastin and their coiled shape.[30] They may also have larger vascular smooth muscle cells (constrictor cells that surround developing vessels).[31]

The superficial layers of the endometrium now demonstrate hematoma formation and concomitant fissure development. Autophagy and heterophagy ensue, as well as apoptosis. This leads to sloughing of the outer two-thirds of the endometrium. This sloughed tissue is what is lost during the menstruation process.

ANGIOGENIC FACTORS

By far the most important components involved in the monitoring of angiogenesis are vascular endothelial growth factor (VEGF), basic fibroblast growth factor (bFGF), epidermal growth factor (EGF) and the angiopoietins (Ang). However, many other angiogenic factors may play a role in the menstrual cycle. Each year, putative factors are being added to that list, including the matrix metalloproteinases (MMP), the prostanoids, endothelin, urokinase-type plasminogen activator (u-PA), angiogenin, and thrombin (Table 3.1).

VEGF AND ITS RECEPTORS

In the endometrium the VEGF family of genes is thought to be crucial in angiogenesis. These factors are highly specific mitogens for vascular

Table 3.1 The angiogenic and antiangiogenic factors

Proangiogenic factors	Antiangiogenic factors
Vascular endothelial growth factors	Angiostatin
A, B, C, D	Thrombospondin
Angiopoietins 1, 2	Endostatin
Placental growth factor	Tumor necrosis factor-α
Granulocyte colony-stimulating factor	Prolactin
Granulocyte–macrophage colony-stimulating factor	Thromboxane A_2
Leptin	
Interleukin-8	
Proliferin	
Insulin-like growth factor-1, -2	
Transforming growth factor-α, β	
Chorionic gonadotropin	
Estrogens	
Prostaglandin E_1, E_2	
Tumor necrosis factor-α	
Hepatocyte growth factor	

Reproduced from Zygmunt et al. Eur J Obstet Gynecol 2003;110:S10–18[45] by permission of the Society for Reproduction and Fertility.

endothelial cells, and can be found in the endometrium throughout the menstrual cycle. The family consists of VEGF-A, B, C, D, E, and placental growth factor (PIGF). These ligands bind to three receptor types, VEGFR-1, 2, and 3. The VEGF members known to be involved in endometrial angiogenesis include VEGF-A, B, and C.

VEGF-A is derived from eight exons located on chromosome 6[32] and has five known splice variants (Figure 3.3). The first four exons are thought to be the most important, as they are common to all of the variants. The isoforms include $VEGF_{206}$ and $VEGF_{189}$, which express all eight exons; $VEGF_{165}$, encompassing all the exons except number 6; $VEGF_{145}$, which lacks only exon 7; and

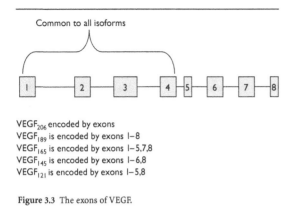

Common to all isoforms

$VEGF_{206}$ encoded by exons
$VEGF_{189}$ is encoded by exons 1–8
$VEGF_{165}$ is encoded by exons 1–5,7,8
$VEGF_{145}$ is encoded by exons 1–6,8
$VEGF_{121}$ is encoded by exons 1–5,8

Figure 3.3 The exons of VEGF.

$VEGF_{121}$, which lacks both exons 6 and 7. Each different exon confers charge to the final product as well, with exons 6 and 7 encoding a relatively higher number of basic amino acids. This leads to differences in the isoelectric points of each isoform, with the smaller proteins being more acidic.[33] The significance of this has yet to be determined.

Within the human endometrium all of the isoforms of VEGF-A have been found, the most common being $VEGF_{121}$ and $VEGF_{165}$. Although all isoforms seem to have the same activity, some of their differences may lie in their ability to bind the extracellular matrix. $VEGF_{121}$ is found most commonly in soluble form, whereas $VEGF_{165}$ and, to a greater extent, $VEGF_{189}$, is regulated by binding to heparin sulfate proteoglycans found in the extracellular matrix.[34,35] It is thought that these larger forms of VEGF provide a reservoir of growth factors available for use throughout the menstrual cycle. Their release could easily be accomplished through heparinases or u-PA.[36,37]

Hypoxia is the most powerful activator of VEGF-A expression. In response to hypoxia, VEGF expression is up regulated at least twofold in glandular tissue and threefold in stromal tissue in in vitro studies.[38] This response has been shown to be affected through at least two distinct pathways. Expression of VEGF mRNA is upregulated, beginning with the heterodimerization of the hypoxia-inducible factor-1α (HIF-1α) transcription factor with the aryl hydrocarbon receptor nuclear translocator.[39,40] The heterodimer

then binds to a site on the promoter region of the VEGF gene approximately 900 base pairs (bp) upstream from the transcription start site. The second pathway involves the decrease in VEGF mRNA degradation through the binding of nuclear proteins that stabilize message.[41]

Both estrogen and progesterone are also involved in the transcription of VEGF-A message.[20,42] The VEGF promoter has at least two estrogen response elements and has been found to be responsive to both estrogen receptor α and estrogen receptor β.[43] It has also been found to increase its expression through progesterone response elements.[42] The list of other factors involved in VEGF expression continues to expand. VEGF-A is also found to be up regulated by EGF, PGE-2, IL-1, IL-6, TGF-β, and hCG.[44]

VEGF-A actions include mitogenesis of endothelial cells, activation of serine proteases (uPA and tPA) and collagenases, increased endothelial cell chemotaxis, and vasodilatation.[45] Thus it is intimately involved in each step of angiogenesis.

VEGF-B has only recently been localized to the endometrium, in the stroma and blood vessels throughout the menstrual cycle. Ovarian hormones do not seem to influence the expression of this growth factor, and it seems to be expressed in a fairly constant fashion during the menstrual cycle.[46,47] The function of VEGF-B is complex. It can form a heterodimer with VEGF-A, and putatively enhances the angiogenic effect of other growth factors.[48] VEGF-B is seen in close proximity to glandular epithelium, as it is known to bind to heparin in the extracellular membrane.[46]

VEGF-C is also a newly detected factor to the endometrium. It is found primarily in the uterine-specific natural killer cell population (uNK). Like VEGF-B, it seems to be expressed in a constant fashion throughout the menstrual cycle and so it seems to have no association with steroid hormones. However, it is regulated by EGF, which is hormonally regulated, so this finding is a bit confusing. It has no HIF-1α region in its promoter sequence, so it also does not respond to hypoxia as VEGF-A does.

VEGF-C stimulates the lymphatic endothelial cell proliferation and migration via the VEGFR-2 and -3 receptors.[49] Other functions of this specific protein are still under investigation. Factors known to increase the expression of VEGF-C are tumor necrosis factor-α (TNF-α) and interleukin-1 (IL-1).

The VEGF receptors include VEGFR-1 (Flt-1), VEGFR-2 (KDR/murine analog Flk-1), and VEGFR-3. These receptors are known to be members of the tyrosine kinase family and are expressed on the surface of endothelial cells as well as in soluble forms during pregnancy (sVEGFR-1).

VEGFR-1 has been localized to endometrial glands, blood vessels, and in scattered areas of the stromal compartment.[50–52] The stromal localization may be due to staining of macrophages.[53,54]

VEGFR-2 has thus far been found only in epithelial cells.[55] VEGFR-2, when bound to its receptor, is known to induce the release of nitric oxide from endothelial cells.[56] This is thought to promote mitogenesis and increase the permeability of vessels, as well as blocking apoptosis. VEGFR-1 antagonizes these effects by binding to its ligand but conferring no activity in regard to mitogenesis or the permeability of vessels. It does, however, increase migration of the endothelial cells.[55] It is also thought to be involved in the regulation of circulating progenitor endothelial cells through its binding of VEGF-B.[58]

VEGFR-3 expression is localized to uNK cells of the endometrium and the vessels themselves.[46,59] The ligand for both VEGFR-2 and -3 is VEGF-C. A new VEGF receptor, neurophilin-1, has recently been discovered. Its role in angiogenesis is still unsolved.

ANGIOPOIETINS

Another angiogenic family of growth factors has been clearly established in the endometrium. Angiopoietins are involved primarily in the survival of endothelial cells, in the remodeling of the capillary plexus during the cycle, and in the stabilization of the plexus once it is remodeled.[60–62] The two angiopoietins thus far identified have been named, appropriately, Ang-1 and Ang-2.

Ang-1 is expressed by vascular smooth muscle cells (the progenitors of which are fibroblast cells interspersed throughout the stromal compart-

ment of the endometrium). Ang-1 promotes smooth muscle cell mitogenesis through the production of platelet-derived growth factor and heparin-binding epidermal growth factor.[63]

Ang-2 is found predominantly in the uNK cells. Approximately 70% of uNK cells secrete Ang-2: those nearest the luminal epithelium of the endometrium, and those about the vascular smooth muscle cells. Ang-2 is the natural antagonist to its family member Ang-1. When bound to its receptor, it leads to vessel destabilization and neovascularization in the presence of VEGF. Without concomitant VEGF, vessels will undergo atrophy and apoptosis.[63]

The major receptor for both the angiopoietins, Tie-2, is found on blood vessel endothelium and initiates the tyrosine kinase intracellular pathway. Ang-1 binds to Tie-2, causing its phosphorylation,[64] which leads to endothelial cell migration,[65] sprouting,[66,67] and the prevention of apoptotic events in vitro.[68,69] In vivo, it increases new vessel growth, branching, and maturation.[67,70] Once the ligand–receptor complex is bound to the developing vessel, stabilization occurs.

Tie-2 has been implicated in intussusceptive angiogenesis of the endometrium, at least in mouse models.[71] It is detected mainly in the vessels and glandular epithelium of normal endometrium. Tie-2 is upregulated by VEGF and bFGF in cultured endothelial cells.[72–74]

Ang-2 also has affinity for the Tie-2 receptor; however, binding does not induce phosphorylation and subsequent activation of the receptor. The lack of phosphorylation is thought to lead to the destabilization or regression that occurs when this ligand and receptor associate.

FIBROBLAST GROWTH FACTORS

The fibroblast growth factors are a family of factors involved in growth and differentiation. The family is composed of 18 members, of which two are known to be involved in angiogenesis (FGF-1 or acidic FGF, and FGF-2 or basic FGF). These molecules stimulate proliferation of endothelial cells and inhibit their apoptosis. Their receptors are present in both high-affinity (FGFR 1–4) and low-affinity forms (heparin sulfate proteoglycans). The high-affinity receptors are of the tyrosine kinase family and induce signaling transduction pathways in the cells. The low-affinity receptors function mainly through sequestration of the ligand for use in the future. These molecules are found predominantly in epithelial cells, although some lesser staining can be found in the stromal fibroblasts.[52]

Although the main action of FGF is unknown, when it binds to either FGFR-1 or FGFR-2, VEGFR-2 expression is upregulated.[75] It is also known to increase the expression of MMP-1, which stimulates endothelial cell migration through the stromal interstitium.[76–78]

EPIDERMAL GROWTH FACTOR

EGF is a known mitogen for a variety of cell types, including human microvascular endothelial cells[79,80] and lymphatic endothelial cells.[81–83] It is found primarily in the stroma of the endometrium, with its receptor being localized to endometrial arteries but not veins.[52]

ENDOTHELIN

This factor is involved in the growth and development of the spiral arterioles during the menstrual cycle. Endothelin is a potent vasoconstrictor, thought to function through its release of $PGF_{2\alpha}$, as well as a vascular smooth muscle and endothelial cell mitogen.[84–88]

PROSTANOIDS

Prostanoids are known vasoconstrictors and are thought to help invoke the ischemic response of the arteries during the late secretory phase of the menstrual cycle, leading to hypoxia and VEGF expression.[87]

ANGIOGENIN

Angiogenin has only recently been described. It is a polypeptide that was initially isolated from colon carcinoma cells[89] and is a member of the pancreatic ribonuclease superfamily. In vitro it has been isolated to both glandular and stromal cells of the endometrium, and its expression seems to be upregulated at least three- to fourfold when comparing proliferative to mid- and late secretory menstrual phases. Interestingly, just as with VEGF and FGF, hypoxia causes increased expression of angiogenin.[12] Further characterization of this factor is necessary to elucidate its role in the growth and regression of the endometrium.

THROMBIN

Thrombin has been shown to indirectly increase angiogenesis by increasing VEGF expression in human endometrial stromal cells.[90] It directly stimulates angiogenesis by increasing endothelial proliferation and increasing VEGFR-2 expression in endothelial cells.[91] Its exact mechanism in the control of the menstrual cycle still is yet unsolved.

MATRIX METALLOPROTEINASES

The MMPs are a family of zinc-dependent enzymes capable of degrading most of the proteins that can be found in the extracellular matrix. These proteins were initially discovered in the endometrium in the early 1990s.[92–94] They have been found both in vitro and in vivo in both stromal and epithelial cells;[93] however, at menstruation most MMP are released from the stromal cell population.[94,95]

MMP mediate angiogenesis by degrading extracellular matrices in preparation for migration and tube formation of endothelial cells. MMP-1–3, -7, and -9–11 are found in the endometrium during the menstrual cycle.[96] Progesterone is known to decrease their expression, and its withdrawal is known to increase their expression. During the menstrual cycle this would correspond with an increase in the MMP as the progesterone levels decrease at the end of the secretory phase. This leads initially to the shedding of the superficial layer of the endometrium, as well as creation of the extracellular space necessary to develop the new vasculature in the early part of the proliferative phase of the cycle.

The endometrium also secretes the tissue inhibitors of MMPs, the TIMPs.[93,97] The levels of the inhibitors are unaffected by ovarian steroid hormones, and they are constitutively expressed throughout the menstrual cycle. They also seem to be degraded at approximately the same rate as the MMPs.[98]

As with all of the factors involved in angiogenesis, the MMPs are also under paracrine regulation. VEGF, as well as hepatocyte growth factor, transforming growth factor-β (TGF-β), and thrombin can upregulate the expression the MMPs and decrease the expression of their inhibitors, the TIMPs.[57,99,100] Activated T cells have also been shown to increase the expression of MMPs from endothelial cells and vascular smooth muscle cells.

PLASMINOGEN ACTIVATOR

It is generally accepted that u-PA and its inhibitor the plasminogen activator inhibitor-1 (PAI-1) are involved in the first phase of angiogenesis, apparently in the remodeling of the extracellular matrix and migration of the endothelial cells.[101–103] u-PA is the enzyme responsible for the conversion of plasminogen into the active serine protease plasmin, which degrades the matrix proteins and activates several of the MMPs.[104–106]

ANTIANGIOGENIC FACTORS

Although there are many factors involved in angiogenesis during the menstrual cycle, there is also a robust antiangiogenic force holding angiogenesis in check. The factors elucidated thus far include the thrombospondins,[106–108] the fragments of thrombospondins,[109] endostatin,[110] angiostatin, platelet factor 4, and TGF-β (see Table 3.1).

THROMBOSPONDIN-1

Thrombospondin-1 (TSP-1) is a glycoprotein that was originally identified in platelet α granules. Its

release is initiated from thrombin activation of the platelet itself.[111] It has also been found to be secreted by vascular smooth muscle cells, endothelial cells, macrophages, fibroblasts, and neutrophils.[111–113]

In endothelial cells this factor has been shown to be antiproliferative,[114] to disrupt the adhesion and migration of endothelial cells,[107,115] and to inhibit angiogenesis.[116–121] Although membrane-bound thrombospondin may have an angiogenic activity, soluble thrombospondin decreases the proliferation of endothelial cells and modulates endothelial cell adhesion.[111] The DNA region responsible for this antiangiogenic activity has been mapped to a procollagen homology sequence; however, the exact mechanism of action is still under investigation. The human TSP gene has two progesterone response elements in its promoter sequence, and so it comes as no surprise that its expression is upregulated by progesterone.[107]

TSP-1 acts upon many other factors involved in the angiogenic pathway. It has been shown to prevent the activation of MMP-2 and -9, known to decompose the extracellular matrix in preparation for the invasion of new blood vessel growth.[122] It also downregulates platelet-derived endothelial cell adhesion molecule-1, and binds to endothelial cell glycoprotein CD-36, both associated with anti-angiogenic activity.[108,123] It promotes endothelial cell apoptosis by upregulating BAX secretion, increasing the activity of caspase-3 (both proapoptotic proteins) and downregulating the antiapoptotic gene product BCL-2.[124]

ANGIOSTATIN

Angiostatin is the proteolytic portion of plasminogen, so it shares the functions of plasminogen. It blocks the proliferation of endothelial cells and suppresses early tumor cell growth in mouse models.[125]

TRANSFORMING GROWTH FACTOR-β

TGF-β has been found in menstrual endometrium by several investigators.[85,126,127] It is thought to inhibit vascular smooth muscle cell proliferation and upregulate smooth muscle cells actin in various cell types. It also upregulates the expression of preproendothelin, the precursor for endothelin.[128–130]

THE FACTORS DURING THE MENSTRUAL CYCLE

Although the results are conflicting for many of the factors, a summary of the factors putatively involved in each stage of the menstrual cycle, and their compartments of origin, will be reviewed (Table 3.2). Because of the conflicting data thus far, it is not feasible to create a working model of the exact steps involved in angiogenesis during the menstrual cycle. Further studies are needed before the complete pathway is established.

THE FACTORS AND THEIR RECEPTORS IN THE PROLIFERATIVE PHASE

The precise cyclic variation of VEGF expression during the menstrual cycle has yet to be defined. Many of the data in regard to the precise timing of expression and to the cell or organ of origin of the protein itself are conflicting. It is clear, however, that VEGF is present in the endometrium in the proliferative phase.

As regards the glandular expression of VEGF, there is no clear consensus as to whether there is a change in the proliferative phase or not, or even in which direction the change occurs.[72,131–137] Similarly, there is no clear consensus as to the expression of stromal VEGF expression, with studies showing both increased and unchanging expression.[72,138,139] The vascular expression of VEGF also has no clear expression pattern during the proliferative phase, having been shown as both increased and unchanged across the phase.[72,131] In circulating leukocytes, such as neutrophils, monocytes and T lymphocytes,[140–146] VEGF has been shown to be both elevated and unchanged in this phase as well.

VEGF receptor expression has been examined in only a few studies. VEGFR-1 has been found in low levels during the midproliferative phase, weakly to moderately in the stroma, and only rarely in endometrial glandular cells.[52,136] VEGFR-2 was found in the endothelial and glandular cells from the midproliferative phase until menstruation.[50,52,136]

Ang-1 is found in the early and midproliferative phase of the cycle in the peristromal vasculature, which speaks to its paracrine function. This is in contrast to Ang-2, which is expressed to a lesser degree during the proliferative phase of the cycle. The Ang-1 and -2 receptor, Tie-2, exhibits its first peak of expression during the early proliferative phase (just like Ang-1), decreasing in the mid–late proliferative phase.[12]

FGF-2 has been found, albeit inconsistently, in the glands, stroma, and basement membrane of the vasculature solely in the proliferative phase of the cycle.[52,76] Interestingly, FGFR-1 is only expressed in glands and stroma, not in the vasculature, during the late proliferative and secretory phases. Conversely, FGFR-2 is expressed throughout the cycle;[52] localization to specific tissue has yet to be determined.

EGF is expressed weakly in epithelium in the midproliferative phase, decreasing in the secretory and menstrual phases. In the stroma its expression is variable, and it has not been localized to vessels. The expression of its receptor has not been established in the proliferative phase.[52]

A subset of MMPs is expressed throughout the menstrual cycle. During the proliferative phase of the cycle, MMP-1–3 and -11 are expressed in the stroma,[94] MMP-7 is found in the glandular epithelium,[94,97] and MMP-9 is found in the polymorphonuclear cells and monocytes confined to the blood vessels.[147] The inhibitor TIMP-1 is found in the stromal cells during this phase.[94,148]

THE FACTORS IN THE SECRETORY PHASE

As with the proliferative phase, the data regarding the expression of VEGF during the secretory

Table 3.2 The factors throughout the menstrual cycle

Factor	Tissue localization
Early proliferative phase	
VEGF	Controversial
Ang-1	Peristromal vasculature
FGF-1, 2	Glands, endothelium, other?
MMP-1, 2, 3, 7, 9, 11	Glands, stroma, white blood cells
Angiogenin	Glands, stroma
Midproliferative phase	
VEGF	Controversial
Ang-1	Peristromal vasculature
FGF-1	Glands, endothelium, other?
EGF	Glands, stroma
MMP-1, 2, 3, 7, 9, 11	Glands, stroma, white blood cells
Angiogenin	Glands, stroma
Late proliferative phase	
VEGF	Controversial
FGF-1	Glands, endothelium, other?
MMP-1, 2, 3, 7, 9, 11	Glands, stroma, white blood cells
Angiogenin	Glands, stroma
Early secretory phase	
VEGF	Controversial
Ang-2	Glands, stroma
Angiogenin	Glands, stroma
TSP-1	Stroma, endothelium, vascular smooth muscle
Midsecretory phase	
VEGF	Controversial
Ang-2	Glands, stroma
Tie-2	Glands, vessels
Endothelin-1	Glands, stroma, endothelium
TGF-β	Glands, stroma, endothelium
Angiogenin	Glands, stroma
MMP-1, 2, 3, 9, 10	Glands, stroma, white blood cells
TSP-1	Stroma, endothelium, vascular smooth muscle
Late secretory phase	
VEGF	Controversial
Ang-2	Glands, stroma
Tie-2	Glands, vessels
Endothelin-1	Glands, stroma, endothelium
TGF-β	Glands, stroma, endothelium
Angiogenin	Glands, stroma
MMP-2, 3, 7, 10, 11	Glands, stroma
TSP-1	Stroma, endothelium, vascular smooth muscle
Menstrual phase	
FGF-2	Vessels
MMP-1, 2, 3, 7, 9, 10, 11	Stroma, vessels, glands, white blood cells

phase are sometimes conflicting with regard to its localization and timing.

In the both glandular and vascular cells VEGF has been shown to increase during the secretory phase.[20,136,137,149] The expression in stromal cells is quite variable, with investigators finding increases, decreases, and no changes in this phase.[131,133,136,149–152]

In the stroma, VEGFR-2 receptors are upregulated. In the epithelium their expression is unchanged throughout the entire cycle.[50,149] In the blood vessels the picture is less clear, with conflicting reports of both increased and decreased expression of VEGFR-2.[50,149] VEGFR-1 stains negligibly throughout the entire menstrual cycle.[149]

Ang-2 has more prominent expression in the secretory phase in both glandular epithelium and stroma.[57,153] Tie-2 elicits a second peak of expression in the mid–late secretory phase of the menstrual cycle in both vessels and glandular tissue.[153] This second rise in Tie-2 expression is found in conjunction with the growth of the spiral arteries.[30,74]

Although FGF-2 is found most commonly during the menstrual and early proliferative phases of the cycle, FGFR-2 is found in the vessels of the endometrium, specifically the arteries, during the late proliferative and secretory phases,[52] with FGFR-1 specifically found only in the late secretory phase.

EGF expression is found only rarely in the secretory phase of the menstrual cycle; however, its receptor, EGFR, stains abundantly in the epithelium, glands, and stroma during this phase.[52]

Endothelin-1 expression has been found during the mid and late secretory phases of the cycle, but has not yet been examined in the proliferative phase. Its expression is found both in the glandular epithelial cells and in the perivascular stroma, endothelial cells, and vessel basement membrane.[30,85,126]

Angiogenin seems to be expressed in an incremental fashion from the proliferative to the secretory phases of the cycle. It is expressed in both glands and stroma.[12]

MMP-2, -3, -10 and -11[94,147,154] are found in the stromal cells during the mid–late secretory phases, and MMP-7 in the glandular epithelium in the late secretory phase.[94,97] MMP-9 is found both in the epithelial glandular cells during the secretory phase – specifically days 19–20[77] – and in the polymorphonuclear cells confined to the vessels.[147] TIMP-1 is found in the periglandular and perivascular spaces,[94,148] and TIMP-3 is found in the stroma during this time.[155]

TSP-1 is found in the basement membrane of the capillary plexus during this phase, as well as in the stromal, epithelial, and vascular smooth muscle cells.[107]

TGF-β is found in a very similar pattern to that of endothelin-1. It is found in the mid–late secretory phases in the glands, the perivascular stroma, and the endothelial cells. However, it also has not been studied at other times during the cycle. The presence of this factor is associated with vessel contractility.[30,128,130]

THE FACTORS IN THE MENSTRUAL PHASE

FGF-2 is found in vessels with the highest intensity during both the proliferative and the menstrual phases of the cycle;[52,73,156] however, its receptors are found mainly during the secretory phase.

Although most EGF is expressed during the proliferative phase, in the vessels EGFR staining occurs in a bimodal fashion, in both the early secretory and the menstrual phase.[52]

TSP-1 is expressed in the endometrial vasculature just prior to the onset of menstruation.[88]

Both endothelin and prostanoids have been found in the premenstrual endometrium. These are the factors associated with vasoconstriction, ischemia, and local hypoxia.[86,87,157]

MMP-1 and -2 are found in the stroma and perivascular space during the menstrual phase of the cycle.[94,154,158-160] MMP-3 is found in the stroma and vessels situated near the superficial endometrium during the premenstrual and menstrual phases.[94,147,158,161]

MMP-7 has been localized to endometrial glandular epithelial cells as well as luminal cells.[97,162] MMP-9 is expressed both in polymorphonuclear cells and monocytic cells, and in the stroma;[94,147] MMP-10 and -11 are expressed in the stroma,[94,162] and TIMP 1 is found in the epithelium and the periglandular stroma[94,148] during this phase.

CONCLUSION

The regulation of angiogenesis is not completely understood. It is clear, however, that many factors are regulated in a temporal fashion throughout the menstrual cycle. These factors include cytokines, hormones, and growth factors.

The expression of these factors can be regulated through hypoxia, hypoglycemia, shear stress and stretch, components of extracellular matrix (laminin and fibronectin) and their receptors (integrins αv and α5), matrix metalloproteinases and their tissue inhibitors, other proteases (urokinase-type and tissue-type plasminogen activators), fibrin, inflammatory cells, and pericytes. Angiogenesis is tightly controlled by the balanced expression of both these inhibitors and activating factors, with an imbalance of factor expression 'flipping the toggle switch' to initiate or suppress angiogenesis.[163]

Although the data thus far are conflicting, each small portion of the menstrual cycle is being elucidated by the concerted efforts of many investigators. With time, as the true pathway of angiogenesis becomes clear, we will understand both normal and abnormal angiogenesis and begin to develop specific therapeutic pharmacologic treatments to normalize the process when it has gone awry.

REFERENCES

1. Folkman J. Tumor angiogenesis. Adv Cancer Res 1985;43:175–203.
2. Rogers PA, Lederman F, Taylor N. Endometrial vascular growth in normal and dysfunctional states. Hum Reprod Update 1998; B4: 503–8.
3. Risau W, Flamme I. Vasculogenesis. Ann Rev Cell Dev Biol 1995;11: 73–91.
4. Takahashi T, Kalka C, Masuda H et al. Ischemia- and cytokine-induced mobilization of bone marrow-derived endothelial progenitor cells for neovascularization. Nature Med 1999;5:434–8.
5. Sadler TW. Langman's Medical Embryology. Baltimore: Williams & Wilkins, 1995.
6. Taylor HS. The role of HOX genes in the development and function of the female reproductive tract. Semin Reprod Med 2000;18:311–20.
7. Moore KL. The Developing Human: Clinically Oriented Embryology. Philadelphia: WB Saunders, 1977.
8. Orsini LF, Salardi S, Pilu G et al. Pelvic organs in premenarchal girls: relation to puberty and sex hormone concentrations. Radiology 1984;153:113–16.
9. Salardi S, Orsini LF, Cacciari E et al. Pelvic ultrasonography in premenarchal girls: relation to puberty and sex hormone concentrations. Arch Dis Child 1985; 60:120–5.
10. Klauber N, Rohan RM, Flynn E, D'Amato RJ. Critical components of the female reproductive pathway are suppressed by the angiogenesis inhibitor AGM-1470. Nature Med 1987;3:443–6.
11. Gambino LS, Wreford NG, Bertram JF et al. Angiogenesis occurs by vessel elongation in proliferative phase human endometrium. Hum Reprod 2002;17: 1199–206.
12. Koga K, Osuga Y, Tsutsumi O et al. Demonstration of angiogenin in human endometrium and its enhanced expression in endometrial tissues in the secretory phase and the decidua. J Clin Endocrinol Metab 2001;86:5609–14.
13. Rogers PAW, Gargett CE. Endometrial angiogenesis. Angiogenesis 1998;2:287–94.
14. Randall JM, Fisk NH, McTavish A et al. Transvaginal ultrasonic assessment of endometrial growth in spontaneous and hyperstimulated menstrual cycles. Br J Obstet Gynaecol 1989;96:954–9.
15. Bakos O, Lundkvist O, Bergh T. Transvaginal sonographic evaluation of endometrial growth and texture in spontaneous ovulatory cycles – a descriptive study. Hum Reprod 1993;8:799–806.
16. Ono M, Shiina Y. Cytological evaluation of angiogenesis in endometrial aspirates. Cytopathology 2001;12:37–43.
17. Hii LLP, Rogers PAW. Endometrial vascular and glandular expression of integrin αvβ3 in women with and without endometriosis. Hum Reprod 1998;13:1030–5.
18. Roberts DK, Parmley H, Walker NJ et al. Ultrastructure of the microvasculature in the human endometrium throughout the normal menstrual cycle. Am J Obstet Gynecol 1992;166:1393–406.
19. Rogers PAW, Abberton KM, Susil B. Endothelial cell migratory signal produced by human endometrium during the menstrual cycle. Hum Reprod 1992;7:1061–6.
20. Bausero P, Cavaille F, Meduri G et al. Paracrine action of vascular endothelial growth factor in the human endometrium: production and target sites, and hormonal regulation. Angiogenesis 1998;22:167–82.
21. Giudice LC. The endometrial cycle. In: Adashi EY, Rock JA Rosenwaks Z, eds. Reproductive Endocrinology, Surgery and Technology. Philadelphia: Lippincott-Raven, 1996; 272–300.
22. Sarker KP, Yamahata H, Nakata M et al. Recombinant thrombomodulin inhibits thrombin-induced vascular endothelial growth factor production in neuronal cells. Haemostasis 1999;29:343–52.
23. Ferenczy A, Bertrand G, Gelfand MM. Proliferation kinetics of human endometrium during the normal menstrual cycle. Am J Obstet Gynecol 1979;133: 859–67.
24. Abberton KM, Taylor NH, Healy DL et al. Vascular smooth muscle α-actin distribution around endometrial arterioles during the menstrual cycle: increased expression during the perimenopause and lack of correlation with menorrhagia. Hum Reprod 1996;11:204–11.
25. Dockery P, Perret S, Rogers PAW et al. Endometrial morphology and the endometrial vascular bed. In: O'Brien S, Cameron I, MacLean A, eds. Disorders of the Menstrual Cycle. London: RCOG Press, 2000; 402.
26. Goodger AM, Rogers PAW. Endometrial endothelial cell proliferation during the menstrual cycle. Hum Reprod 1994;9:399–405.
27. Morgan KG, Wilkinson N, Buckley CH. Angiogenesis in normal, hyperplastic, and neoplastic endometrium. J Pathol 1996;179:317–20.
28. Sheppard BL, Bonner J. The development of vessels of the endometrium during the menstrual cycle. In: Diczfalusy E, Fraser IS, Webb FTG, eds. Endometrial Bleeding and Steroidal Contraception. Bath: Pitman Press, 1979; 65–85.
29. Kaiserman-Abramof IR, Padykula HA. Angiogenesis in the postovulatory primate endometrium: the coiled arteriolar system. Anat Rec 1989;224:479–89.
30. Abberton KM, Taylor NH, Healy DL et al. Vascular smooth muscle cell proliferation in arterioles of the human endometrium. Hum Reprod 1999;14:1072–9.

31. Ramsey E. Vascular anatomy. In: Wynn RM, ed. Biology of the Uterus. New York: Plenum Press, 1977; 59–76.

32. Vincenti V, Cassano C, Rocchi M et al. Assignment of the vascular endothelial growth factor gene to human chromosome 6p21.3. Circulation 1996;93:1493–5.

33. Tischer E, Mitchell R, Hartmen T et al. The human gene for vascular endothelial growth factor: multiple protein forms are encoded through alternative exon splicing. J Biol Chem 1991;266:11947–54.

34. Ferrara N, Davis-Smyth T. The biology of vascular endothelial growth factor. Endocrinol Rev 1997;181:4–25.

35. Gitay-Goren H, Soker S, Vlodavsky I et al. The binding of vascular endothelial growth factor to its receptors is dependent on cell surface-associated heparin-like molecules. J Biol Chem 1992;267:6093–8.

36. Houck KA, Leung DW, Rowland AM et al. Dual regulation of vascular endothelial growth factor bioavailability by genetic and proteolytic mechanisms. J Biol Chem 1992;267:26031–7.

37. Plouet J, Moro F, Bertagnoli S et al. Extracellular cleavage of the vascular endothelial growth factor 189-amino acid form by urokinase is required for its mitogenic effect. J Biol Chem 1997; 2722:13390–6.

38. Sharkey AM, Day K, McPherson A et al. Vascular endothelial growth factor expression in human endometrium is regulated by hypoxia. J Clin Endocrinol Metab 2000;85:402–9.

39. Levy AP, Levy NS, Wegner S et al. Transcriptional regulation of the rat vascular endothelial growth factor gene by hypoxia. J Biol Chem 1995;270:13333–40.

40. Forsythe JA, Jiang BH, Iyer NV et al. Activation of vascular endothelial growth factor gene transcription by hypoxia-inducible factor 1. Mol Cell Biol 1996;16: 4604–13.

41. Claffey KP, Shih SC, Mullen A et al. Identification of a human VPF/VEGF 3′ untranslated region mediating hypoxia-induced mRNA stability. Mol Biol Cell 1998;9:469–81.

42. Shifren JL, Tseng JF, Zaloudek CJ et al. Ovarian steroid regulation of vascular endothelial growth factor in the human endometrium: implications for angiogenesis during the menstrual cycle and in the pathogenesis of endometriosis. J Clin Endocrinol Metab 1996;81:3112–18.

43. Hyder SM, Stancel GM. Identification of functional estrogen response elements in the gene coding for the potent angiogenic factor vascular endothelial growth factor. Cancer Res 2000;6012:3183–90.

44. Zygmunt M, Mazzuca D, Han V. Human chorionic gonadotropin (hCG) induces VEGF expression in vitro. Placenta 2000;31:A23.

45. Zygmunt M, Herr F, Münstedt K et al. Angiogenesis and vasculogenesis in pregnancy. Euro J Obstet Gynecol Reprod Biol 2003;110:S10–S18.

46. Möller B, Lindblom B, Olovsson M. Expression of the vascular endothelial growth factors B and C and their receptors in human endometrium during the menstrual cycle. Acta Obstet Gynecol Scand 2002;81:817–24.

47. Laitinen M, Ristimaki A, Honkasalo M et al. Differential hormonal regulation of vascular endothelial growth factors VEGF, VEGF-B, and VEGF-C messenger ribonucleic acid levels in cultured human granulosa–luteal cells. Endocrinology 1997;138:4748–56.

48. Olofsson B, Pajusola K, von Euler G et al. Genomic organization of the mouse and human genes for vascular endothelial growth factor B (VEGF-B) and characterization of a second splice isoform. J Biol Chem 1996;271:19310–17.

49. Joukov V, Pajusola K, Kaipainen A et al. A novel vascular endothelial growth factor, VEGF-C, is a ligand for the Flt4 (VEGFR-3) and KDR (VEGFR-2; receptor tyrosine kinases. EMBO J 1996;15:290–8.

50. Meduri G, Bausero P, Perrot-Applanat M. Expression of vascular endothelial growth factor receptors in the human endometrium: modulation during the menstrual cycle. Biol Reprod 2000;62:439–47.

51. Nayak NR, Critchley HOD, Slayden OD et al. Progesterone withdrawal up-regulates vascular endothelial growth factor receptor type 2 in the superficial zone stroma of the human and macaque endometrium: potential relevance to menstruation. J Clin Endocrinol Metab 2000;85:3442–52.

52. Möller B, Rasmussen C, Lindblom B et al. Expression of the angiogenic growth factors VEGF, FGF-2, EGF and their receptors in normal human endometrium during the menstrual cycle. Mol Hum Reprod 2001;71:65–72.

53. Ahmed A, Li XF, Dunk C et al. Co-localization of vascular endothelial growth factor and its Flt-1 receptor in human placenta. Growth Factors 1995;12:235–43.

54. Clauss M, Weich H, Breier G et al. The vascular endothelial growth factor receptor Flt-1 mediates biological activities. Implications for a functional role of placenta growth factor in monocyte activation and chemotaxis. J Biol Chem 1996;271:17629–34.

55. Krüssel JS, Casan EM, Raga F et al. Expression of mRNA for vascular endothelial growth factor transmembranous receptors Flt1 and KDR, and the soluble receptor s-flt in cycling human endometrium. Mol Hum Reprod 1999;5:452–8.

56. Kroll J and Waltenberger J. A novel function of VEGF receptor-2 (KDR) rapid release of nitric oxide in response to VEGF-A stimulation in endothelial cells. Biochem Biophys Res Commun 1999;265:636–9.

57. Smith S. Regulation of angiogenesis in the endometrium. Trends Endocrinol Metab 2001;12:147–51.

58. Fong GH, Zhang L, Bryce DM et al. Increased hemangioblast commitment, not vascular disorganization, is the primary defect in lft-1 knock-out mice. Development 1999;126:3015–25.

59. Kaipainen A, Korhonen J, Mustonen T et al. Expression of the fms-like tyrosine kinase 4 gene becomes restricted to lymphatic endothelium during development. Proc Natl Acad Sci USA 1995;92:3566–70.

60. Sato TN, Tozawa Y, Deutsch U et al. Distinct roles of the receptor tyrosine kinases Tie-1 and Tie-2 in blood vessel formation. Nature 1995;376:70–4.

61. Suri C, McClain J, Thurston G et al. Increased vascularization in mice overexpressing angiopoietin-1. Science 1998;282:468–71.

62. Hayes AJ, Huang WQ, Mallah J et al. Angiopoietin-1 and its receptor Tie-2 participate in the regulation of capillary-like tubule formation and survival of endothelial cells. Microvasc Res 1999;58:224–37.

63. Hanahan D. Signaling vascular morphogenesis and maintenance. Science 1997;277:48–50.

64. Davis S, Aldrich TH, Jones PF et al. Isolation of angiopoietin-1, a ligand for the TIE2 receptor, by secretion-trap expression cloning. Cell 1996;87:1161–69.

65. Witzenbichler B, Maisonpierre PC, Jones P et al. Chemotactic properties of angiopoietin-1 and –2, ligands for the endothelial-specific receptor tyrosine kinase Tie-2. Biol Chem 1998;273:18514–521.

66. Koblized TL, Weiss C, Yancopoulos GD et al. Angiopoietin-1 induces sprouting angiogenesis in vitro. Curr Biol 1998;8:529–532.

67. Kim I, Kim HG, Moon S-O et al. Angiopoietin-1 induces endothelial cell sprouting through the activation of focal adhesion kinase and plasmin secretion. Circ Res 2000;86:952–959.

68. Papapetropoulos A, Fulton D, Mahboubi K et al. Angiopoietin-1 inhibits endothelial cell apoptosis via the Akt/surviving pathway. J Biol Chem 2000;275:9102–9105.

69. Kim I, Kim HG, So JN et al. Angiopoietin-1 regulates endothelial cell survival through the phosphatidylinositol 3′-kinase/Akt signal transduction pathway. Circ Res 2000;86:24–29.

70. Thurston G, Suri C, Smith K et al. Leakage-resistant blood vessels in mice transgenically over-expressing angiopoietin-1. Science 1999;286:2511–2514.

71. Patan S. TIE1 and TIE2 receptor tyrosine kinases inversely regulate embryonic angiogenesis by the mechanism of intussusceptive microvascular growth. Microvasc Res 1998;56:1–21.

72. Li XF, Gregory J, Anmed A. Immunolocalization of vascular endothelial growth factor in human endometrium. Growth Factors 1994;11:277–82.

73. Sangha RK, Li XF, Shams M et al. Fibroblast growth factor receptor-1 is a critical component for endometrial remodeling: localization and expression of basic fibroblast growth factor and FGF-R1 in human endometrium during the menstrual cycle and decreased FGF-R1 expression in menorrhagia. Lab Invest 1997;77:389–402.

74. Weston G, Rogers PAW. Endometrial angiogenesis. Baillière's Clin Obstet Gynaecol 2000;14:919–36.

75. Friesel R, Burgess WH, Maciag T. Heparin-binding growth factor 1 stimulates tyrosine phosphorylisation in NIH 3T3 cells. Mol Cell Biol 1989;9:1857–65.

76. Ferriani RA, Charnock-Jones DS, Prentice A et al. Immuno-histochemical localization of acidic and basic fibroblast growth factors in normal human endometrium and endometriosis and the detection of their mRNA by polymerase chain reaction. Hum Reprod 1993;81:11–16.

77. Dong J-C, Dong H, Campana A et al. Matrix metalloproteinases and their specific tissue inhibitors in menstruation. Reproduction 2002;123:621–31.

78. Partridge CR, Hawker JR Jr, Forough R. Overexpression of a secretory form of FGF-1 promotes MMP-1 mediated endothelial cell migration. J Cell Biochem 2000;78:487–99.

79. Nezu E, Ohashi Y, Kinoshita S et al. Recombinant human epidermal growth factor and corneal neovascularization. Jpn J Ophthalmol 1992;36:401–6.

80. Ushiro S, Ono M, Izumi H et al. Heparin-binding epidermal growth factor-like growth factor: p91 activation induction of plasminogen activator/inhibitor, and tubular morphogenesis in human microvascular endothelial cells. Jpn J Cancer Res 1996;87:68–77.

81. Imai T, Kurachi H, Adachi K et al. Changes in epidermal growth factor receptor and the levels of its ligands during menstrual cycle in human endometrium. Biol Reprod 1995;52:928–38.

82. Niikura H, Sasano H, Kaga K et al. Expression of epidermal growth factor family proteins and epidermal growth factor receptor in human endometrium. Hum Pathol 1996;27:282–9.

83. McBean JH, Brumsted JR, Stirewalt WS. In vivo estrogen regulation of epidermal growth factor receptor in human endometrium. J Clin Endocrinol Metab 1997;82:1467–71.

84. Giudice LC. Growth factors and growth modulators in human uterine endometrium: their potential relevance to reproductive medicine. Fertil Steril 1994;61:1–17.

85. Marsh MM, Malakooti N, Taylor NH et al. Endothelin and neutral endopeptase in the endometrium of women with menorrhagia. Hum Reprod 1997;12:2036–40.

86. Casey ML, MacDonald PC. Modulation of endometrial blood flow: regulation of endothelin-1 biosynthesis and degradation in human endometrium. In: Alexander NJ, d'Arcangues C, eds. Steroid Hormones and Uterine Bleeding. Washington DC: AAAS Press, 1992; 209.

87. Markee JE. Morphological basis for menstrual bleeding. Bull NY Acad Med 1948;24:253–268.

88. Cameron IT, Davenport AP, Brown MJ et al. Endothelin-1 stimulates prostaglandin F2 alpha release from human endometrium. Prost Leuk Essen Fatty Acids 1991;42:155–157.

89. Fett JW, Strydom DJ, Lobb RR et al. Isolation and characterization of angiogenin, an angiogenic protein from human carcinoma cells. Biochem 1985;24:5480–5486.

90. Lockwood C, Krikun G, Chang Koo AB et al. Differential effects of thrombin and hypoxia on endometrial stromal and glandular epithelial cell vascular endothelial growth factor expression. J Clin Endocrinol Metab 2002;87:4280–4286.

91. Bassus S, Herkert O, Kronemann N et al. Thrombin causes vascular endothelial growth factor expression in vascular smooth muscle cells: role of reactive oxygen species. Arterioscler Thromb Vasc Biol 2001;21:1550–1555.

92. Marbaix E, Donnez J, Courtoy PJ et al. Progesterone regulates the activity of collagenase and related gelatinases A and B in human endometrial explants. Proceed Natl Acad Sci USA 1992;8911:11789–11793.

93. Martelli M, Campana A and Bischof P. Secretion of matrix metalloproteinases by human endometrial cells in vitro. J Reprod Fert 1993;98:67–76.

94. Rodgers WH, Matrisian LM, Giudice LC et al. Patterns of matrix metalloproteinase expression in cycling endometrium imply differential functions and regulation by steroid hormones. J Clin Inv 1994;94:946–953.

95. Rawdanowicz TJ, Hampton AL, Nagase H et al. Matrix metalloproteinase production by cultured human endometrial stromal cells: identification of interstitial collagenase, gelatinase-A, gelatinase-B, and stromelysin-1 and their differential regulation by interleukin-1 alpha and tumor necrosis factor-alpha. J Clin Endocrinol Metab 1994;79:530–6.

96. Hulboy DL, Rudolph LA, Matrisian LM. Matrix metalloproteinases as mediators of reproductive function. Mol Hum Reprod 1997;31:27–45.

97. Rodgers WH, Osteen KG, Matrisian LM et al. Expression and localization of matrilysin, a matrix metalloproteinase, in human endometrium during the reproductive cycle. Am J Obstet Gynecol 1993;168:253–60.

98. Salamonsen LA, Woolley DE. Matrix metalloproteinases in normal menstruation. Hum Reprod 1996;112:124–33.

99. Lamoreaux WJ, Fitzgerald ME, Reiner A et al. Vascular endothelial growth factor increases release of gelatinase A and decreases release of tissue inhibitor of metalloproteinases by microvascular endothelial cells in vitro. Microvasc Res 1998;55:29–42.

100. Wang H, Keiser JA. Vascular endothelial growth factor upregulates the expression of matrix metalloproteinases in vascular smooth muscle cells: role of flt-1. Circul Res 1998;83:832–40.

101. Pepper MS. Manipulating angiogenesis: from basic science to the bedside. Arterioscler Thromb Vasc Biol 1997;17:605–19.

102. van Hinsbergh VWM. Impact of endothelial activation on fibrinolysis and local proteolysis in tissue repair. Ann NY Acad Sci 1992;667:151–62.

103. Vassalli J-D, Pepper MS. Membrane proteases in focus. Nature 1994;370:14–15.

104. Okumura Y, Sato H, Seiki M et al. Proteolytic activation of the precursor of membrane type 1 matrix metalloproteinase by human plasmin: a possible cell surface activator. FEBS Lett 1997;402:181–4.

105. Santibanez JF, Martinez J. Membrane-associated procollagenase of leukemic cells Is activated by urokinase-type plasminogen activator. Leukemia Res 1993;17:1057–62.
106. Murphy G, Stanton H, Cowell S et al. Mechanisms for pro matrix metalloproteinase activation. APMIS 1999;107:38–44.
107. Iruela-Arispe ML, Porter P, Bornstein P et al. Thrombospondin-1, an inhibitor of angiogenesis, is regulated by progesterone in the human endometrium. J Clin Invest 1996;972:403–12.
108. Sheibani N et al. Thrombospondin-1, a natural inhibitor of angiogenesis, regulates platelet-endothelial cell adhesion molecule-1 expression and endothelial cell morphogenesis. Mol Biol 1997;8:1329–41.
109. Guo NH, Krutzch HC, Inman IK et al. Thrombospondin 1 and type I repeat peptides of thrombospondin 1 specifically induce apoptosis of endothelial cells. Cancer Res 1997;57:1735–42.
110. O'Reilly MS, Boehm T, Shing Y et al. Endostatin: an endogenous inhibitor of angiogenesis and tumor growth. Cell 1997;88:277–85.
111. DiPietro LA, Polverini PJ. Angiogenic macrophages produce the angiogenic inhibitor thrombospondin 1. Am J Pathol 1993;143:678–84.
112. Mosher DF. Physiology of thrombospondin. Annu Rev Med 1990;41:85–97.
113. Bornstein P, Sage EH. The thrombospondins: structure and regulation of expression. Meth Enzymol 1994;245:63–85.
114. Bagavandoss P, Wilks JW. Specific inhibition of endothelial cell proliferation by thrombospondin. Biochem Biophys Res Commun 1990;170:867–72.
115. Murphy-Ullrich JE, Höök M. Thrombospondin modulates focal adhesions in endothelial cells. J Cell Biol 1989;109:1309–19.
116. Good DJ, Polverini PJ, Rastinejad F et al. A tumor suppressor-dependent inhibitor of angiogenesis is immunologically and functionally indistinguishable from a fragment of thrombospondin. Proc Natl Acad Sci USA 1990;87:6624–8.
117. Rastinejad F, Polverini PJ, Bouck NP. Regulation of the activity of a new inhibitor of angiogenesis by a cancer suppressor gene. Cell 1989;56:345–55.
118. Iruela-Arispe ML, Bornstein P, Sage H. Thrombospondin exerts an antiangiogenic effect on tube formation by endothelial cells in vitro. Proc Natl Acad Sci USA 1991;88:5026–30.
119. DiPietro LA, Nebgen DR, Polverini PJ. Downregulation of endothelial cell thrombospondin 1 enhances in vitro angiogenesis. J Vasc Res 1994;31:178–85.
120. Tolsma SS, Volpert OV, Good DJ et al. Peptides derived from two separate domains of the matrix protein thrombospondin 1 have anti-angiogenic activity. J Cell Biol 1993;122:497–511.
121. Dameron KM, Volpert OV, Tainsky MA et al. Control of angiogenesis in fibroblasts by p53 regulation of thrombospondin-1. Science 1994;265:1582–4.
122. Bein K, Simons M. Thrombospondin type 1 repeats interact with matrix metalloproteinase 2. Regulation of metalloproteinase activity. J Biol Chem 2000;275:32167–73.
123. Dawson DW, Pearce SF, Zhong R et al. CD36 mediates the in vitro inhibitory effects of thrombospondin-1 on endothelial cells. J Cell Biol 1997;138:707–17.
124. Nor JE, Mitra RS, Sutorik MM et al. Thrombospondin-1 induces endothelial cell apoptosis and inhibits angiogenesis by activating the caspase death pathway. J Vasc Res 2000;37:209–18.
125. O'Reilly MS, Holmgren L, Shing Y et al. Angiostatin: a novel angiogenesis inhibitor that mediates the suppression of metastases by a Lewis lung carcinoma. Cell 1994;792:315–28.
126. Salamonsen LA, Butt AR, Macpherson AM et al. Immunolocalization of the vasoconstrictor endothelin in the human endometrium during the menstrual cycle and in umbilical cord at birth. Am J Obstet Gynecol 1992;167:163–7.
127. Gold LI, Saxena B, Mittal KR et al. Increased expression of transforming growth factor β isoforms and basic fibroblast growth factor in complex hyperplasia and adenocarcinoma of the endometrium: evidence for paracrine and autocrine action. Cancer Res 1994;54:2347–58.
128. Schwartz SM, Liaw L. Growth control and morphogenesis in the development and pathology of arteries. J Cardiovasc Pharmacol. 1993;21(Suppl 1):S31–S49.
129. Grainger DJ, Kemp PR, Lui AC et al. Activation of transforming growth factor β is inhibited in transgenic apolipoprotein a mice. Nature 1994;370:460–2.
130. Polli V, Bulletti C, Galassi A et al. Transforming growth factor- β1 in the human endometrium. Gynecol Endocrinol 1996;10:297–302.
131. Maas JWM, Groothuis PA, Dunselman GAJ et al. Endometrial angiogenesis throughout the human menstrual cycle. Hum Reprod 2001;16:1557–61.
132. Naresh B, Sengupta J, Bhargava V et al. Immunohistological localization of vascular endothelial growth factor in human endometrium. Indian J Physiol Pharmacol 1999;432:165–70.
133. Macpherson AM, Archer DF, Leslie S et al. The effect of etonorgestrel on VEGF, estrogen and progesterone receptor immunoreactivity and endothelial cell number in human endometrium. Hum Reprod 1999;1412:3080–7.
134. Gargett CE, Lederman FL, Lau TM et al. Lack of correlation between vascular endothelial growth factor production and endothelial cell proliferation in the human endometrium. Hum Reprod 1999;14:2080–8.
135. Wang H, Chen G. Expression of vascular endothelial growth factor and its receptors, flt-1 and kinase insert domain-containing receptor in normal human endometrium during menstrual cycle. Zhonghua Fu Chan Ke Za Zhi 2002;3712:729–32.
136. Torry DS, Holt VJ, Keenan JA et al. Vascular endothelial growth factor expression in cycling human endometrium. Fertil Steril 1996;661:72–80.
137. Charnock-Jones DS, Macpherson AM, Archer DF et al. The effect of progestins on vascular endothelial growth factor, estrogen receptor and progesterone receptor immunoreactivity and endothelial cell density in human endometrium. Hum Reprod 2000;15(Suppl 3): 85–95.
138. Torry DS, Torry RJ. Angiogenesis and the expression of vascular endothelial growth factor in endometrium and placenta. Am J Reprod Immunol 1997;37:21–9.
139. Lau TM, Affandi B, Rogers PAW. The effects of levonorgestrel implants on vascular endothelial growth factor expression in the endometrium. Mol Hum Reprod 1998;51:57–63.
140. Gargett Ce, Lederman F, Heryanto B et al. Focal vascular endothelial growth factor correlates with angiogenesis in human endometrium. Hum Reprod 2001;16:1065–75.
141. Gargett CE, Rogers PA. Human endometrial angiogenesis. Reproduction 2001;1212:181–6.
142. Gaudry M, Bregerie O, Andrieu V et al. Intracellular pool of vascular endothelial growth factor in human neutrophils. Blood 1997;90:4153–61.
143. Taichman NS, Young S, Cruchley AT et al. Human neutrophils secrete vascular endothelial growth factor. J Leukocyte Biol 1997;62:397–400.
144. Freeman MR, Schneck FX, Gagnon ML et al. Peripheral blood T lymphocytes and lymphocytes infiltrating human cancers express vascular endothelial growth factor: a potential role for T cells in angiogenesis. Cancer Res 1995;55:4140–5.

145. Harmey JH, Dimitriadis E, Kay E et al. Regulation of macrophage production of vascular endothelial growth factor (VEGF; by hypoxia and transforming growth factor β-1. Ann Surg Oncol 1998;5:271–8.

146. Song JY, Russell P, Markham R et al. Effects of high dose progestogens on white cells and necrosis in human endometrium. Hum Reprod 1996;11:1713–18.

147. Jeziorska M, Nagase H, Salamonsen LA et al. Immunolocalization of the matrix metalloproteinases gelatinase B and stromelysin-1 in human endometrium throughout the menstrual cycle. J Reprod Fertil 1996;107:43–51.

148. Hampton AL, Butt AR, Riley SC et al. Tissue inhibitors of metalloproteinases in endometrium of ovariectomized steroid treated ewes and during the estrous cycle and early pregnancy. Biol Reprod 1995;53:302–11.

149. Sugino N, Kashida S, Karube-Harada A et al. Expression of vascular endothelial growth factor (VEGF) and its receptors in human endometrium throughout the menstrual cycle and in early pregnancy. Reproduction 2002;123:379–87.

150. Li XF, Charnock-Jones DS, Zhang E. Angiogenic growth factor messenger ribonucleic acids in uterine natural killer cells. J Clin Endocrinol Metab 2001;86:1823–34.

151. Charnock-Jones DS, Sharkey AM, Rajput-Williams J et al. Identification and localization of alternately spliced mRNAs for vascular endothelial growth factor in human uterus and estrogen regulation in endometrial carcinoma cell lines. Biol Reprod 1993;48:1120–8.

152. Hornung D, Lebovic DI, Shifren JL et al. Vectorial secretion of vascular endothelial growth factor by polarized human endometrial epithelial cells. Fertil Steril 1998;69:909–15.

153. Hewett P, Nijjar S, Shams M et al. Short communication: downregulation of angiopoietin-1 expression in menorrhagia. Am J Pathol 2002;160:773–80.

154. Irwin JC, Kirk D, Gwatkin RBL et al. Human endometrial matrix metalloproteinase-2, a putative menstrual proteinase. J Clin Invest 1996;97:438–47.

155. Higuchi T, Kanzaki H, Nakayama H et al. Induction of tissue inhibitor of metalloproteinase-3 gene expression during in vitro decidualization of human endometrial stromal cells. Endocrinology 1995;136:4973–81.

156. Rusnati M, Casarotti G, Pecorelli S et al. Estro-progestinic replacement therapy modulates the levels of basic fibroblast growth factor (FGF-2) in postmenopausal endometrium. Gynecol Oncol 1993;48:88–93.

157. Ohbuchi H, Nagai K, Yamaguchi M et al. Endothelin-1 and big endothelin-1 increase in human endometrium during menstruation. Am J Obstet Gynecol 1995;173:1483–90.

158. Hampton AL, Salamonsen LA. Expression of messenger ribonucleic acid encoding matrix metalloproteinases and their tissue inhibitors is related to menstruation. J Endocrinol 1994;141:R1–R3.

159. Marbaix E, Kokorine I, Henriet P et al. The expression of interstitial collagenase in human endometrium is controlled by progesterone and by estradiol and is related to menstruation. Biochem J 1995; 305: 1027–30.

160. Kokorine I, Marbaix E, Henriet P et al. Focal cellular origin and regulation of interstitial collagenase (matrix metalloproteinase-1) are related to menstrual breakdown in the human endometrium. J Cell Sci 1996;109:2151–60.

161. Freitas S, Meduri G, Le Nestour E et al. Expression of metalloproteinases and their inhibitors in blood vessels in human endometrium. Biol Reprod 1999;61:1070–82.

162. Brenner RM, Rudolph LA, Matrisian LM et al. Nonhuman primate models: Artificial menstrual cycles, endometrial matrix metalloproteinases and subcutaneous endometrial grafts. Hum Reprod 1996;11(Suppl 2):150–64.

163. Hanahan D, Folkman J. Patterns and emerging mechanisms of the angiogenic switch during tumorigenesis. Cell 1996;86:353–64.

4. Epidemiology of Endometriosis

Stacey A. Missmer and Daniel W. Cramer

Because few well-designed epidemiologic studies exist, the incidence, prevalence, and risk factors for endometriosis remain uncertain. However, despite the relative paucity of studies, some consistent observations have emerged – findings that have led to several hypotheses regarding the pathogenesis of endometriosis. This chapter will discuss the methodologic issues that have limited the study of endometriosis to date, summarize the current pathophysiologic hypotheses, and review the body of epidemiologic evidence as it applies to these hypotheses.

METHODOLOGIC ISSUES

Several methodologic issues have proved problematic for epidemiologic studies of endometriosis, especially those related to case–control studies.[1,2] First, the current clinical definition of the disease includes a wide spectrum of symptoms and pathologic findings. Second, no strategy for control selection appears entirely satisfactory, partly because factors that might determine which women come to a diagnosis of endometriosis could be related to exposures of interest. Third, although pinpointing the exact onset of disease is impossible when the pathologic changes specific to endometriosis are unclear and perhaps unobservable, incident rather than prevalent cases should be enrolled in epidemiologic studies whenever possible.

Traditionally, endometriosis has been defined as the presence of functional endometrial glands and stroma outside the uterus but still within the pelvic cavity. This definition allows women found to have asymptomatic disease at the time of unrelated surgery (e.g. tubal ligation) to be included as cases. However, from a public health standpoint we are interested in disease that produces symptoms resulting in morbidity that affects the lives of those who are diagnosed. Thus, some gynecol-

ogists have suggested that endometriosis be defined not only by the presence of ectopic endometrium, but also by evidence that the lesions are active cellularly, or have affected normal physiology.[3] Examples of cellular activity or physiologic effect might include evidence that the lesions are deep (>5 mm), manifest as ovarian endometriomas, or are associated with pelvic adhesions not attributable to other causes. Indeed, because it has been hypothesized that ovarian-related endometriosis may have an underlying etiology distinct from that of peritoneal endometriosis, we suggest that when sample size permits, researchers should consider conducting subanalyses distinguishing between cases with and without a history of endometriomas.

Holt and Weiss have encouraged epidemiologists to operationalize these definitions in case selection, asserting that continuing the use of varied case definitions prevents the comparison of study results.[4] At the very least, it would seem that asymptomatic endometriosis found at tubal ligation should not be included in studies where most cases are symptomatic. Zondervan and colleagues[2] argue that the relatively high prevalence of minimal or mild endometriosis in asymptomatic women may represent a normal physiologic process, and that study cases should be limited to women who present with severe or at least symptomatic disease. Further, to reduce the magnitude of misclassification, analyses of the incident diagnosis of endometriosis might be restricted to those who have laparoscopic confirmation of the disease, as this has long been considered the gold standard.[5,6] The inclusion of cases diagnosed at hysterectomy may also be appropriate, but comparison of the case and noncase groups may be confounded by the indication for hysterectomy.

However, by limiting our case definition to those with surgical confirmation of disease, we may be introducing selection bias. It is possible that patients with more frequent utilization of the medical system, those of higher socioeconomic class, or those with the most severe/aggressive disease may be more likely to undergo investigative laparoscopy. It is also possible that those with endometriosis whose symptoms are improved by less invasive, more generic treatments (e.g. anti-inflammatory medications or oral contraceptives) may never 'need' an invasive, albeit confirmatory, diagnosis. However, in several studies the severity of endometriosis in women with laparoscopic confirmation does not appear to be skewed toward more extensive disease.[7-10]

Additionally, the invasive nature of diagnosis may introduce detection bias; the thoroughness of examination may differ between cases identified during a work-up for infertility or pelvic symptoms and controls who were declared to be free of endometriosis during a tubal ligation or other surgical procedure not initiated by symptoms.[11] Approximately 20% of all women who have been unsuccessful in conceiving after more than 12 months of unprotected intercourse are found to have endometriosis.[12] The selection of cases who come to diagnosis on the basis of a work-up for infertility may undersample those who are symptomatic with pelvic pain and discomfort. Had these women not attempted to become pregnant, a large proportion might never have received a laparoscopic diagnosis of endometriosis. We may also assume that cases who do not report infertility but who have had a laparoscopic diagnosis are 'symptomatic', otherwise a surgical evaluation would not have been conducted. Because endometriosis with infertility is typically indicative of asymptomatic disease secondary to other primary causes of infertility, the risk factors for endometriosis with infertility could be different from those for symptomatic endometriosis without concurrent infertility. Also, when the study population is comprised only of infertile women (common in the epidemiologic literature), comparing infertile cases with a comparison or control group comprised of infertile women without endometriosis may yield results that differ not only in direction and magnitude of effect, but also in interpretation

from those that would be observed when comparisons are made with fertile women without endometriosis.[11] This is particularly true when the exposures of interest, such as menstrual cycle characteristics or reproductive history, are correlated with both endometriosis and infertility.

The ideal design would be a prospective cohort study of endometriosis in which women at risk for disease are enrolled and followed over time. At baseline, the population should be restricted to women who are premenopausal and have intact uteri, as the occurrence of endometriosis after hysterectomy or menopause is rare. Also, prevalent cases cannot be included in the study population and – depending on the minimum age of the cohort – may be women who were diagnosed at a younger age owing to more severe disease, had greater access to medical care, or experienced symptoms that were not improved by generic treatment. Therefore, cohorts should be assembled that include healthy women who are young enough to pick up those diagnosed with endometriosis at an early age.

When the design and conduct of a cohort study is not possible, a case–control study provides a valid estimate of the rate of disease associated with an exposure (rate ratio) – provided that the cases and controls are validly chosen.[13] The selection of controls, in particular, is key to assuring the validity of any case–control design. Controls must represent the exposure distribution of the population from which the cases arose, and sampling must be independent of that exposure. Any restriction or exclusion applied to cases must also be applied to controls. Finally, to require that a control be matched to a case on the basis of both symptoms and diagnostic procedures would lead to an overmatched control group, which would not allow many factors of potential interest to be studied.

Alternatively, purely population-based selection of controls has also been argued against, because women with undiagnosed disease may be selected, thus attenuating the association between exposure and disease. However, as Zondervan et al demonstrate, the likely community prevalence of severe/symptomatic endometriosis is less than 2%.[2] It does seem reasonable to match on factors influencing the likelihood of receiving medical attention, such as the availability of medical insurance, and access to gynecologic services. Researchers may also consider adjusting for healthcare use in analytic models, if only through a dichotomous proxy variable created from questions regarding the frequency of physical examinations, Pap smears, pelvic examinations, or breast examinations conducted by a clinician.

Ideally, case–control studies should focus on incident rather than prevalent cases.[2] The proportion of those with long-term disease will be greatest among prevalent cases, and self-reported or clinical data collected from cases after the onset of symptoms may represent changes in exposure or recall that occurred in response to disease. However, with chronic diseases such as endometriosis that are typically diagnosed only after a threshold of symptoms is reached, it may be impossible to know exactly when disease onset occurred. Misdiagnoses are common, and years may pass between the onset of symptoms and a confirmed diagnosis.[14–17] Consequently, all analyses are really estimating the incidence of endometriosis diagnosis, rather than the incidence of disease onset, and the temporal relation between exposure and outcome may be inaccurately modeled. In any case, when prevalent cases are included a priori, it must be noted that the odds ratio is a valid estimate of the underlying rate ratio only if the outcome is rare – usually defined as a prevalence of 10% or less in the general population.[13]

Although the ideal epidemiologic study has not yet been performed, it is worth describing the current pathogenic hypotheses and reviewing the epidemiologic evidence accumulated to date.

PATHOGENIC HYPOTHESES

Figure 4.1 illustrates a model for the pathogenesis of endometriosis that attempts to integrate the diverse hypotheses described in detail below. This model emphasizes the importance of retrograde

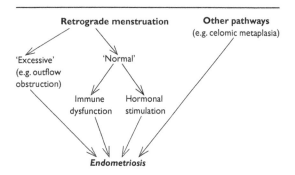

Figure 4.1 A summary of the pathogenic hypotheses for endometriosis. (Reproduced from Missmer and Cramer. Obstet Gynecol Clin N Am 2003;30:1–9 with permission from Elsevier.)

menstruation in disease pathogenesis. In some cases, retrograde menstruation alone might be sufficient to cause disease, such as when it is excessive – for instance because of outflow obstruction owing to, for example, vaginal or cervical stenosis, or a non-communicating uterine horn. In other cases, a 'normal degree' of retrograde menstruation might operate in conjunction either with immune factors that might affect the clearing of the material from the pelvis and/or with hormonal stimuli that might affect its growth. We must also consider the contributions of other pathways, such as that of coelomic metaplasia, which we do not yet fully understand or whose epidemiologic correlates have not yet been identified.

RETROGRADE MENSTRUATION

In most women the majority of menstrual blood flow occurs in an 'antegrade' direction, i.e. from the endometrium, through the cervix and into the vagina. 'Retrograde' menstruation describes endometrial blood flow from the uterus, through the fallopian tubes and into the peritoneal cavity. In 1927, Sampson argued that subsequent implantation and growth of endometrial tissue on extrauterine structures leads to the development of endometriosis.[18] This hypothesis was supported by clinical findings that lesions tended to be clustered around structures in close proximity to the distal ends of the fallopian tubes.

Case reports identify endometriosis in women with müllerian anomalies, such as a non-communicating uterine horn, where the only menstrual egress is through the fallopian tube.[19–22] Similarly, surgical interventions that may alter the natural flow of menstrual fluid, such as cesarean section or cervical conization, may also be related to the risk of endometriosis.[23,24] Women with endometriosis are more likely to present with gross anatomical complications, such as vaginal or cervical stenosis, that, based upon mathematical modeling of the fluid dynamics of menstrual flow, may increase the likelihood and volume of retrograde menstruation.[25] In addition, compatible with case series that have suggested an increased prevalence of mitral valve prolapse[26] and pyloric stenosis[27] among women with endometriosis, decreased elasticity of the reproductive system may impede menstrual flow through the cervix and vagina.[27]

Clinical work has shown that growth factors and viable endometrial cells can be found in menstrual and peritoneal fluid,[28] and endometrium has been experimentally implanted and grown within the peritoneal cavity.[29] However, because laparoscopy during menses has shown that up to 90% of women have retrograde menstruation, the reasons for differences in implantation rates between women remain unclear.[30] Risk may be associated with factors that increase the volume, frequency, and duration of retrograde menstruation and promote the implantation and growth of endometrial plaques.[31]

HORMONAL MILIEU

There is strong circumstantial evidence that endometriosis is dependent on circulating steroid hormones. Endometriosis plaques have been shown to have estrogen, progesterone, and androgen receptors and to grow in the presence of estrogen, but to atrophy when exposed to androgens.[17,32,33] The disease has not been reported in premenarcheal girls, and the rare cases in postmenopausal women have been largely in those who were exposed to hormone replacement therapy.[34] Interventions that reduce estradiol production, either surgical (oophorectomy) or hormonal (GnRH agonist analogs), are both the most reliable way to cause atrophy of endometriosis lesions and the most effective in treating pain symptoms. Interventions that stimulate the androgen receptor (danazol, methyl testosterone) are also effective in the treatment of pain caused by endometriosis. High-dose synthetic progestins are effective in the treatment of endometriosis through multiple mechanisms of action: (1) suppression of LH and FSH secretion, which in turn suppresses estradiol production; (2) direct antiestrogenic effects on endometriosis lesions; and (3) induction of terminal differentiation in endometriosis lesions ('pseudodecidualization'). Once endometriosis tissue undergoes pseudodecidualization, it can no longer grow. Thus it has been hypothesized that conditions altering steroid hormone levels may influence the incidence of endometriosis, perhaps by increasing the proliferation of endometrial cells or promoting the survival of extrauterine implants.

IMMUNE SYSTEM MORBIDITY

For more than a decade, anecdotal, laboratory, and population-based evidence has suggested that women with endometriosis have a higher prevalence of immune system morbidity.[35] It is possible that women with endometriosis developed the disease because of immune system abnormalities that prevent the 'clearing' of endometrial tissue from the peritoneal environment, thereby allowing retrograde menstruation to establish lesions within the peritoneal cavity.[31] Several studies have shown decreased natural killer cell activity in the peripheral blood mononuclear cells of women with endometriosis, although this finding has not been consistently confirmed.[17,33,36] Other studies have shown an increased concentration of leukocytes (particularly macrophages, T lymphocytes, and natural killer cells) in the peritoneal fluid of women with endometriosis.[16,17,33,36] Halme et al compared the peritoneal macrophage secretions of women with and without endometriosis and found that cases demonstrated increased secretion of growth factors and proinflammatory cytokines.[29] Other authorities believe that the observed immunologic changes are the result of endometriosis lesions causing a chronic pelvic inflammation and an increase of immune cells in the peritoneal fluid.[37] Interestingly, factors secreted by these immune cells appear to cause endometriosis lesions to grow. It is likely that there is 'cross-talk' between the immune system and endometriosis lesions. For example, endometriosis lesions cause inflammation, inducing immune cells to enter the peritoneal environment, and in turn, immune cells secrete factors that can stimulate the growth of endometriosis lesions.

COELOMIC METAPLASIA

Another debated pathogenic hypothesis is that some plaques, particularly those involving the ovaries, are generated by monoclonal tumors that arise from a somatic mutation of ovarian epithelium or pelvic peritoneal mesothelium.[38] Evidence to support metaplastic pathogenesis includes the observation of rare cases of endometriosis among men who have received estrogen treatments for a long period.[39–41] To our knowledge there have been no reports of endometriosis among transgender men undergoing treatment for female reassignment, although discovery of endometriosis in this population would also support this pathogenic hypothesis. Pathways to the initiation of coelomic metaplasia remain unclear, although it has been hypothesized that inflammatory response may play a role.[16,42] It is possible that what we today define clinically as endometriosis may in fact have heterogeneous origins, one arising from retrograde menstruation and the other from metaplasia, both influenced by the hormonal milieu and immune system abnormalities.

EPIDEMIOLOGIC EVIDENCE

PREVALENCE AND INCIDENCE

As described above, determining the prevalence and incidence of endometriosis is difficult.

Published estimates of prevalence have varied by mode of diagnosis. Among women seeking tubal ligation, the prevalence of endometriosis was found in two studies to range from 2 to 18%.[43,44] The prevalence within infertile populations has been reported to range from 5 to 50%.[16,45–49] The range of prevalence for women admitted to a hospital because of pelvic pain is 5–21%.[46–49] A group that appears to be at considerable risk for endometriosis is adolescents with intractable dysmenorrhea or pelvic pain, among whom about 50% are found to have the diagnosis.[50,51] This observation suggests that adolescents with severe dysmenorrhea (generally defined as requiring analgesics and bed rest) have a high likelihood of endometriosis and require particular attention for efforts at early detection or prevention. No autopsy data for any age group have ever been published.

Incidence data in the general population are less readily available. Houston et al reported that the incidence rate of histologically confirmed endometriosis among white women 15–49 years old in Rochester, Minnesota, from 1970 to 1979 was 160/100 000 woman-years.[34,52] Incidence increased with age, from 17/100 000 woman-years among those aged 15–19 to 285/100 000 woman-years among those aged 40–44. Among women aged 45–49 the incidence rate fell to 184/100 000 woman-years. A more recent study based on hospital discharges found endometriosis to be the first listed diagnosis in 1.3 per 1000 discharges in women aged 15–44.[53] Thus, endometriosis appears confined to the childbearing and immediately postmenopausal years, providing demographic support for the idea that pathogenesis involves the estrogen milieu.

RISK FACTORS

MENSTRUAL AND REPRODUCTIVE FACTORS

Menstrual cycle characteristics and reproductive history may reflect between-person variation in hormonal milieu. In some studies[54,55] higher levels of estradiol[56–58] and estrone[56] have been observed among adult women who had earlier menarche. Estradiol levels have also been observed to be higher among nulliparous women than among parous women,[59,60] whereas androgen levels have the opposite association with parity.[61]

In addition to their relation to the hormonal milieu, menstrual cycle characteristics and reproductive history may influence the total volume of endometrial cells released into the peritoneal cavity.[62] The risk of endometriosis appears to be increased in the presence of reproductive factors associated with increased exposure to menstruation, such as earlier age at menarche, shorter menstrual cycle length, longer duration of flow, greater menstrual volume of flow, and reduced parity.[63] Although several studies have found that an early menarche (often defined as age 11) increases the risk for endometriosis, sample sizes were small, and a significant linear trend has not been reported.[11,24,64-67] Most of these same studies and others have found that risk is also increased with a shorter cycle length.[10,24,64-69] In a hospital-based case–control study of 286 women with primary infertility and 3794 who had delivered a liveborn infant, cases were more likely than controls to have shorter menstrual cycle lengths ($\leq$27 days versus $\geq$38 days) (OR = 2.1, 95% CI = 1.5–2.9), and a non-significant increase in risk was found with cycle irregularity.[64]

There is less consistent evidence related to the duration and heaviness of menstrual flow and tampon use. Darrow et al reported that cases under the age of 30 compared with friend controls of the same age were significantly more likely to have menstrual flow for 6 or more days per month, heavy flow, severe cramps, increasing symptoms, and to have used tampons for more than 14 years.[9] However, Cramer et al observed no correlation with exclusive tampon use.[64] A recent study reported that women who used tampons exclusively were less likely to have endometriosis, although this may be because case women experience greater flow volume and must use a combination of tampon and feminine napkin.[70,71] This study also observed that women with endometriosis are less likely to engage in intercourse during menses, suggesting that sexu-

al activity or orgasm during menstruation 'may confer protection' from the disease. Although we concur with critics who argue that cases are likely to experience chronic pelvic pain and dyspareunia that peaks during menstruation, and therefore are less likely to report having sex at this time,[71,72] we agree with the authors' assertion that further study to establish the temporal relation between patterns of sexual activity and symptom onset is needed.[73]

Dysmenorrhea is a strong risk factor for endometriosis but has generally been considered simply a symptom of existing disease, as it is easy to imagine that monthly bleeding from pelvic lesions is painful. However, because dysmenorrhea may correlate with stronger uterine contractility,[74] an alternate interpretation is that dysmenorrhea is associated with some degree of outflow obstruction, stronger uterine cramping, and an increased propensity toward retrograde menstruation.

There is similar difficulty in discovering the relation between childbearing and endometriosis. Although the disruption of pelvic anatomy and ovarian function leading to infertility or decreased sexual activity as the result of severe chronic pelvic pain and dyspareunia may be clearly a consequence of endometriosis, it is also reasonable to propose that delayed childbearing could also be a cause. A case-control study among multiparous women diagnosed with endometriosis during a tubal ligation suggested that higher parity is associated with a lower risk of endometriosis.[10] This relation was also observed in a case–control study comparing cases with women admitted for acute conditions at the same hospital.[66] Because each pregnancy decreases the lifetime number of months during which a woman is exposed to menstrual fluid, the mechanism of risk may be similar to that of women with longer menstrual cycles, who are exposed to the sloughing of endometrial tissue less frequently than women with shorter cycles. In addition, permanent cervical dilation occurs with labor and vaginal delivery,[75] possibly reducing the resistance to menstrual flow and decreasing the likelihood of retrograde menstruation.

Also, the decidual reaction that occurs on the ovarian and pelvic surface attributed to high hormone levels during pregnancy might result in decreased susceptibility to endometriosis implantation or growth.

Finally, the epidemiologic data have consistently reflected a protective effect of current oral contraceptive (OC) use, whereas former use seems to increase risk.[6,10,76,77] Risk among past users has been observed to be greatest with more recent time since last use.[63,76-78] Biologic hypotheses compatible with protection include the possibility that OCs decrease risk by stopping ovulation and decreasing the volume of menstrual flow, thereby reducing the likelihood of retrograde menstruation or monoclonal mutation.[79] In patients with endometriosis, treatment with OCs has been shown to suppress cell proliferation and increase apoptosis of eutopic endometrial tissue.[80]

However, because OC are often prescribed as a first line of treatment when patients present with menstrual cycle irregularity, heavy menstrual flow, or dysmenorrhea, it is impossible to determine whether those who are taking oral contraceptives and are subsequently diagnosed with endometriosis developed the disease before or after the exposure. In addition, it is probable that the diagnosis of endometriosis is delayed in OC users. OCs have been shown to decrease symptoms in the short-term, but symptoms re-emerge once use is discontinued or the disease progresses in severity.[63] This intractable confounding by indication makes interpretation of these studies difficult.[63,76] A true underlying effect of oral contraceptives is also less likely, as no study has reported a dose–response effect for lifetime duration of use.[10,63,76] Future studies addressing this association must include data that explicitly describe the reasons for the initiation of oral contraceptive use and preceding gynecologic symptoms.

BODY HABITUS

Weak inverse associations between endometriosis and weight and BMI (body mass index, kg/m^2) have been found.[9,11,64] Women with higher BMI have more irregular menstrual cycles and are believed to have increased rates of anovulatory infertility. The greater prevalence of oligomenorrhea among obese women may explain both their increased risk of infertility and their decreased risk of endometriosis. Conversely, an increased risk with greater height has been reported for endometriosis.[11,64] Taller women may have higher follicular-phase estradiol levels.[60] Also, a study of laparoscopically confirmed endometriosis cases compared with friend controls matched on age (88 cases, 88 controls) reported that for women aged 30 or younger, the odds of endometriosis were inversely related to waist-to-hip ratio (OR = 6.18 for women with a ratio of 0.61–0.72 compared with women with a ratio of 0.76–1.01, 95% CI = 2.01–19.01).[8] A high waist-to-hip ratio is reflective of peripheral fat accumulation that is associated with a high estrogen-to-androgen profile.

In addition to these anthropometric risk factors, the literature supports hypotheses that endometriosis may be associated with red hair.[81] Studies have also suggested that Asian women are at higher risk of endometriosis than women of other races, but that African-American women are at lower risk.[10,34,63] It has been argued that the relation with African-American ancestry is spurious, owing to decreased access to health care and misclassification of the outcome, because racial minority women are often misdiagnosed as having pelvic inflammatory disease rather than endometriosis. The biologic basis for the decreased incidence rates among racial minority women remains unclear, particularly given data suggesting that African-American women experience greater exposure to endogenous estrogens unopposed by progesterone.[82,83]

ENVIRONMENTAL AND LIFESTYLE FACTORS

Environmental exposure to phytoestrogens or hormone disruptors such as polychlorinated biphenyl (PCB) or dioxin have been hypothesized. There is strong animal study evidence, with a relation between dioxin exposure and endometriosis observed in rhesus monkeys

(Macaca mulata),[84,85] rats,[86] and mice.[86,87] However, human epidemiologic studies based on serum levels of dioxin or PCB have been contradictory.[88-92] Most recently, a well-designed case–control and retrospective cohort study have found a non-significant elevation in risk as high as fourfold. However, in both studies sample sizes were small and the confidence intervals about these estimates were wide; thus a null association cannot be excluded.[7,93]

Lifestyle exposures such as cigarette smoking are also known to have an effect on the hormonal milieu. Studies of the effect of smoking on endometriosis have produced conflicting results.[9,64,67,76] Comparing infertile cases with fertile controls, Cramer et al reported an inverse association with cigarette smoking in heavy smokers (≥1 pack per day) who had begun before the age of 17 (OR = 0.5, 95% CI = 0.3–0.9).[64] In addition, a study that used friend controls found a decrease in risk among those who began smoking before age 16 and were currently younger than 30 (OR = 0.3, 95% CI = 0.1–0.9).[9] However, neither a case–control study conducted among parous women[10] nor a cohort study of 17 302 women attending family clinics[76] found an association. These inconsistent findings could result from the fact that although smokers are relatively estrogen deficient, they are also exposed to higher levels of exogenous estrogen in the form of dioxin. Although data vary by tobacco source, it is estimated that a person who smokes one pack of cigarettes per day takes in about 4.3 pg of polychlorinated dibenzodioxins per kilogram body weight per day.[15,94] Perhaps the underlying association is complex – U-shaped or modified by infertility status or other comorbidity.

Studies of endometriosis in infertile populations have suggested a direct relation with both caffeine[95,96] and moderate (one drink or less per day) alcohol consumption,[97] but another study comparing cases with both fertile and infertile controls detected no association with alcohol.[11] Endometriosis patients have higher scores than controls on the Michigan Alcoholism Screening Test and tended to consume more alcohol on a yearly basis.[15] Grodstein et al reported that among women with infertility due solely to endometriosis, and excluding women with additional causes of infertility (158 cases, 3833 controls), the odds ratio for endometriosis was 1.7 (95% CI = 1.2–2.5) for moderate drinkers and 1.8 (95% CI = 1.0–3.2) for heavy drinkers compared with women who did not drink, after adjusting for age, number of sexual partners, cigarette smoking, and caffeine intake.[97] Although it is possible that the cases were self-medicating owing to the painful symptoms of endometriosis, the relation reported by Grodstein was unchanged when analyses were restricted to women who experienced no pain symptoms. Moderate alcohol intake has been shown to increase total and bioavailable estrogen levels.[98,99] Hypotheses relating alcohol consumption to endometriosis may also include disruption of a critical pathway of tissue containment/immune response during the menstrual cycle in adults, or of a critical pathway of physiologic development during adolescence.

Regular exercise, which may lower estrogen levels,[100] has been associated with a reduced risk of endometriosis.[11,64,69,101] However, valid study of this relation may be complicated by the effect of disease symptoms on physical activity. Physical activity may reduce the risk of the disease, but once symptoms begin women may be less likely to exercise, hiding the true effect.

For lifestyle exposures there is the possibility of confounding by factors such as menstrual symptoms or socioeconomic status. However, because of the importance of these exposures, they should continue to be examined in epidemiologic and experimental studies, taking this potential confounding into consideration.

IMMUNE DISORDER COMORBIDITY

Sinaii and colleagues report that within their study population of 3680 cases – all members of the US-based Endometriosis Association who completed a self-administered questionnaire – they observed a statistically significantly greater prevalence of physician-diagnosed rheumatoid arthritis (1.8% compared with 1.2% in the general population), systemic lupus erythematosus (0.8% compared with 0.04%), hypothyroidism (9.6% compared with 1.5%), and multiple sclerosis (0.5% compared with 0.07%).[35] Allergies and asthma were also significantly more common among these women with endometriosis. However, the general population prevalences used for comparison were not limited to women, nor to those of reproductive age. Also, despite presenting a significant difference in the age and education distributions between the survey and general populations, the comorbidity comparisons were not adjusted for any potential confounders.

If such relations do exist, however, they would support hypothesis that the etiology of endometriosis includes abnormalities of immune system function – potentially bidirectionally. Autoimmune disorders may allow the growth and implantation of endometrial tissue outside the uterus. However, in the presence of endometriosis, there may be an increased risk of autoimmune or chronic inflammatory response to the presence of endometriosis that leads to multi-system immune dysfunction.

Table 4.1 shows a summary of the risk factors for endometriosis.

CONCLUSION

As estimated by the Endometriosis Association, millions of women are severely affected by endometriosis; millions more are likely to have asymptomatic disease.[26] Limited study suggests that menstrual and reproductive history, anthropometrics, and both lifestyle and environmental exposures, may play a role in disease etiology. Although a prospective study in a cohort of premenopausal women with adequate healthcare access and visually confirmed endometriosis cases (with subanalyses stratified by infertility status or symptom history) is the ideal design, case–control studies with enrollment of incident cases – perhaps matched on proxies for healthcare access (i.e. likelihood of diagnosis) –

Table 4.1 A summary of risk factors for endometriosis

Risk factor	Direction and consistency of effect*
Menstrual and reproductive factors	
Earlier age at menarche	↑, consistent
Shorter menstrual cycle length	↑↑, consistent
Heavier menstrual volume	↑, limited study
Irregular cycle duration	–, inconsistent
Tampon use	–, inconsistent
Oral contraceptive use	–, inconsistent
Greater parity	↓↓, consistent
Body habitus	
Greater height	↑, inconsistent
Greater weight	↓, inconsistent
Greater body mass index	↓, consistent
Greater waist-to-hip ratio	↓↓, limited study
Red hair	↑, limited study
Caucasian race	↑↑, limited study
Lifestyle and environmental factors	
Regular exercise	↓, consistent
Cigarette smoking	↓, inconsistent
Alcohol use	↑, limited study
Caffeine intake	↑, limited study
PCB, dioxin exposure	↑, consistent in primates but inconsistent in women
Immune disorder comorbidity	
Diagnosis with an autoimmune disorder	↑↑, extremely limited study
Diagnosis with allergen hypersensitivity/asthma	↑↑, extremely limited study

* Arrows indicate the approximate magnitude of the relation: ↑, slight to moderate increase in risk; ↑↑, moderate to large increase in risk; ↓, slight to moderate decrease in risk; ↓↓, moderate to large decrease in risk; –, no association
Reproduced from Missmer and Cramer. Obstet Gynecol Clin N Am 2003;30:1–9 with permission from Elsevier.

compared to both infertile and fertile controls may contribute greatly to the endometriosis literature.

The result of future valid epidemiologic studies of endometriosis will broaden our understanding of the pathogenesis as well as the early signs and symptoms of the disease. Early diagnosis and perhaps even prevention of endometriosis may be possible, but researchers must gather much more detailed data on the epidemiologic characteristics of women who have been diagnosed.

REFERENCES

1. Cramer DW, Missmer SA. The epidemiology of endometriosis. Ann NY Acad Sci 2002;955:11–22.

2. Zondervan KT, Cardon LR, Kennedy SH. What makes a good case-control study? Design issues for complex traits such as endometriosis. Hum Reprod 2002;17:1415–23.

3. Audebert A, Backstrom T, Barlow DH et al Endometriosis 1991: a discussion document. Hum Reprod 1992;7:432–5.

4. Holt VL, Weiss NS. Recommendations for the design of epidemiologic studies of endometriosis. Epidemiology 2000;11:654–9.

5. Pardanani S, Barbieri RL. The gold standard for the surgical diagnosis of endometriosis: visual findings or biopsy results. J Gynecol Tech 1998;4:121–4.

6. Duleba AJ. Diagnosis of endometriosis. Obstet Gyn Clin North Am 1997;24:331–45.

7. Pauwels A, Schepens PH, D'Hooghe T et al. The risk of endometriosis and exposure to dioxins and polychlorinated biphenyls: a case-control study of infertile women. Hum Reprod 2001;16:2050–5.

8. McCann SE, Freudenheim JL, Darrow SL et al. Endometriosis and body fat distribution. Obstet Gynecol 1993;82:545–9.

9. Darrow SL, Vena JE, Batt RE et al. Menstrual cycle characteristics and the risk of endometriosis. Epidemiology 1993;4:135–42.

10. Sangi-Haghpeykar H, Poindexter AN. Epidemiology of endometriosis among parous women. Obstet Gynecol 1995;85:983–92.

11. Signorello LB, Harlow BL, Cramer DW et al. Epidemiologic determinants of endometriosis: a hospital-based case-control study. Ann Epidemiol 1997;7:267–74.

12. Tanahatoe S, Hompes PG, Lambalk CB. Accuracy of diagnostic laparoscopy in the infertility work-up before intrauterine insemination. Fertil Steril 2003;79:361–6.

13. Rothman KJ, Greenland S. Modern Epidemiology, 2nd edn. Philadelphia: Lippincott-Raven, 1998.

14. Hadfield R, Mardon H, Barlow DH, Kennedy S. Delay in diagnosis of endometriosis: a survey of women from the USA and the UK. Hum Reprod 1996;11:878–80.

15. Abdalla H, Rizk B. Fast Facts - Endometriosis. Oxford: Health Press Unlimited, 1998.

16. Hornstein MD, Barbieri RL. Endometriosis. In: Ryan KJ, Berkowitz RS, Barbieri RL et al., eds. Kistner's Gynecology and Women's Health. Missouri: Mosby, 1999.

17. Witz CA, Schenken RS. Pathogenesis. Semin Reprod Endocrinol 1997;15:199–208.

18. Sampson JA. Peritoneal endometriosis due to the menstrual dissemination of endometrial tissue into the peritoneal cavity. Am J Obstet Gynecol 1927;14:422.

19. Fallas RE. Endometriosis. Demonstration for the Sampson theory by a human anomaly. Am J Obstet Gynecol 1956;72:556.

20. Hanton EM, Malkasian GD, Docherty MD, Pratt JH. Endometriosis associated with complete or partial obstruction of menstrual egress. Obstet Gynecol 1966;28:626.

21. Carpenter RG, Jameson WJ. Uterus bicornis with rudimentary horn. Am J Obstet Gynecol 1973;116:973.

22. Schifrin BS, Erez S, Moore JG. Teen-age endometriosis. Am J Obstet Gynecol 1973;116:973–80.

23. Ismail SM. Cone biopsy causes cervical endometriosis and tubo-endometrioid metaplasia. Histopathology 1991;18:107–14.

24. Moen MH, Schei B. Epidemiology of endometriosis in a Norwegian county. Acta Obstet Gynecol Scand 1997;76:559–62.

25. Barbieri RL. Stenosis of the external cervical os: an association with endometriosis in women with chronic pelvic pain. Fertil Steril 1998;70:571–3.

26. Ballweg ML. Overcoming Endometriosis: New Help from the Endometriosis Association. New York: Congdon & Weed, 1987.

27. Liede A, Pal T, Mitchell M, Narod SA. Delineation of a new syndrome: clustering of pyloric stenosis, endometriosis, and breast cancer in two families. J Med Genet 2000;37:794–6.

28. Koninckx PR, Ide P, Vandenbroucke W. New aspects of the pathophysiology of endometriosis and associated infertility. J Reprod Med 1980;24:257–64.

29. Halme J, Becker S, Haskill S. Altered maturation and function of peritoneal macrophages: possible role in pathogenesis of endometriosis. Am J Obstet Gynecol 1987;16:783–9.

30. Halme J, Hammond MG, Hulka JF et al. Retrograde menstruation in healthy women and in patients with endometriosis. Obstet Gynecol 1984;64:151–6.

31. Oral E, Arici A. Pathogenesis of endometriosis. Obstet Gynecol Clin North Am 1997;24:219–33.

32. Barbieri RL. Endometriosis and the estrogen threshold theory: relation to surgical and medical treatment. J Reprod Med 1998;43:287–92.

33. Witz CA. Current concepts in the pathogenesis of endometriosis. Clin Obstet Gynecol 1999; 42:566–85.

34. Houston DE. Evidence for the risk of pelvic endometriosis by age, race and socioeconomic status. Epidemiol Rev 1984;6:167–91.

35. Sinaii N, Cleary SD, Ballweg ML et al. High rates of autoimmune and endocrine disorders, fibromyalgia, chronic fatigue syndrome and atopic diseases among women with endometriosis: a survey analysis. Hum Reprod 2002;17:2715–24.

36. Rier SE, Yeaman GR. Immune aspects of endometriosis: relevance of the uterine mucosal immune system. Semin Reprod Endocrinol 1997;15:209–20.

37. Hill JA. Immunology and endometriosis: fact, artifact, or epiphenomenon? Obstet Gynecol Clin North Am 1997;24:291–306.

38. Jimbo H, Hitomi Y, Yoshikawa H et al. Evidence for monoclonal expansion of epithelial cells in ovarian endometrial cysts. Am J Pathol 1997;150:1173–8.

39. Pinkert TC, Catlow CE, Straus R. Endometriosis of the urinary bladder in a man with prostatic carcinoma. Cancer 1979;43:1562–7.

40. Schrodt GR, Alcorn MO, Ibanez J. Endometriosis of the male urinary system: a case report. J Urol 1980;124:722–3.

41. Martin JD, Hauck AE. Endometriosis in the male. Am Surg 1985;51:426–30.

42. Tamura M, Fukaya T, Murakami T et al. Analysis of clonality in human endometriotic cysts based on evaluation of X chromosome inactivation in archival formalin-fixed, paraffin-embedded tissue. Lab Invest 1998;78:213–18.

43. Strathy JH, Molgaard CA, Coulam CB, Melton LJ 3rd. Endometriosis and infertility: a laparoscopic study of endometriosis among fertile and infertile women. Fertil Steril 1982;38:667–72.

44. Moen MH. Endometriosis in monozygotic twins. Acta Obstet Gynecol Scand 1994;73:59–62.

45. Peterson EP, Behrman SJ. Laparoscopy of the infertile patient. Obstet Gynecol 1970;36:363–70.

46. Duignan NM, Jordan JA, Coughlan BM, Logan-Edwards R. One thousand consecutive cases of diagnostic laparoscopy. J Obstet Gynaecol Br Commonw 1972;79:1016–20.

47. Liston WA, Bradford WP, Downie J, Kerr MG. Laparoscopy in a general gynecologic unit. Am J Obstet Gynecol 1972;113:672–5.

48. Kleppinger RK. One thousand laparoscopies at a community hospital. J Reprod Med 1976;13:13–17.

49. Hasson HM. Incidence of endometriosis in diagnostic laparoscopy. J Reprod Med 1976;16:135–40.

50. Bullock JL, Massey FM, Gambrell RD. Symptomatic endometriosis in teenagers: a reappraisal. Obstet Gynecol 1974;43: 896.

51. Goldstein DP, de Cholnoky C, Emans SJ et al. Laparoscopy on the diagnosis and management of pelvic pain in adolescents. J Reprod Med 1980;24:251.

52. Houston DE, Noller KL, Melton LJ 3rd et al. Incidence of pelvic endometriosis in Rochester, Minnesota, 1970-1979. Am J Epidemiol 1987;125:959–69.

53. National Center for Health Statistics. Ambulatory and inpatient procedures in the United States, 1994. Vital Health Stat 1997;132:1–113.

54. Hill P, Garbaczewski L, Kasumi K, Wynder EL. Plasma hormones in parous, nulliparous and postmenopausal Japanese women. Cancer Lett 1986;33:131–6.

55. Verkasalo PK, Thomas HV, Appleby PN, Davey GK, Key TJ. Circulating levels of sex hormones and their relation to risk factors for breast cancer: a cross-sectional study in 1092 pre- and postmenopausal women (United Kingdom). Cancer Causes Control 2001;12:47–59.

56. MacMahon B, Trichopoulos D, Brown J et al. Age at menarche, urine estrogens and breast cancer risk. Int J Cancer 1982;30:427–31.

57. Apter D, Reinila M, Vihko R. Some endocrine characteristics of early menarche, a risk factor for breast cancer, are preserved into adulthood. Int J Cancer 1989;44:783–7.

58. Moore JW, Key TJA, Wang DY et al. Blood concentrations of estradiol and sex hormone binding globulin in relation to age at menarche in premenopausal British and Japanese women. Breast Cancer Res Treat 1991;18:S47–50.

59. Bernstein L, Pike MC, Ross RK et al. Estrogen and sex hormone binding globulin levels in nulliparous and parous women. J Natl Cancer Inst 1985;74:741–5.

60. Dorgan JF, Reichman ME, Judd JT et al. Relationships of age and reproductive characteristics with plasma estrogens and androgens in premenopausal women. Cancer Epidemiol Biomarkers Prev 1995;4:381–6.

61. Musey VC, Collins DC, Brogan DR et al. Long term effects of a first pregnancy on the hormonal environment: estrogens and androgens. J Clin Endocrinol Metab 1987;64:111–18.

62. Cramer DW. Epidemiology of endometriosis. In: Tilson EA, ed. Endometriosis. New York: Liss, 1987.

63. Eskenazi B, Warner ML. Epidemiology of endometriosis. Obstet Gynecol Clin North Am 1997;24:235–58.

64. Cramer DW, Wilson E, Stillman RJ et al. The relation of endometriosis to menstrual characteristics, smoking, and exercise. JAMA 1986;255:1904–8.

65. Candiani GB, Danesino V, Gastaldi A et al. Reproductive and menstrual factors and risk of peritoneal and ovarian endometriosis. Fertil Steril 1991;56:230–4.

66. Parazzini F, Ferraroni M, Fedele L et al. Pelvic endometriosis: reproductive and menstrual risk factors at different stages in Lombardy, northern Italy. J Epidemiol Commun Health 1995;49:61–4.

67. Matorras R, Rodiquez F, Pijoan JI et al. Epidemiology of endometriosis in infertile women. Fertil Steril 1995;63:34–8.

68. Parazzini F, La Vecchia C, Franeschi S et al. Risk factors for endometrioid, mucinous, and serous benign ovarian cysts. Int J Epidemiol 1989;18:108–12.

69. Arumugam K, Lim JM. Menstrual characteristics associated with endometriosis. Br J Obstet Gynaecol 1997;104:948–50.

70. Meaddough EL, Olive DL, Gallup P et al. Sexual activity, orgasm, and tampon use are associated with a decreased risk for endometriosis. Gynecol Obstet Invest 200253:163–9.

71. Ballweg ML, Quinn BW. Concerning the article by Meaddough et al: Sexual activity, orgasm and tampon use are associated with a decreased risk for endometriosis. Gynecol Obstet Invest 2002;54:63.

72. Guidone HC, Marvel ME. Concerning the article by Meaddough et al: Sexual activity, orgasm and tampon use are associated with a decreased risk for endometriosis. Gynecol Obstet Invest 2002;54:64–5.

73. Kliman HJ, Olive DL. Authors' response to the Letters to the Editors concerning the article by Meaddough et al: Sexual activity, orgasm and tampon use are associated with a decreased risk for endometriosis. Gynecol Obstet Invest 2002;54:65–6.

74. Schulman H, Duviverr R, Blattner MS. The uterine contractility index: a research and diagnostic tool in dysmenorrhea. Am J Obstet Gynecol 1983;45:1049–58.

75. Krantz KE. The anatomy of the human cervix, gross and histologic. In: Moghissi K, ed. The Biology of the Cervix. Chicago: University of Chicago, 1973;1–60.

76. Vessey MP, Villard-Mackintosh L, Painter R. Epidemiology of endometriosis in women attending family planning clinics. Br Med J 1993;306:182–4.

77. Parazzini F, Ferraroni M. Epidemiology of endometriosis. Br Med J 1993;306:930–1.

78. Parazzini F, Di Cintio E, Chatenoud L et al. Oral contraceptive use and risk of endometriosis, Italian Endometriosis Study Group. Br J Obstet Gynaecol 1999;106:695–9.

79. Vercellini P, Ragni G, Trespidi L et al. Does contraception modify the risk of endometriosis? Hum Reprod 1993;8:547–51.

80. Meresman GF, Auge L, Baranao RI et al. Oral contraceptives suppress cell proliferation and enhance apoptosis of eutopic endometrial tissue from patients with endometriosis. Fertil Steril 2002;77:1141–7.

81. Woodworth SH, Singh M, Yussman MA et al. A prospective study on the association between red hair color and endometriosis in infertile patients. Fertil Steril 1995;64:651–2.

82. Witherspoon JT, Butler VW. The etiology of uterine fibroids with special reference to the frequency of their occurrence in the Negro: an hypothesis. Surg Gynecol Obstet 1934;58:57–61.

83. Haiman CA, Pike MC, Bernstein L et al. Ethnic differences in ovulatory function in nulliparous women. Br J Cancer 2002;86:367–71.

84. Fanton JW, Golden JG. Radiation-induced endometriosis in *Macaca mulatta*. Radiat Res 1991;126:141–6.

85. Rier SE, Martin DC, Bowman RE et al. Endometriosis in rhesus monkeys (*Macaca mulatta*) following chronic exposure to 2,3,7,8-tetrachlorodibenzo-p-dioxin. Fund Appl Toxicol 1993;21:433–41.

86. Cummings AM, Metcalf JL, Birnbaum L. Promotion of endometriosis by 1,2,7,8-tetrachlorodibenzo-p-dioxin in rats and mice: time–dose dependence and species comparison. Toxicol Appl Pharmacol 1996;138:131–9.

87. Osteen KG, Bruner KL, Sierra-Rivera E et al. Dioxin (TCDD) can block the protective effect of progesterone in nude mouse model of experimental endometriosis. Fifty-second Annual Meeting of the American Society for Reproductive Medicine; O-068. Boston, MA, 1996:S35.

88. Ahlborg UG, Lipworth L, Titus-Ernstoff L et al. Organochlorine compounds in relation to breast cancer, endometrial cancer, and

endometriosis: an assessment of the biological and epidemiological evidence. Crit Rev Toxicol 1995;25:463–531.

89. Mayani A, Barel S, Soback S, Almagor M. Dioxin concentrations in women with endometriosis. Hum Reprod 1997;12:373–5.

90. Lebel G, Dodin S, Ayotte P et al. Organochlorine exposure and the risk of endometriosis. Fertil Steril 1998;69:221–8.

91. Yoshida K, Ikeda S, Nakanishi J. Assessment of human health risk of dioxins in Japan. Chemosphere 2000;40:177–85.

92. Birnbaum LS, Cummings AM. Dioxins and endometriosis: a plausible hypothesis. Environ Health Perspect 2002;110:15–21.

93. Eskenazi B, Mocarelli P, Warner M et al. Serum dioxin concentrations and endometriosis: a cohort study in Seveso, Italy. Environ Health Perspect 2002;110:629–34.

94. Zeyneloglu HB, Arici A, Olive DL. Environmental toxins and endometriosis. Obstet Gynecol Clin North Am 1997;24:307–29.

95. Grodstein F, Goldman MB, Ryan L, Cramer DW. Relation of female and infertility to consumption of caffeinated beverages. Am. J Epidemiol 1993;137:133–6.

96. Berube S, Marcoux S, Maheux R. Characteristics related to the prevalence of minimal or mild endometriosis in infertile women. Epidemiology 1998;9:504–10.

97. Grodstein F, Goldman MB, Cramer DW. Infertility in women and moderate alcohol use. Am J Public Health 1994;84:1429–32.

98. Reichman ME, Judd JT, Longcope C et al. Effects of alcohol consumption on plasma and urinary hormone concentrations in premenopausal women. J Natl Cancer Inst 1993;85:722–7.

99. Hankinson SE, Hunter DJ. Epidemiology of breast cancer. In: Adami H-O, Hunter D, Trichopoulos D, eds. Textbook of Cancer Epidemiology. Oxford: Oxford University Press, 2002.

100. Baker ER, Mathur RS, Kirk RF et al. Female runners and secondary amenorrhea: correlation with age, parity mileage, and plasma hormonal and sex hormone-binding globulin concentrations. Fertil Steril 1981;36:183–7.

101. Dhillon PK, Holt VL. Recreational physical activity and endometrioma risk. Am J Epidemiol 2003;158:156–64.

5. Pathogenesis of Endometriosis

Craig A. Witz

INTRODUCTION

Endometriosis was described as a disease process over 300 years ago. In the late 17th century it was recognized as peritoneal 'ulcers' occurring on the surface of the bladder, intestine, and surface of the uterus.[1] In the 18th century physicians associated endometriosis with scarring, tissue damage, and pelvic pain. With improvements in microscopy, 19th century investigators identified the growth of ectopic endometrial tissue as the cause of these lesions. However, although it has been extensively investigated, the cause of growth of ectopic endometrial tissue (i.e. glands and stroma) outside the uterus has remained undefined.

In the last century various theories were promulgated to explain the histogenesis of the endometriotic lesion. Most recently, investigators have addressed aspects of the immune system and local peritoneal factors that may be involved with both the histogenesis of endometriosis and its sequelae. This chapter will consider the evidence for different theories of histogenesis and review the current understanding of the contribution of the immune system to the etiology of endometriosis. In addition, recent investigations regarding mechanisms involved in endometrial attachment to the peritoneum will be discussed.

THEORIES REGARDING HISTOGENESIS OF THE ENDOMETRIOTIC LESION

IMPLANTATION THEORY

The implantation theory, usually referred to as Sampson's theory, proposes that endometrial tissue passes through the fallopian tubes during menstruation, then attaches and proliferates at ectopic sites in the peritoneal cavity.[2] Recent studies using laparoscopy have demonstrated that retrograde menstruation is a nearly universal phenomenon in women with patent fallopian tubes.[3,4]

Classic studies performed in the 1950s demonstrated the viability of sloughed endometrial cells and their capacity to implant at ectopic sites. Keettel and Stein demonstrated that endometrial cells could be cultured from menstrual endometrium.[5] In addition, Ridley and Edwards showed that endometrial tissue collected from menstrual endometrium could attach and proliferate in ectopic locations. In their study, menstrual effluent was collected during the second day of menstruation from women scheduled for surgery. The material was injected into the subcutaneous abdominal fat and patients subsequently underwent laparotomy 90–180 days after implantation. The site of injection was excised for histologic study and several patients had viable endometrial glands and stroma at the site of implantation.[6]

Primate animal models have also demonstrated the ability of menstrual endometrium to proliferate in the peritoneal cavity. In another classic study, TeLinde and Scott performed surgery to invert the uterus and divert menstrual flow into the peritoneal cavity. Five of 10 monkeys developed extensive pelvic adhesions and microscopic evidence of endometriosis.[7] In addition, models of endometriosis have been developed in the baboon by injecting menstrual endometrium into the retroperitoneum.[8] Interestingly, endometriosis has been reported to occur naturally in baboons in captivity.[9–11]

Several 'natural experiments' from humans support the implantation model of peritoneal endometriosis. Patients with müllerian anomalies and obstructed menstrual flow through the vagina may have an increased risk of endometriosis.[12,13] The anatomic distribution of endometriosis also provides support for Sampson's theory. Jenkins et al demonstrated an increased frequency of endometriotic implants in the dependent areas of the pelvis where pooling of menstrual debris is expected.[14]

COELOMIC METAPLASIA THEORY

The theory of coelomic metaplasia proposes that endometriosis may develop from metaplasia of cells lining the pelvic peritoneum.[15] Iwanoff and Meyer are recognized as originators of this theory. A prerequisite of the coelomic metaplasia theory is that mesothelial cells lining the ovary and pelvic peritoneum contain cells capable of differentiating into endometrium. An attractive component of the theory is that it can account for the occurrence of endometriosis anywhere that mesothelium is found. This includes reports of endometriosis occurring in the pleural cavity.[16-20] Pleural endometriosis could result from local metaplasia of pleural mesothelium. On the other hand, it could also result from transdiaphragmatic passage of peritoneal fragments of endometrium,[17] as well as vascular metastasis of endometrium.

Coelomic metaplasia is thought to account for the rare occurrences of endometriosis reported in males.[21,22] In these reports the men were all undergoing estrogen therapy. Although coelomic metaplasia was a possibility, estrogen stimulation of müllerian rests could not be excluded. Likewise, the occurrence of endometrial carcinoma in males is thought to arise from müllerian remnants.[23,24]

Still further support for the coelomic metaplasia theory may be found in the study of benign and malignant epithelial ovarian tumors, both of which are considered to be derivatives of germinal epithelium. The presence of ovarian surface endometriosis could be accounted for by this type of transformation.

INDUCTION THEORY

The induction theory is an extension of the coelomic metaplasia theory. This theory proposes that menstrual endometrium produces substances that induce peritoneal tissues to form endometriotic lesions.

EMBRYONIC RESTS THEORY

Von Recklinghausen and Russell[25,26] are credited with the theory that endometriosis results from embryonic cell rests which, when stimulated, could differentiate into functioning endometrium. As described above, rare cases of endometriosis have been reported in men. Transformation of embryonic rests is a plausible explanation for this phenomenon.

LYMPHATIC AND VASCULAR METASTASIS THEORIES

The lymphatic metastasis theory of endometriosis is often referred to as Halban's theory. Halban[27] reported that endometriosis could arise in the retroperitoneum and in sites not directly opposed to peritoneum. Sampson had also suggested that endometriosis could result from lymphatic and hematogenous dissemination of endometrial cells.[28]

An extensive communication of lymphatics has been demonstrated between the uterus, ovaries, tubes, pelvic and vaginal lymph nodes, kidney, and umbilicus.[29] Metastasis of endometrial cells via the lymphatic system to these areas is therefore anatomically possible. In 1952, Javert[30] reported the presence of endometrial tissue in 6.5% of 153 cases of pelvic lymphadenectomy. In patients with endometriosis, the incidence of lymph node endometriosis was 29%. These findings are consistent with a literature review showing a 6.7% incidence of lymph node endometriosis in 178 autopsy cases.[30]

Lymphatic and vascular metastasis of endometrium has been offered as an explanation for rare cases of endometriosis occurring in locations remote from the peritoneal cavity. In addition to pleural tissue, endometriosis has been reported in pulmonary parenchyma.[17,18,20] Vascular or lymphatic metastasis may also explain cases of endometriosis that have been reported in bone, biceps muscle, peripheral nerves, and the brain.[20]

COMPOSITE THEORY

Javert[31] proposed a composite theory of the histogenesis of endometriosis which combines implantation and vascular/lymphatic metastasis, as well as a theory of direct extension of endometrial tissue through the myometrium. Along similar lines, Nisolle and Donnez[32] have recently argued that the histogenesis of endometriosis depends on the location and 'type' of the endometriotic implant. For example, peritoneal endometriosis can be explained by the implantation theory. Ovarian endometriomas could be the result of coelomic metaplasia of invaginated ovarian epithelial inclusions. Rectovaginal endometriosis, which often resembles adenomyosis, could result from metaplasia of müllerian remnants located in the rectovaginal septum.[32]

These composite theories are attractive in that they recognize a multifaceted mechanism of histogenesis. It seems logical that a disease with such variable manifestations may originate via several mechanisms.

GENETIC FACTORS

It has long been thought that endometriosis has a genetic basis. Although there does not seem to be an association with HLA haplotypes,[33,34] there is an increased prevalence of endometriosis in first-degree relatives of affected women compared with the general population.[35-37] In addition, a study of 16 pairs of monozygotic twins found that 14 were concordant for endometriosis.[38] Some authors have suggested that endometriosis may be a genetically transmitted disorder that results in an altered immune surveillance that allows for the attachment and growth of ectopic endometrium.[39]

ENVIRONMENTAL EXPOSURE TO TOXINS

Environmental exposure to polyhalogenated aromatic hydrocarbons (PHAH), including dioxins, and polychlorinated biphenyls (PCB) has been implicated in the pathogenesis of endometriosis. These molecules are ubiquitous in the environment. Currently, dioxins are formed during the combustion of organic materials and are also produced as trace contaminants in various industrial processes. Most exposure to humans occurs via accumulation in the food chain.[40] PCB are found in commercial products, including electrical equipment, paints, and pesticides. There is evidence that the action of dioxins and PCB is mediated through an interaction with the aryl hydrocarbon receptor (AhR). This is a nuclear receptor with an unknown natural ligand that acts as a transcription factor. In addition, PCB may act independently of the AhR and may influence estrogen activity.[41,42]

Using a model involving rhesus monkeys, Rier et al[41] reported an increased prevalence of endometriosis in animals that had been chronically exposed to dioxins and PCB. This group of investigators also reported alterations in immune competent cells exposed to these compounds. Exposure to dioxin increased the production of TNF-α and decreased NK cytolytic activity (see below) from stimulated peripheral blood mononuclear cells (PBMC).[41]

A cause-and-effect relationship in humans is less clear. Eskinazi and co-workers performed a population-based cohort study in Seveso, Italy, where a factory explosion led to the highest known population exposure to 2,3,7,8-tetrachlorodibenzo-p-dioxin (TCDD). In women with high serum levels of dioxin the relative risk of endometriosis was 2.1 compared to women with low levels. However, this difference was not statistically significant (90% CI = 0.5–8.0).[43] In an in vitro study, Zhao et al reported the expression of the AhR by endometrial stromal cells (ESC) and endometriotic stromal cells. Following exposure to dioxin there was increased transcription of RANTES (see below) demonstrated in both stromal cells types.[42]

LOCAL PERITONEAL AND IMMUNE FACTORS

Alterations in the immunologic response to retrograde menstruation have been implicated in the genesis and maintenance of the endometriotic lesion. This defective immunosurveillance may lead to decreased clearance of menstrual debris from the peritoneal cavity and may allow for the attachment of ectopic endometrium to peritoneal surfaces. Moreover, an abnormal immune response could actually promote the persistence and growth of ectopic endometrial tissue.[44]

PERITONEAL FLUID (PF) LEUKOCYTES

To evaluate the role of the immune system in the pathogenesis of endometriosis, investigators have evaluated immune cells and their secretory products in peritoneal fluid (PF), peripheral blood (PB), and in the endometriotic lesion itself. Examination of the cellular and biochemical composition of PF has revealed differences between women with and without endometriosis. Under normal conditions PF cell concentrations are greater than 1×10^6 cells per cubic centimeter. Macrophages are the predominant cell type,[45–47] the remainder being desquamated mesothelium and lymphocytes.

Hill et al found increased concentrations of leukocytes in the PF of patients with stages I and II endometriosis compared to fertile controls. The most significant increases were in the concentration of macrophages, helper T lymphocytes, and natural killer (NK) cells. Interestingly, similar increases were seen in patients with unexplained infertility and no evidence of endometriosis.[46] Haney et al reported an inverse relationship between the extent of endometriosis and the total cell count of the PF.[48] Olive et al also demonstrated increased cell counts in PF from infertile women with endometriosis compared to other infertile women. However, when controlling for other confounding factors, the best correlation with increased macrophage number was non-mechanical infertility, including patients with endometriosis.[49]

MACROPHAGES AND CYTOKINE PRODUCTION

Macrophages are key components of natural immunity. These cells are involved in recognizing foreign cells and processing them for presentation to T lymphocytes. In the peritoneal cavity these cells are involved in the removal of both foreign and damaged cells.

Paradoxically, in patients with endometriosis, growth factors and cytokines produced by peritoneal leukocytes may contribute to the survival of endometriotic implants.[44,50] Halme et al was one of the first to suggest this phenomenon. These investigators demonstrated an increased secretion of macrophage-derived growth factor from peritoneal macrophages in women with endometriosis compared to women with normal pelvic anatomy or with pelvic adhesions.[51] Similarly, increases in PF concentrations of the proinflammatory macrophage-derived cytokines interleukin-1 (IL-1)[52,53] and tumor necrosis factor-α (TNF-α)[53–58] have been described in patients with endometriosis. TNF-α activates inflammatory leukocytes and stimulates macrophages to produce other cytokines, such as IL-1, IL-6, and more TNF-α. Interleukin-1 also acts on mononuclear cells to increase further production of IL-1 and IL-6.[59]

Increased PF concentrations and in vitro production of other macrophage secretory products, such as IL-6[58,60] and interleukin-8 (IL-8),[56,61–63] have also been described in patients with endometriosis. Both of these cytokines are produced by many different cell types.[64,65] IL-6 is involved in the growth and differentiation of many immunocompetent cells.[59] IL-8 is a chemoattractor and activator of neutrophils, and is a potent angiogenic agent.[66,67]

T LYMPHOCYTES AND CYTOKINE PRODUCTION

An imbalance in the secretory products of T helper lymphocytes has also been implicated in the pathogenesis of endometriosis. Following activation, helper T cells may differentiate into two different subsets that produce cytokines with dichotomous results. T helper cells type 1 (Th1) produce cytokines that are promoters of cell-mediated immunity. These cytokines, including IL-2, γ-interferon, and IL-12, are principle mediators of cell-mediated immunity. T helper type 2

(Th2) cytokines include IL-4, IL-5, IL-10, and IL-13,[68] and are involved in B-lymphocyte differentiation as well as the suppression of cell-mediated immunity.[68,69] Several investigations have reported increased levels of Th2 cytokines and decreased Th1 cytokines in PF and PB in patients with endometriosis.[70,71]

Hsu et al examined the expression of IL-2, γ-interferon, IL-4, and IL-10 of mononuclear cells from PF and PB. These investigators found increased levels of IL-4 mRNA in mononuclear cells, as well as increased levels of IL-4 protein in the PF and PB of patients with endometriosis. However, the concentration of IL-4 in the PF was similar in patients with pelvic adhesions. The concentration of IL-10 was increased in PF, but decreased in PB of patients with endometriosis. In contrast, the secretion of Th1 cytokines, IL-2, and γ-interferon, was decreased in the PF of patients with endometriosis. Interestingly, the PF concentrations of IL-2 and γ-interferon were also decreased in patients with pelvic adhesions.[70]

Similar to the findings of Hsu et al, Ho et al found increased levels of IL-10 in PF of patients with early-stage endometriosis compared to those with advanced stages and to controls. These investigators postulate that increased levels of Th2 cytokines result in the decreased numbers of PF Th1 cells found in their study.[72] In contrast, on examining patients with advanced endometriosis, Rana et al failed to demonstrate increased levels of IL-10 in PF. However, this group did find increased basal and stimulated synthesis of IL-10 by cultured peritoneal mononuclear cells.[56] Similarly, other investigators have not demonstrated differences in PF IL-10 levels.[71]

Transforming growth factor-β (TGF-β), a T-cell and macrophage-derived cytokine, is also found in greater concentrations in the peritoneal fluid of women with endometriosis than in fertile and infertile women without the disease.[73] TGF-β is highly pleiotropic. Depending on culture conditions, it can stimulate the growth of some cells and inhibit the growth of others. It is potentially important in endometriosis as it antagonizes many responses of lymphocytes. For example, TGF-β can inhibit T-cell proliferation following stimulation by polyclonal mitogens, and can inhibit the maturation of cytotoxic lymphocytes.[59]

Along a similar line, Mclaren et al demonstrated decreased levels of IL-13, a Th2-produced cytokine, in PF of patients with endometriosis.[71] IL-13 has the capacity to inhibit proinflammatory cytokine synthesis by activated macrophages. In this study, T cells and macrophages isolated from PF did not seem to express IL-13, whereas glandular and stromal cells from eutopic and ectopic endometrium were immunohistochemically positive.

Increased apoptosis of T lymphocytes via activation of the Fas-Fas ligand signaling pathway could also contribute to an altered immune response in endometriosis.[74,75] Fas is a receptor for Fas ligand. Fas-bearing cells undergo apoptosis when they interact with Fas ligand. Fas ligand is expressed predominately on activated T cells. It is also expressed by endometrial glandular and stromal cells. Soluble Fas ligand may be produced by enzymatic cleavage of the membrane-bound form of the molecule. Garcia-Velasco and coworkers found increased serum and PF levels of soluble Fas ligand in patients with stage III and IV endometriosis compared to fertile controls and patients with early-stage disease.[75] Moreover, Selam et al observed increased Fas ligand expression by endometrial stromal cells (ESC) and glandular cells exposed to IL-8. Treatment of ESC with IL-8, when co-cultured with Jurkhat T lymphocytes, led to increased apoptosis of the Jurkhat T lymphocytes.[74] Thus, increased concentration of soluble Fas ligand in the peritoneal fluid or serum could lead to apoptosis of immune cells that are involved with the clearance of retrograde menstruum.

DISCORDANCE OF RESULTS

The results of studies concerning cytokine activity in patients with endometriosis have often been inconsistent.[76-78] The reasons for these discrepancies are not entirely clear, but may reflect differences in methodology. Likewise, differences in control groups may affect results. For example, failure to include infertile patients without endometriosis as part of a control group could lead to the erroneous conclusion that a specific finding is associated with endometriosis when, in fact, this finding is more closely related to infertility than it is to endometriosis.[79]

MACROPHAGE RECRUITMENT

Increased PF concentrations of cytokines that lead to the migration, proliferation, and activation of macrophages have been reported in patients with endometriosis.[80,81] Endometriotic lesions may contribute to the recruitment of macrophages. The macrophage products IL-1β and TNF-α stimulate endometrial epithelial and mesothelial cells to produce the chemokine monocyte chemotactic protein-1 (MCP-1).[82,83] Increased PF concentrations of MCP-1 have been reported in patients with endometriosis.[82,83] In addition, increased expression of MCP-1 in eutopic endometrium has been demonstrated in patients with endometriosis compared to fertile controls.[84]

Another small molecular weight cytokine, RANTES (regulated upon activation, normal T-cell expressed and secreted), has also been implicated in the pathogenesis of endometriosis. RANTES is a T-lymphocyte product that is involved in macrophage recruitment and activation. Increased PF concentrations of RANTES have been found in patients with endometriosis.[85] Stromal cells from both eutopic and ectopic endometrium have also been shown to produce RANTES, and this production is increased by tumor necrosis factor-α and interferon-γ in culture.[86]

In addition to increased recruitment, PF macrophages in patients with endometriosis may have an altered lifecycle. McLaren et al reported that PF macrophages from patients with endometriosis might be resistant to apoptosis secondary to an increased expression of Bcl-2 and decreased expression of Bax.[87] Bcl-2 protein is a cell survival factor that acts by preventing apoptosis. On the other hand, the cell survival-promoting ability of Bcl-2 is opposed by Bax secondary to the formation of Bax-Bcl-2 heterodimers.[88]

CYTOKINES AND ENDOMETRIOSIS

Possible effects of PF cytokines on endometriotic lesions have been extrapolated from studies concerning the growth and differentiation of endometrial cells in culture. These PF cytokines may be responsible for the proliferation and differentiation of attached fragments of ectopic endometrium. Also, it is likely that PF cytokines contribute to the formation of adhesions often found in patients with endometriosis.[89]

ANGIOGENESIS

It has been estimated that growth beyond a critical tissue volume of 1×10^6 cells will require a new vascular supply. The production of angiogenic growth factors by endometriotic lesions is a hypothesized mechanism by which established implants ensure their continued growth. Oosterlynck et al demonstrated an increased concentration of angiogenic factors in PF from women with endometriosis.[90] More specifically, vascular endothelial growth factor (VEGF), a potent angiogenic factor involved in neovascularization, has been found in PF of patients with endometriosis during the proliferative phase of the cycle.[91,92] Macrophages present in both peritoneal fluid and the stroma of the endometriotic implant appear to be a major source of VEGF. Macrophage estrogen and progesterone receptors have been demonstrated, and stimulation with both steroids leads to increased VEGF production.[93]

Not surprisingly, VEGF production has been described in eutopic endometrium. It is expressed in endometrial glandular epithelium, and more diffusely in endometrial stroma. It is expressed in increasing amounts throughout the cycle.[92,94] Similar expression is seen in endometriotic implants. Like macrophages, endometrial stromal cells increase expression of VEGF in response to estrogen and progesterone.[92] Thus, VEGF which is produced by macrophages and endometrial cells may play a role in promoting the growth of the endometriotic lesion.

Therapies targeting VEGF in a mouse model of endometriosis support this concept. In a xenograft model of endometriosis in which human endometrium was transplanted into the peritoneum of the nude mouse, Hull et al demonstrated that antibodies to human VEGF inhibited the growth of ectopic endometrium.[95] In a similar model, Dabrosin et al reported eradication of endometriotic lesions using gene transfer. In this study, 14 mice with established endometriosis had eradication of endometriotic lesions following intraperitoneal administration of an adenovirus transfected with angiostatin, a natural inhibitor of angiogenesis.[96]

NATURAL KILLER CELL ACTIVITY

Decreased natural killer cell (NK) activity has been implicated in the pathogenesis of endometriosis.[97-100] NK cells are large granular lymphocytes that possess the ability to kill certain tumor cells and cells infected by virus.[101] NK cell activity is increased by the macrophage and T-cell products IL-1, IL-2, IL-12, IFN-γ, and TNF-α.[101,102] With regard to endometriosis, decreased NK activity is suggested to impair the clearance of retrograde menstruated endometrium from the peritoneal cavity. This theory also assumes that endometriotic cells are NK targets.[102]

Studies have revealed decreased NK cell activity in peripheral blood mononuclear cells (PBMC) of women with endometriosis. Several authors have reported decreased NK cell activity of PBMC in patients with endometriosis to K562 cells (a target cell lysed by NK cells in vitro). This decreased activity seems to correlate with the severity of the disease.[97-100] In addition, decreased NK activity of PBMC seems to correlate with increasing estrogen concentrations[99,103] whereas GnRH analogs increase NK activity in

PBMC in women with advanced endometriosis.[104] The decreased NK activity seems to be a qualitative defect and is not caused by decreased numbers of NK cells. In contrast to these findings, D'Hooghe et al failed to demonstrate a similar decrease in PBMC NK cell activity against the K562 cell line in a study of endometriosis using a baboon model.[105]

For the hypothesis of impaired NK activity to be plausible, NK cells of patients with endometriosis should have decreased cytotoxicity to autologous endometrium. This more specific decrease in the cytotoxicity of PBMC to endometrial antigens has been reported by several investigators.[97,106] The work of Vigano et al demonstrated cytotoxicity to endometrial cells, but no difference in NK toxicity to K562 cells in patients with endometriosis. Thus, the defect in NK activity was thought to be specific for the endometrial target cell.[106]

Decreased NK cytotoxicity to K562 cells has also been described in PF mononuclear cells from women with endometriosis.[98,107,108] Oosterlynck et al found that peritoneal fluid from women with endometriosis had significantly reduced NK-mediated cytotoxicity to K562 cells and decreased proliferation in response to phytohemagglutinin compared to fertile women without endometriosis. When compared to the PF of infertile women without endometriosis, significant differences were only seen in cases of severe endometriosis.[109] There are conflicting results regarding NK activity following NK cell exposure to serum from patients with endometriosis.[109,110]

The cause of the supposed decreased NK cytotoxicity in endometriosis is not known. TGF-β which, as previously stated, is found in increased concentrations in PF of women with endometriosis, inhibits NK activity.[73] However, the increased concentrations of peritoneal macrophages secreting IL-1 and TNF-α would be expected to increase NK activity. To reconcile this paradox, Hill has speculated that a possible mechanism could involve stimulation of antibodies in response to ectopic endometrium. The resultant immune complexes could inhibit NK activity by binding Fc receptors on NK cells. Also, prostaglandin E production by activated macrophages could suppress NK activity.[102,111]

More recently, Mazzeo et al demonstrated increased levels of the IL-12 p40 subunit in PF of patients with endometriosis. In vitro, the free p40 subunit leads to decreased cytotoxicity of autologous endometrium by NK cells that were incubated with IL-12. The p40 inhibitory effect was thought to be a result of downregulation of the NK cell IL-12 receptor.[112] Another recent investigation has demonstrated an increased proportion of NK cells in PF and in PB that express killer inhibitory receptors (KIR) in patients with endometriosis. Defects in this type of receptor could explain why these NK cells may not be toxic to target cells that express major histocompatibility determinates that are characteristic of 'self' (i.e. to the patients' own sloughed endometrium, or endometrium growing at ectopic sites).[113]

Like the associated increase in peritoneal macrophage and cytokine concentration, it is unclear whether decreased NK activity leads to the formation of the endometriotic lesion, or whether it is merely a result of the disease. As decreased NK activity has been described in cancer patients with large tumor burdens, it is possible that advanced endometriosis could have a similar effect. A more complete understanding of the role of NK cells in the pathogenesis of endometriosis may ultimately depend on further definition of specific NK target molecules.

RESIDENT LEUKOCYTES IN ENDOMETRIOSIS

Resident leukocytes in endometriotic implants may contribute to the persistence and growth of the implant. In eutopic endometrium, leukocytes comprise up to 25% of the stroma. The majority of these cells are macrophages and T cells.[114,115] Studies of ectopic endometrium have revealed increased concentrations of stromal leukocytes compared to eutopic endometrium. This is accounted for by increases in macrophages, T helper–inducer (CD4), and T cytolytic–suppressor

(CD8) cells.[116-119] In addition, there is an increased proportion of activated T cells[118] as well as T cells and macrophages that express greater amounts of interferon-γ in endometriotic implants compared to eutopic endometrium.[120] Furthermore, the number of NK cells is decreased in ectopic endometrium.[116-118] It is hypothesized that resident leukocytes in endometriosis, by responding to and by producing cytokines, may help account for differential growth and persistence of implants.

ABNORMALITIES IN EUTOPIC ENDOMETRIUM

AROMATASE PRODUCTION

The expression of aromatase in endometriotic implants has been described.[121] Using RT-PCR, Noble et al also reported that aromatase transcripts were detected in endometriotic implants. In addition, the eutopic endometrium from endometriosis patients demonstrated aromatase transcription. In contrast, aromatase transcription was not detectable in eutopic endometrium from disease-free women.[122] Although it was hoped that eutopic endometrial expression of aromatase could be used as a screening test for endometriosis, this notion has recently been discounted. Like Noble et al, Dheenadayalu and co-workers[123] found a high degree of correlation of aromatase transcription with endometriosis. However, in this study the investigators found that the transcription of aromatase mRNA was not confined to women with endometriosis. Twenty-five percent of women without endometriosis had expression of aromatase in eutopic endometrium. Moreover, 32% (6/19) of patients without detectable aromatase transcripts in eutopic endometrium had endometriosis.[123]

PRODUCTION AND RESPONSE TO GROWTH FACTORS

Hepatocyte growth factor (HGF) secretion was found to be significantly increased in cultured endometrial stromal cells from infertile patients with endometriosis compared to those without endometriosis.[124] HGF has also been reported to be elevated in peritoneal fluid of patients with endometriosis.[125] HGF was first described as a mitogen for hepatocytes. It is also reported to have mitogenic effects on endometrial epithelium.[126] The HGF receptor is the c-Met proto-oncogene product. Using immunohistochemistry, Khan and co-workers[126] found increased eutopic endometrial expression of HGF and c-Met in patients with endometriosis compared with controls. The authors hypothesize that increased HGF activity may lead to increased migration and proliferation of ectopic endometrium. Increased HGF activity also leads to increased vascularity by causing increases in VEGF.[126]

In a study using cultured ESC and EEC, Braun et al recently compared the response of eutopic endometrium from patients with and without endometriosis to TNF-α. These investigators demonstrated proliferation of eutopic endometrium from endometriosis patients. In contrast, TNF-α failed to enhance – and often inhibited – the proliferation of eutopic endometrial cells from women without endometriosis. The authors hypothesize that this differential effect could be due to altered expression of TNF-α receptors in eutopic endometrium. TNF-α regulates both cellular proliferation and apoptosis through two distinct receptors (TNFR1 and TNFR2, respectively).[127]

Similar disparate responses of eutopic endometrium following IL-8 and IL-12 exposure have been demonstrated in patients with and without endometriosis. Gazvani et al found that IL-12 significantly inhibited the survival of endometrial cells from women without endometriosis compared to endometrial cells from women with endometriosis.[128] Likewise, IL-1 has been shown to increase the production of MCP-1 by eutopic endometrial cells in women with endometriosis compared to women without endometriosis.[129] Three receptors for IL-1 have been designated. IL-1 receptor I and receptor III (IL-1RI and IL-1RIII, respectively) may induce cell activation. In contrast, binding to IL-1RII may

inhibit these effects. Recently, Kharfi et al reported decreased IL-1RII transcription in eutopic endometrium of patients with endometriosis. This decreased transcription was greatest in patients with early-stage disease.[130]

REACTIVE OXYGEN SPECIES

Some investigators have suggested that reactive oxygen species (ROS) may play a role in the pathogenesis of endometriosis. Reactive oxygen species are produced during normal oxygen metabolism in the respiratory cycle when an electron is transferred to oxygen, producing a superoxide anion (O_2^-).[131] Through the action of superoxide dismutase, hydrogen peroxide is formed (H_2O_2). Hydrogen peroxide is detoxified by glutathione peroxidase or converted to H_2O and O_2 by catalase.[132] ROS may be damaging to lipids, proteins, and nucleic acids. Lipid peroxidation is particularly harmful as it leads to cell membrane damage. In addition, these reactions often involve catalysis by transition metals. The ferrous iron, interacting with hydrogen peroxide, leads to the liberation of a hydroxyl radical.[131] Hence the presence of iron in the peritoneal cavity resulting from retrograde menstruation has been implicated in the pathogenesis of endometriosis.[132]

Wang et al reported no difference in ROS when comparing the peritoneal fluid from patients with endometriosis to fertile controls.[133] In contrast, Shanti et al reported increases in serum autoantibodies directed against oxidatively modified proteins in patients with endometriosis.[134] Other investigators have reported increased concentrations of oxidatively modified lipid–protein complexes in the peritoneal fluid of endometriosis patients.[135] These substances presumably arise from oxidation of lipoproteins and other proteins. Certain oxidized lipoproteins may act as monocyte and T-lymphocyte chemoattractants and activators.[136] For example, Rong et al have reported increased production of MCP-1 from cultured peritoneal mesothelial cells (PMC) and endometrial cells exposed to oxidized low-density lipoproteins (LDL).[137]

CHARACTERIZING INITIAL ATTACHMENT OF ECTOPIC ENDOMETRIUM

According to the implantation theory of endometriosis, intraperitoneal endometrial cells must have the ability to implant outside the uterus. Several crucial questions concerning the initial interaction of endometrial cells with the peritoneum remain unsettled. Until recently, it was unclear which endometrial cells – stroma or epithelium – attach to the peritoneum. It now appears that both endometrial stromal cells (ESC) and epithelial cells (EEC) are able to attach to the peritoneal membrane.[138] In addition, the manner of attachment to the peritoneum by endometrial cells remains controversial. Specifically, it is debated whether endometrial cells attach to intact, viable mesothelium (i.e. the epithelium lining of the peritoneum).

Some have postulated that peritoneal mesothelial cells (PMC) are a barrier to the attachment of ectopic cells to the peritoneum.[139,140] These investigators hypothesize that trauma to the mesothelial lining is a prerequisite for endometrial adhesion.[141,142] In contrast, Witz and co-workers have demonstrated that EEC and ESC rapidly adhere to intact PMC.[138,143,148] Within 1 hour these cells from proliferative, secretory, and menstrual-phase endometria adhere to explants of peritoneal mesothelium and to mesothelial cells grown in monolayer culture.

Following attachment to the peritoneum, the early endometriotic lesion is locally invasive.[144,145] Using peritoneal explants, Witz and colleagues found that there is disruption of PMC within 24 hours and invasion into the extracellular matrix.[146] Invasion of PMC grown in monolayer culture followed a similar time course.[147]

Whether the presence of intact fragments of endometrium in the peritoneal cavity is necessary for the formation of endometriosis is not yet certain. Witz et al demonstrated that menstrual endometrium, and dispersed ESC and EEC, have the ability to attach and invade the peritoneal mesothelium. In contrast, cultured human myometrial cells attach to peritoneal mesothelium but do not invade into the peritoneal stroma.[148,149] In a xenograft model using the nude mouse as a recipient of human endometrial transplantation, Belliard demonstrated that peritoneal administration of both cultured ESC and EEC that were pre-exposed to estrogen is necessary for the formation of endometriotic implants. Injection of cell suspensions of either ESC or EEC alone did not result in the formation of endometriotic lesions.[150] Nap et al performed a similar experiment to determine the formation of endometriotic-like lesions using the chicken chorioallantoic membrane as a recipient of grafted human endometrium. These investigators reported that endometriosis-like lesions developed only when intact fragments of endometrium invaded the chorioallantoic membrane. Collagenase-digested endometrium did not form these lesions.[151] These data suggest that individual endometrial cells are capable of invading the mesothelium. The formation of typical endometriotic lesions (i.e. with glands and stroma), at least in short-term experiments, seems to require the interaction of both ESC and EEC.

CELL ADHESION MOLECULES (CAM) AND MESOTHELIAL–ENDOMETRIAL ADHESION

Several recent investigations have focused on CAM that could be involved in the initial adhesion of endometrial cells to PMC. CD44, the principal receptor for hyaluronic acid (HA), is expressed by ESC and EEC.[152-154] Dechaud and colleagues have demonstrated that CD44 is expressed by ESC and EEC in cell culture.[155] In addition, the CD44 ligand HA is synthesized by mesothelial cells.[156-158] In vitro studies have demonstrated that disruption of HA at the surface of mesothelial cells inhibits binding of ESC and EEC to mesothelium.[155]

Integrin expression has also been the focus of numerous studies addressing the genesis of the endometriotic lesion. Integrins are a family of glycosylated heterodimeric transmembrane adhesion receptors that consist of non-covalently bound α and β subunits. These molecules are the major receptor by which cells attach to components of the ECM. Some integrins also mediate cell–cell adhesion.[159] The name 'integrin' refers to the function of integrating the cells' exterior (i.e. the ECM and other cell surface CAM) with the cells' interior.[160] Adhesive interactions via integrins, both cell–cell and cell–matrix, provide physical support and lead to the transduction of signals that regulate movement and alter gene expression.[159] When integrins interact with the ECM there is downstream signaling through molecules such as the Rho-like GTPases, phospholipase C, ERK, and JNK cascades.[159]

Integrins can exist in low- and high-affinity states.[159,161] Changes in integrin affinity for ECM proteins are modulated by intracellular signals.[161] This process is termed 'inside-out signaling'.

Immunohistochemical studies have demonstrated that the $\alpha2\beta1$ (collagen and laminin receptor) and $\alpha3\beta1$ (collagen, laminin, and fibronectin receptor) integrins are present on the apical surface (i.e. towards the peritoneal cavity) of mesothelial cells.[162,163] However, function blocking anti-integrin antibodies do not inhibit the adhesion of endometrial cells to mesothelial cells, suggesting that integrins are not involved in the initial adhesion of endometrial cells to mesothelium.[164]

INVASION OF THE EXTRACELLULAR MATRIX OF THE PERITONEUM

The early endometriotic lesion invades the peritoneal stroma. Hence, knowledge of the composition of the peritoneal ECM is important in evaluating the histogenesis of endometriosis. Studies of the peritoneal membrane using electron microscopy demonstrate PMC lying over a continuous basement membrane (BM). Beneath the BM there is dense connective tissue consisting mainly of collagen fibrils organized into thick bundles.[165]

Recently, several groups of investigators have suggested that mesothelial cells express ECM proteins such as collagen (Col), fibronectin (FN), and laminin (LM) at their surface (i.e. towards the peritoneal cavity).[166,167] These investigators have suggested that these PMC surface ECM proteins are involved in the initial attachment of ovarian cancer cells to the mesothelium. Investigations

using confocal laser scanning microscopy (CLSM) have refuted this hypothesis. With CLSM it is possible to discriminate details of the ECM composition immediately surrounding PMC. This work demonstrated that the basement membrane underlying PMC consists largely of Col IV and LM. However, there is overlap of underlying FN and Col I with these basement membrane proteins. Col I is a major component of the peritoneal ECM, extending in a diffuse, reticular pattern throughout the submesothelial stroma. At the apical surface of the peritoneal membrane there is a more dense layer of Col I that extends 10–15 μm from the BM to the underlying loose connective tissue. Furthermore, ECM proteins are not seen at the surface of PMC (i.e. towards the peritoneal cavity).[168]

IMPORTANCE OF MATRIX METALLOPROTEINASES (MMP)

To evaluate the process of peritoneal invasion there has been great interest in the production of matrix metalloproteinases (MMP) by endometrial cells. Matrix metalloproteinases play an important role in remodeling the ECM of many tissues. Together, this multigene family of enzymes has the ability to degrade essentially all of the components of the extracellular matrix. The action of MMP is inhibited by specific tissue inhibitors of metalloproteinases (TIMP).[169–171]

Not surprisingly, MMP have been implicated in the pathogenesis of endometriosis. In a model of endometriosis using nude mice and human endometrium, estrogen treatment of endometrium increased MMP production and led to the implantation of ectopic endometrium. In contrast, progesterone treatment of endometrium, which inhibits MMP production, or the addition of TIMP-1, decreased ectopic implantation.[172]

INTEGRINS AND BINDING TO THE PERITONEAL EXTRACELLULAR MATRIX

There are many studies evaluating and comparing the expression of integrins in eutopic and ectopic endometrium.[173-175] It is likely that the unique integrin expression by ectopic endometrium, compared with eutopic endometrium, is a response to existence in an environment that differs from that of the endometrial cavity.

Function-blocking integrin antibodies have been shown to decrease the binding of ESC and EEC to ECM components of the peritoneum.[164,176] Cytokines implicated in the pathogenesis of endometriosis (see above) influence endometrial integrin expression. Epidermal growth factor (EGF) and transforming growth factor-β (TGF-β) induce expression of α1β1 integrin by ESC. There is decreased expression of the α6 subunit in response to interleukin-1α (IL-1α), IL-1β, and tumor necrosis factor-α (TNF-α). An increase in α1β1 integrin was accompanied by increased adhesion to collagen, but there was no change in binding to FN and VN.[177] In a similar study, Garcia-Velasco and co-workers demonstrated a dose-dependent increase of adhesion of ESC to FN with IL-8 treatment. This group of investigators also demonstrated that ESC binding to FN, LM, and Col IV leads to increased production of MCP-1 mRNA. This increased production was dependent on binding to the β1 integrin subunit. In addition, IL-8 production increased when ESC were plated on ECM components.[178,179]

CADHERINS

Cadherins are transmembrane calcium-dependent CAM that are involved in homophilic adhesion (i.e. binding of like cadherins on two different cells).[180] Cadherins are the major component of the zonula adherens (ZA).

Recently, cadherins have gained attention as 'tumor suppressors'.[181-183] Animal models have indicated that the loss of E-cadherin (epithelial cadherin) is involved in the formation of epithelial cancers.[182,183] In addition, a 'switch' involving the replacement of E-cad by mesenchymal cadherins such as N-cadherin has been reported in carcinomas. N-cadherin may allow the dissociation of single cells from a tumor mass and provide interactions with endothelial and stromal components.[182,183]

Investigations by Gaetje and co-workers demonstrated that endometriotic implants contain an invasive cell type with an ability to invade collagen gels. In contrast, cultures from eutopic endometrium contained very few invasive cells.[184] Further work demonstrated that the majority (>90%) of invasive cells from endometriotic lesions were cytokeratin positive (i.e. epithelioid) and E-cad negative. Immunohistochemical evaluation revealed that 5–25% of epithelial cells in ectopic endometrium were E-cad negative, whereas in eutopic endometrium less than 1% of the epithelial cells were E-cad negative.[185] These findings suggest that N-cadherin is a 'pathfinding' cadherin that allows invasion and migration.[186]

CONCLUSION

No single theory can explain all cases of endometriosis. As endometriosis has multiple manifestations it is likely that several mechanisms are involved in its pathogenesis. Recently, evidence has been presented suggesting that components of the immune system contribute to the pathophysiology of endometriosis. An understanding of these alterations in immune function should help guide diagnosis and therapy in the future. For instance, a recent pilot study performed by Bedaiwy et al suggests that alterations in serum cytokine levels could be used to predict the presence of endometriosis.[187] In addition, it is hoped that new information gained from technologies such as cDNA microarrays will help generate novel hypotheses regarding the pathogenesis and pathophysiology of endometriosis.[188-191] At present, large gaps remain in our current understanding of factors controlling cell attachment, growth, and differentiation of ectopic endometrium.

REFERENCES

1. Knapp VJ. How old is endometriosis? Late 17th- and 18th-century European descriptions of the disease. Fertil Steril 1999;72:10–14.

2. Sampson J. Peritoneal endometriosis due to the menstrual dissemination of endometrial tissue into the peritoneal cavity. Am J Obstet Gynecol 1927;14:422–69.

3. Halme J, Hammond MG, Hulka JF et al. Retrograde menstruation in healthy women and in patients with endometriosis. Obstet Gynecol 1984;64:151–4.

4. Liu DT, Hitchcock A. Endometriosis: its association with retrograde menstruation, dysmenorrhoea and tubal pathology. Br J Obstet Gynecol 1986;93:859–62.

5. Keettel WC, Stein RJ. The viability of the cast-off menstrual endometrium. Am J Obstet Gynecol 1951;61:440–2.

6. Ridley JH, Edwards IK. Experimental endometriosis in the human. Am J Obstet Gynecol 1958;76:783–90.

7. TeLinde RW, Scott RB. Experimental endometriosis. Am J Obstet Gynecol 1950;60:1147–73.

8. D'Hooghe TM, Bambra CS, Raeymaekers BM et al. Intrapelvic injection of menstrual endometrium causes endometriosis in baboons (Papio cynocephalus and Papio anubis). Am J Obstet Gynecol 1995;173:125–34.

9. Merrill JA. Spontaneous endometriosis in the Kenya baboon (Papio doguera). Am J Obstet Gynecol 1968;101:569–70.

10. Moore CM, Hubbard GB, Leland MM et al. Spontaneous ovarian tumors in twelve baboons: a review of ovarian neoplasms in non-human primates. J Med Primatol 2003;32:48–56.

11. Dick EJ Jr, Hubbard GB, Martin LJ et al. Record review of baboons with histologically confirmed endometriosis in a large established colony. J Med Primatol 2003;32:39–47.

12. Olive DL, Henderson DY. Endometriosis and müllerian anomalies. Obstet Gynecol 1987;69:412–15.

13. Sanfilippo JS, Wakim NG, Schikler KN et al. Endometriosis in association with uterine anomaly. Am J Obstet Gynecol 1986;154:39–43.

14. Jenkins S, Olive DL, Haney AF. Endometriosis: pathogenetic implications of the anatomic distribution. Obstet Gynecol 1986;67:335–8.

15. Ridley JH. The histogenesis of endometriosis: a review of facts and fancies. Obstet Gynecol Surv 1968;23:1–35.

16. Hobbs JE, Bortnick AR. Endometriosis of the lungs; experimental and clinical study. Am J Obstet Gynecol 1940;40:832–43.

17. Cassina PC, Hauser M, Kacl G et al. Catamenial hemoptysis. Diagn MRI Chest 1997;111:1447–50.

18. Van Schil PE, Vercauteren SR, Vermeire PA et al. Catamenial pneumothorax caused by thoracic endometriosis. Ann Thorac Surg 1996;62:585–6.

19. Bhatia DS, McFadden PM, Kline RC. Recurrent catamenial hemopneumothorax. South Med J 1998;91:398–401.

20. Jubanyik KJ, Comite F. Extrapelvic endometriosis. Obstet Gynecol Clin North Am 1997;24:411–40.

21. Pinkert TC, Catlow CE, Straus R. Endometriosis of the urinary bladder in a man with prostatic carcinoma. Cancer 1979;43:1562–7.

22. Schrodt GR, Alcorn MO, Ibanez J. Endometriosis of the male urinary system: a case report. J Urol 1980;124:722–3.

23. Sufrin G, Gaeta J, Staubitz WJ et al. Endometrial carcinoma of prostate. Urology 1986;27:18–23.

24. Melicow MM, Pachter MR. Endometrial carcinoma of prostatic utricle (uterus masculinus). Cancer 1967;20:1715–22.

25. Von Recklinghausen F. Adenomyomas and cystadenomas of the wall of the uterus and tube: their origin as remnants of the wolffian body. Wien Klin Wochenschr 1896;8:530.

26. Russell WW. Aberrant portions of the müllerian duct found in an ovary. Ovarian cysts of müllerian origin. Bull Johns Hopkins Hosp 1899;10:8–10.

27. Halban J. Metastatic hysteroadenosis. Wien Klin Wochenschr 1924;37:1205–6.

28. Sampson JA. Heterotopic or misplaced endometrial tissue. Am J Obstet Gynecol 1925;10:649–64.

29. Schenken RS. Pathogenesis. In: Schenken RS, ed. Endometriosis: Contemporary Concepts in Clinical Management. Philadelphia: JB Lippincott, 1989.

30. Javert CT. The spread of benign and malignant endometrium in the lymphatic system with a note of coexisting vascular involvement. Am J Obstet Gynecol 1952;64:780–806.

31. Javert CT. Pathogenesis of endometriosis based on endometrial homeoplasia, direct extension, exfoliation and implantation, lymphatic and hematogenous metastasis. Including five case reports of endometrial tissue in pelvic lymph nodes. Cancer 1949; 2: 399–410.

32. Nisolle M, Donnez J. Peritoneal endometriosis, ovarian endometriosis, and adenomyotic nodules of the rectovaginal septum are three different entities. Fertil Steril 1997;68:585–96.

33. Simpson JL, Malinak LR, Elias S et al. HLA associations in endometriosis. Am J Obstet Gynecol 1984;148:395–7.

34. Maxwell C, Kilpatrick DC, Haining R et al. No HLA–DR specificity is associated with endometriosis. Tissue Antigens 1989;34:145–7.

35. Kennedy S, Mardon H, Barlow D. Familial endometriosis. J Assist Reprod Genet 1995;12:32–34.

36. Simpson JL, Elias S, Malinak LR et al. Heritable aspects of endometriosis. I. Genetic studies. Am J Obstet Gynecol 1980;137:327–31.

37. Moen MH, Magnus P. The familial risk of endometriosis. Acta Obstet Gynecol Scand 1993;72:560–4.

38. Hadfield RM, Mardon HJ, Barlow DH et al. Endometriosis in monozygotic twins. Fertil Steril 1997;68:941–2.

39. Oral E, Arici A. Pathogenesis of endometriosis. Obstet Gynecol Clin North Am 1997;24:219–33.

40. Hays SM, Aylward LL. Dioxin risks in perspective: past, present, and future [see comment]. Regul Toxicol Pharmacol 2003;37:202–17.

41. Rier SE. The potential role of exposure to environmental toxicants in the pathophysiology of endometriosis. Ann NY Acad Sci 2002;955:201–12.

42. Zhao D, Pritts EA, Chao VA et al. Dioxin stimulates RANTES expression in an in-vitro model of endometriosis. Mol Hum Reprod 2002;8:849–54.

43. Eskenazi B, Mocarelli P, Warner M et al. Serum dioxin concentrations and endometriosis: a cohort study in Seveso, Italy. Environ Health Perspect 2002;110:629–34.

44. Lebovic DI, Mueller MD, Taylor RN. Immunobiology of endometriosis. Fertil Steril 2001;75:1–10.

45. Haney AF, Muscato JJ, Weinberg JB. Peritoneal fluid cell populations in infertility patients. Fertil Steril 1981;35:696–8.

46. Hill JA, Faris HM, Schiff I et al. Characterization of leukocyte subpopulations in the peritoneal fluid of women with endometriosis. Fertil Steril 1988;50:216–22.

47. Halme J, Becker S, Wing R. Accentuated cyclic activation of peritoneal macrophages in patients with endometriosis. Am J Obstet Gynecol 1984;148:85–90.

48. Haney AF, Jenkins S, Weinberg JB. The stimulus responsible for the peritoneal fluid inflammation observed in infertile women with endometriosis. Fertil Steril 1991;56:408–13.

49. Olive DL, Weinberg JB, Haney AF. Peritoneal macrophages and infertility: the association between cell number and pelvic pathology. Fertil Steril 1985;44:772–7.

50. Martinez–Roman S, Balasch J, Creus M et al. Transferrin receptor (CD71) expression in peritoneal macrophages from fertile and

infertile women with and without endometriosis. Am J Reprod Immunol 1997;38:413-17.

51. Halme J, White C, Kauma S et al. Peritoneal macrophages from patients with endometriosis release growth factor activity in vitro. J Clin Endocrinol Metab 1988;66:1044-9.

52. Fakih H, Baggett B, Holtz G et al. Interleukin-1: a possible role in the infertility associated with endometriosis. Fertil Steril 1987;47:213-17.

53. Taketani Y, Kuo TM, Mizuno M. Comparison of cytokine levels and embryo toxicity in peritoneal fluid in infertile women with untreated or treated endometriosis. Am J Obstet Gynecol 1992;167:265-70.

54. Eisermann J, Gast MJ, Pineda J et al. Tumor necrosis factor in peritoneal fluid of women undergoing laparoscopic surgery. Fertil Steril 1988;50:573-9.

55. Halme J. Release of tumor necrosis factor-alpha by human peritoneal macrophages in vivo and in vitro. Am J Obstet Gynecol 1989;161:1718-25.

56. Rana N, Braun DP, House R et al. Basal and stimulated secretion of cytokines by peritoneal macrophages in women with endometriosis. Fertil Steril 1996;65:925-30.

57. Overton C, Fernandez-Shaw S, Hicks B et al. Peritoneal fluid cytokines and the relationship with endometriosis and pain. Hum Reprod 1996;11:380-6.

58. Harada T, Yoshioka H, Yoshida S et al. Increased interleukin-6 levels in peritoneal fluid of infertile patients with active endometriosis. Am J Obstet Gynecol 1997;176:593-7.

59. Abbas AK, Lichtman AH, Pober JS. Cellular and Molecular Immunology. Philadelphia: WB Saunders, 1994.

60. Rier SE, Parsons AK, Becker JL. Altered interleukin-6 production by peritoneal leukocytes from patients with endometriosis. Fertil Steril 1994;61:294-9.

61. Ryan IP, Tseng JF, Schriock ED et al. Interleukin-8 concentrations are elevated in peritoneal fluid of women with endometriosis. Fertil Steril 1995;63:929-32.

62. Arici A, Tazuke SI, Attar E et al. Interleukin-8 concentration in peritoneal fluid of patients with endometriosis and modulation of interleukin-8 expression in human mesothelial cells. Mol Hum Reprod 1996;2:40-5.

63. Iwabe T, Harada T, Tsudo T et al. Pathogenetic significance of increased levels of interleukin-8 in the peritoneal fluid of patients with endometriosis. Fertil Steril 1998;69:924-30.

64. Tseng JF, Ryan IP, Milam TD et al. Interleukin-6 secretion in vitro is upregulated in ectopic and eutopic endometrial stromal cells from women with endometriosis. J Clin Endocrinol Metab 1996;81:1118-22.

65. Arici A, Seli E, Zeyneloglu HB et al. Interleukin-8 induces proliferation of endometrial stromal cells: a potential autocrine growth factor. J Clin Endocrinol Metab 1998;83:1201-5.

66. Oral E, Arici A. Peritoneal growth factors and endometriosis. Semin Reprod Endocrinol 1996;14:257-67.

67. Arici A. Local cytokines in endometrial tissue: the role of interleukin-8 in the pathogenesis of endometriosis. Ann NY Acad Sci 2002;955:101-9.

68. Hill JA. Immunology and endometriosis. Fact, artifact, or epiphenomenon? Obstet Gynecol Clin North Am 1997;24:291-306.

69. Abbas AK, Lichtman AH, Pober JS. Cellular and Molecular Immunology. Philadelphia: WB Saunders, 1994.

70. Hsu CC, Yang BC, Wu MH et al. Enhanced interleukin-4 expression in patients with endometriosis. Fertil Steril 1997;67:1059-64.

71. McLaren J, Dealtry G, Prentice A et al. Decreased levels of the potent regulator of monocyte/macrophage activation, interleukin-13, in the peritoneal fluid of patients with endometriosis. Hum Reprod 1997;12:1307-10.

72. Ho HN, Wu MY, Chao KH et al. Peritoneal interleukin-10 increases with decrease in activated CD4+ T lymphocytes in women with endometriosis. Hum Reprod 1997;12:2528-33.

73. Oosterlynck DJ, Meuleman C, Waer M et al. Transforming growth factor-beta activity is increased in peritoneal fluid from women with endometriosis. Obstet Gynecol 1994;83:287-92.

74. Selam B, Kayisli UA, Garcia-Velasco JA et al. Regulation of fas ligand expression by IL-8 in human endometrium. J Clin Endocrinol Metab 2002;87:3921-7.

75. Garcia-Velasco JA, Mulayim N, Kayisli UA et al. Elevated soluble Fas ligand levels may suggest a role for apoptosis in women with endometriosis. Fertil Steril 2002;78:855-9.

76. Keenan JA, Chen TT, Chadwell NL et al. IL-1 beta, TNF-alpha, and IL-2 in peritoneal fluid and macrophage-conditioned media of women with endometriosis. Am J Reprod Immunol 1995;34:381-5.

77. Vercellini P, De Benedetti F, Rossi E et al. Tumor necrosis factor in plasma and peritoneal fluid of women with and without endometriosis. Gynecol Obstet Invest 1993;36:39-41.

78. Awadalla SG, Friedman CI, Haq AU et al. Local peritoneal factors: their role in infertility associated with endometriosis, Am J Obstet Gynecol 1987;157:1207-14.

79. Martinez-Roman S, Balasch J, Creus M et al. Immunological factors in endometriosis-associated reproductive failure: studies in fertile and infertile women with and without endometriosis. Hum Reprod 1997;12:1794-9.

80. Weil SJ, Wang S, Perez MC et al. Chemotaxis of macrophages by a peritoneal fluid protein in women with endometriosis. Fertil Steril 1997;67:865-9.

81. Sharpe-Timms KL, Bruno PL, Penney LL et al. Immunohistochemical localization of granulocyte–macrophage colony-stimulating factor in matched endometriosis and endometrial tissues. Am J Obstet Gynecol 1994;171:740-5.

82. Akoum A, Lemay A, McColl S et al. Elevated concentration and biologic activity of monocyte chemotactic protein-1 in the peritoneal fluid of patients with endometriosis. Fertil Steril 1996;66:17-23.

83. Arici A, Oral E, Attar E et al. Monocyte chemotactic protein-1 concentration in peritoneal fluid of women with endometriosis and its modulation of expression in mesothelial cells. Fertil Steril 1997;67:1065-72.

84. Jolicoeur C, Boutouil M, Drouin R et al. Increased expression of monocyte chemotactic protein-1 in the endometrium of women with endometriosis. Am J Pathol 1998;152:125-33.

85. Khorram O, Taylor RN, Ryan IP et al. Peritoneal fluid concentrations of the cytokine RANTES correlate with the severity of endometriosis. Am J Obstet Gynecol 1993;169:1545-9.

86. Hornung D, Ryan IP, Chao VA et al. Immunolocalization and regulation of the chemokine RANTES in human endometrial and endometriosis tissues and cells. J Clin Endocrinol Metab 1997;82:1621-8.

87. McLaren J, Prentice A, Charnock-Jones DS et al. Immunolocalization of the apoptosis regulating proteins Bcl-2 and Bax in human endometrium and isolated peritoneal fluid macrophages in endometriosis. Hum Reprod 1997;12:146-52.

88. Spencer SJ, Cataldo NA, Jaffe RB. Apoptosis in the human female reproductive tract. Obstet Gynecol Surv 1996;51:314-23.

89. Haney AF. Endometriosis, macrophages, and adhesions. Prog Clin Biol Res 1993;381:19-44.

90. Oosterlynck DJ, Meuleman C, Sobis H et al. Angiogenic activity of peritoneal fluid from women with endometriosis. Fertil Steril 1993;59:778-82.

91. McLaren J, Prentice A, Charnock-Jones DS et al. Vascular endothelial growth factor (VEGF) concentrations are elevated in peritoneal fluid of women with endometriosis. Hum Reprod 1996;11:220–3.

92. Shifren JL, Tseng JF, Zaloudek CJ et al. Ovarian steroid regulation of vascular endothelial growth factor in the human endometrium: implications for angiogenesis during the menstrual cycle and in the pathogenesis of endometriosis. J Clin Endocrinol Metab 1996;81:3112–18.

93. McLaren J, Prentice A, Charnock-Jones DS et al. Vascular endothelial growth factor is produced by peritoneal fluid macrophages in endometriosis and is regulated by ovarian steroids. J Clin Invest 1996;98:482–9.

94. Torry DS, Holt VJ, Keenan JA et al. Vascular endothelial growth factor expression in cycling human endometrium. Fertil Steril 1996;66:72–80.

95. Hull ML, Charnock-Jones DS, Chan CL et al. Antiangiogenic agents are effective inhibitors of endometriosis. J Clin Endocrinol Metab 2003;88:2889–99.

96. Dabrosin C, Gyorffy S, Margetts P et al. Therapeutic effect of angiostatin gene transfer in a murine model of endometriosis. Am J Pathol 2002;161:909–18.

97. Oosterlynck DJ, Cornillie FJ, Waer M et al. Women with endometriosis show a defect in natural killer activity resulting in a decreased cytotoxicity to autologous endometrium. Fertil Steril 1991;56:45–51.

98. Oosterlynck DJ, Meuleman C, Waer M et al. The natural killer activity of peritoneal fluid lymphocytes is decreased in women with endometriosis. Fertil Steril 1992;58:290–5.

99. Garzetti GG, Ciavattini A, Provinciali M et al. Natural killer cell activity in endometriosis: correlation between serum estradiol levels and cytotoxicity. Obstet Gynecol 1993;81:665–8.

100. Wilson TJ, Hertzog PJ, Angus D et al. Decreased natural killer cell activity in endometriosis patients: relationship to disease pathogenesis. Fertil Steril 1994;62:1086–8.

101. Abbas AK, Lichtman AH, Pober JS. Cellular and Molecular Immunology. Philadelphia: WB Saunders, 1994.

102. Hill JA. Immunology and endometriosis. Fertil Steril 1992;58:262–4.

103. Di Stefano G, Provinciali M, Muzzioli M et al. Correlation between estradiol serum levels and NK cell activity in endometriosis. Ann NY Acad Sci 1994;741:197–203.

104. Garzetti GG, Ciavattini A, Provinciali M et al. Natural cytotoxicity and GnRH agonist administration in advanced endometriosis: positive modulation on natural killer activity. Obstet Gynecol 1996;88:234–40.

105. D'Hooghe TM, Scheerlinck JP, Koninckx PR et al. Anti-endometrial lymphocytotoxicity and natural killer cell activity in baboons (Papio anubis and Papio cynocephalus) with endometriosis. Hum Reprod 1995;10:558–62.

106. Vigano P, Vercellini P, Di Blasio AM et al. Deficient antiendometrium lymphocyte-mediated cytotoxicity in patients with endometriosis. Fertil Steril 1991;56:894–9.

107. Ho HN, Chao KH, Chen HF et al. Peritoneal natural killer cytotoxicity and CD25+ CD3+ lymphocyte subpopulation are decreased in women with stage III–IV endometriosis. Hum Reprod 1995;10:2671–5.

108. Wu MY, Chao KH, Chen SU et al. The suppression of peritoneal cellular immunity in women with endometriosis could be restored after gonadotropin releasing hormone agonist treatment. Am J Reprod Immunol 1996;35:510–16.

109. Oosterlynck DJ, Meuleman C, Waer M et al. Immunosuppressive activity of peritoneal fluid in women with endometriosis. Obstet Gynecol 1993;82:206–12.

110. Kanzaki H, Wang HS, Kariya M et al. Suppression of natural killer cell activity by sera from patients with endometriosis. Am J Obstet Gynecol 1992;167:257–61.

111. Garzetti GG, Ciavattini A, Provinciali M et al. Decrease in peripheral blood polymorphonuclear leukocyte chemotactic index in endometriosis: role of prostaglandin E2 release. Obstet Gynecol 1998;91:25–9.

112. Mazzeo D, Vigano P, Di Blasio AM et al. Interleukin-12 and its free p40 subunit regulate immune recognition of endometrial cells: potential role in endometriosis. J Clin Endocrinol Metab 1998;83:911–16.

113. Maeda N, Izumiya C, Yamamoto Y et al. Increased killer inhibitory receptor KIR2DL1 expression among natural killer cells in women with pelvic endometriosis. Fertil Steril 2002;77:297–302.

114. Kamat BR, Isaacson PG. The immunocytochemical distribution of leukocytic subpopulations in human endometrium. Am J Pathol 1987;127:66–73.

115. Marshall RJ, Jones DB. An immunohistochemical study of lymphoid tissue in human endometrium. Int J Gynecol Pathol 1988;7:225–35.

116. Oosterlynck DJ, Cornillie FJ, Waer M et al. Immunohistochemical characterization of leucocyte subpopulations in endometriotic lesions. Arch Gynecol Obstet 1993;253:197–206.

117. Jones RK, Bulmer JN, Searle RF. Immunohistochemical characterization of stromal leukocytes in ovarian endometriosis: comparison of eutopic and ectopic endometrium with normal endometrium. Fertil Steril 1996;66:81–9.

118. Witz CA, Montoya IA, Dey TD et al. Characterization of lymphocyte subpopulations and T cell activation in endometriosis. Am J Reprod Immunol 1994;32:173–9.

119. Klein NA, Pergola GM, Tekmal RR et al. Cytokine regulation of cellular proliferation in endometriosis. Ann NY Acad Sci 1994;734:322–32.

120. Klein NA, Pergola GM, Rao-Tekmal R et al. Enhanced expression of resident leukocyte interferon gamma mRNA in endometriosis. Am J Reprod Immunol 1993;30:74–81.

121. Kitawaki J, Noguchi T, Amatsu T et al. Expression of aromatase cytochrome P450 protein and messenger ribonucleic acid in human endometriotic and adenomyotic tissues but not in normal endometrium. Biol Reprod 1997;57:514–19.

122. Noble LS, Simpson ER, Johns A et al. Aromatase expression in endometriosis. J Clin Endocrinol Metab 1996;81:174–9.

123. Dheenadayalu K, Mak I, Gordts S et al. Aromatase P450 messenger RNA expression in eutopic endometrium is not a specific marker for pelvic endometriosis. Fertil Steril 2002;78:825–9.

124. Sugawara J, Fukaya T, Murakami T et al. Increased secretion of hepatocyte growth factor by eutopic endometrial stromal cells in women with endometriosis. Fertil Steril 1997;68:468–72.

125. Osuga Y, Tsutsumi O, Okagaki R et al. Hepatocyte growth factor concentrations are elevated in peritoneal fluid of women with endometriosis. Hum Reprod 1999;14:1611–13.

126. Khan KN, Masuzaki H, Fujishita A et al. Immunoexpression of hepatocyte growth factor and c-Met receptor in the eutopic endometrium predicts the activity of ectopic endometrium. Fertil Steril 2003;79:173–81.

127. Braun DP, Ding J, Dmowski WP. Peritoneal fluid-mediated enhancement of eutopic and ectopic endometrial cell proliferation is dependent on tumor necrosis factor-alpha in women with endometriosis. Fertil Steril 2002;78:727–32.

128. Gazvani R, Smith L, Fowler PA. Effect of interleukin-8 (IL-8), anti-IL-8, and IL-12 on endometrial cell survival in combined endometrial gland and stromal cell cultures derived from women with and without endometriosis. Fertil Steril 2002;77:62–7.

129. Akoum A, Lemay A, Brunet C et al. Secretion of monocyte chemotactic protein-1 by cytokine-stimulated endometrial cells of women with endometriosis. Le Groupe d'Investigation en Gynécologie. Fertil Steril 1995;63:322–8.

130. Kharfi A, Boucher A, Akoum A. Abnormal interleukin-1 receptor type II gene expression in the endometrium of women with endometriosis. Biol Reprod 2002;66:401–6.

131. Imlay JA. Pathways of oxidative damage. Annu Rev Microbiol 2003;57:395–418.

132. Van Langendonckt A, Casanas-Roux F, Donnez J. Oxidative stress and peritoneal endometriosis. Fertil Steril 2002;77:861–70.

133. Wang Y, Sharma RK, Falcone T et al. Importance of reactive oxygen species in the peritoneal fluid of women with endometriosis or idiopathic infertility. Fertil Steril 1997;68:826–30.

134. Shanti A, Santanam N, Morales AJ et al. Autoantibodies to markers of oxidative stress are elevated in women with endometriosis. Fertil Steril 1999;71:1115–18.

135. Murphy AA, Palinski W, Rankin S et al. Macrophage scavenger receptor(s) and oxidatively modified proteins in endometriosis. Fertil Steril 1998;69:1085–91.

136. Murphy AA, Santanam N, Morales AJ et al. Lysophosphatidyl choline, a chemotactic factor for monocytes/T lymphocytes is elevated in endometriosis. J Clin Endocrinol Metab 1998;83:2110–13.

137. Rong R, Ramachandran S, Santanam N et al. Induction of monocyte chemotactic protein-1 in peritoneal mesothelial and endometrial cells by oxidized low-density lipoprotein and peritoneal fluid from women with endometriosis. Fertil Steril 2002;78:843–8.

138. Witz CA, Thomas MR, Montoya-Rodriguez IA et al. Short-term culture of peritoneum explants confirms attachment of endometrium to intact peritoneal mesothelium. Fertil Steril 2001;74:385–90.

139. van der Linden PJ, de Goeij AF, Dunselman GA et al. Endometrial cell adhesion in an in vitro model using intact amniotic membranes [see comments]. Fertil Steril 1996;65:76–80.

140. Groothuis PG, Koks CA, de Goeij AF et al. Adhesion of human endometrium to the epithelial lining and extracellular matrix of amnion in vitro: an electron microscopic study. Hum Reprod 1998;13:2275–81.

141. Groothuis PG, Koks CA, de Goeij AF et al. Adhesion of human endometrial fragments to peritoneum in vitro. Fertil Steril 1999;71:1119–24.

142. Koks CA, Groothuis PG, Dunselman GA et al. Adhesion of shed menstrual tissue in an in-vitro model using amnion and peritoneum: a light and electron microscopic study. Hum Reprod 1999;14:816–22.

143. Witz CA, Montoya-Rodriguez IA, Schenken RS. Adhesion of antegrade shed menstrual endometrium to intact peritoneal mesothelium. Presented at the 57th Annual Meeting of the American Society for Reproductive Medicine, Orlando, Florida, 20–25 October 2001.

144. Spuijbroek MD, Dunselman GA, Menheere PP et al. Early endometriosis invades the extracellular matrix. Fertil Steril 1992;58:929–33.

145. Sillem M, Hahn U, Coddington CC 3rd et al. Ectopic growth of endometrium depends on its structural integrity and proteolytic activity in the cynomolgus monkey (Macaca fascicularis) model of endometriosis [see comments]. Fertil Steril 1996;66:468–73.

146. Witz CA, Montoya-Rodriguez IA, Schenken RS. Whole peritoneal explants – a novel model of the early endometriosis lesion. Fertil Steril 1999;71:56–60.

147. Witz CA, Cho S, Centonze VE et al. Time series analysis of transmesothelial invasion by endometrial stromal and epithelial cells using three-dimensional confocal microscopy. Fertil Steril 2003;79:770–8.

148. Witz CA, Allsup KT, Montoya-Rodriguez IA et al. Culture of menstrual endometrium with peritoneal explants and mesothelial monolayers confirms attachment to intact mesothelial cells. Hum Reprod 2002;17:2832–8.

149. Witz CA, Montoya-Rodriguez IA, Centonze VE et al. Menstrual endometrium and individual endometrial stromal and epithelial cells are unique in their ability to adhere to and invade peritoneal mesothelium. Presented at the 58th Annual Meeting of the American Society of Reproductive Medicine, Seattle, WA, 2002.

150. Beliard A, Noel A, Goffin F et al. Role of endocrine status and cell type in adhesion of human endometrial cells to the peritoneum in nude mice. Fertil Steril 2002;78:973–8.

151. Nap AW, Groothuis PG, Demir AY et al. Tissue integrity is essential for ectopic implantation of human endometrium in the chicken chorioallantoic membrane. Hum Reprod 2003;18:30–4.

152. Behzad F, Seif MW, Campbell S et al. Expression of two isoforms of CD44 in human endometrium. Biol Reprod 1994;51:739–47.

153. Saegusa M, Hashimura M, Okayasu I. CD44 expression in normal, hyperplastic, and malignant endometrium. J Pathol 1998;184:297–306.

154. Yaegashi N, Fujita N, Yajima A et al. Menstrual cycle dependent expression of CD44 in normal human endometrium. Hum Pathol 1995;26:862–5.

155. Dechaud H, Witz CA, Montoya-Rodriguez IA et al. Mesothelial cell-associated hyaluronic acid facilitates endometrial stromal and epithelial cell binding to mesothelium. Fertil Steril 2001;76:1012–18.

156. Jones LM, Gardner MJ, Catterall JB et al. Hyaluronic acid secreted by mesothelial cells: a natural barrier to ovarian cancer cell adhesion. Clin Exp Metastasis 1995;13:373–80.

157. Yung S, Thomas GJ, Stylianou E et al. Source of peritoneal proteoglycans. Human peritoneal mesothelial cells synthesize and secrete mainly small dermatan sulfate proteoglycans. Am J Pathol 1995;146:520–9.

158. Laurent TC, Fraser JR. Hyaluronan. FASEB J 1992;6:2397–404.

159. Humphries MJ. Integrin cell adhesion receptors and the concept of agonism. Trends Pharmacol Sci 2000;21:29–32.

160. van der Flier A, Sonnenberg A. Function and interactions of integrins. Cell Tissue Res 2001;305:285–98.

161. Brakebusch C, Bouvard D, Stanchi F et al. Integrins in invasive growth. J Clin Invest 2002;109:999–1006.

162. Witz CA, Montoya-Rodriguez IA, Miller DM et al. Mesothelium expression of integrins in vivo and in vitro. J Soc Gynecol Invest 1998;5:87–93.

163. Witz CA, Takahashi A, Montoya-Rodriguez IA et al. Expression of the α2β1 and α3β1 integrins at the surface of mesothelial cells: a potential attachment site of endometrial cells. Fertil Steril 2000;74:579–84.

164. Witz CA, Cho S, Montoya-Rodriguez IA et al. The alpha(2)beta(1)and alpha(3)beta1 integrins do not mediate attachment of endometrial cells to peritoneal mesothelium. Fertil Steril 2002;78:796–803.

165. Slater NJ, Raftery AT, Cope GH. The ultrastructure of human abdominal mesothelium. J Anat 1989;167:47–56.

166. Lessan K, Aguiar DJ, Oegema T et al. CD44 and beta1 integrin mediate ovarian carcinoma cell adhesion to peritoneal mesothelial cells. Am J Pathol 1999;154:1525–37.

167. Strobel T, Cannistra SA. Beta1-integrins partly mediate binding of ovarian cancer cells to peritoneal mesothelium in vitro. Gynecol Oncol 1999;73:362–7.

168. Witz CA, Montoya-Rodriguez IA, Cho S et al. Composition of the extracellular matrix in the peritoneum. J Soc Gynecol Invest 2001;8:299–30.

169. Martelli M, Campana A, Bischof P. Secretion of matrix metallo-proteinases by human endometrial cells in vitro. J Reprod Fertil 1993;98:67–76.

170. Rawdanowicz TJ, Hampton AL, Nagase H et al. Matrix metallo-proteinase production by cultured human endometrial stromal cells: identification of interstitial collagenase, gelatinase-A, gelati-nase-B, and stromelysin-1 and their differential regulation by interleukin-1-alpha and tumor necrosis factor-alpha. J Clin Endocrinol Metab 1994;79:530–6.

171. Osteen KG, Bruner KL, Sharpe-Timms KL. Steroid and growth factor regulation of matrix metalloproteinase expression and endometriosis. Semin Reprod Endocrinol 1996;14:247–55.

172. Bruner KL, Matrisian LM, Rodgers WH et al. Suppression of matrix metalloproteinases inhibits establishment of ectopic lesions by human endometrium in nude mice. J Clin Invest 1997;99:2851–7.

173. Bridges JE, Prentice A, Roche W et al. Expression of integrin adhesion molecules in endometrium and endometriosis. Br J Obstet Gynaecol 1994;101:696–700.

174. Rai V, Hopkisson J, Kennedy S et al. Integrins alpha 3 and alpha 6 are differentially expressed in endometrium and endometriosis. J Pathol 1996;180:181–7.

175. Beliard A, Donnez J, Nisolle M et al. Localization of laminin, fibronectin, E-cadherin, and integrins in endometrium and endometriosis. Fertil Steril 1997;67:266–72.

176. Koks CA, Groothuis PG, Dunselman GA et al. Adhesion of men-strual endometrium to extracellular matrix: the possible role of integrin alpha(6)beta(1) and laminin interaction. Mol Hum Reprod 2000;6:170–7.

177. Grosskinsky CM, Yowell CW, Sun J et al. Modulation of integrin expression in endometrial stromal cells in vitro. J Clin Endocrinol Metab 1996;81:2047–54.

178. Garcia-Velasco JA, Arici A. Interleukin-8 expression in endome-trial stromal cells is regulated by integrin-dependent cell adhe-sion. Mol Hum Reprod 1999;5:1135–40.

179. Garcia-Velasco JA, Seli E, Arici A. Regulation of monocyte chemotactic protein-1 expression in human endometrial stromal cells by integrin-dependent cell adhesion. Biol Reprod 1999;61:548–52.

180. Pollard TD, Earnshaw WC. Cell biology. Philadelphia: Elsevier Science, 2002.

181. Gumbiner BM. Cell adhesion: the molecular basis of tissue archi-tecture and morphogenesis. Cell 1996;84:345–57.

182. Cavallaro U, Schaffhauser B, Christofori G. Cadherins and the tumour progression: is it all in a switch? Cancer Lett 2002;176:123–8.

183. Conacci-Sorrell M, Zhurinsky J, Ben-Ze'ev A. The cadherin-catenin adhesion system in signaling and cancer. J Clin Invest 2002;109:987–91.

184. Gaetje R, Kotzian S, Herrmann G et al. Invasiveness of endometri-otic cells in vitro. Lancet 1995;346:1463–4.

185. Gaetje R, Kotzian S, Herrmann G et al. Nonmalignant epithelial cells, potentially invasive in human endometriosis, lack the tumor suppressor molecule E-cadherin. Am J Pathol 1997;150:461–7.

186. Zeitvogel A, Baumann R, Starzinski-Powitz A. Identification of an invasive, N-cadherin-expressing epithelial cell type in endometriosis using a new cell culture model. Am J Pathol 2001;159:1839–52.

187. Bedaiwy MA, Falcone T, Sharma RK et al. Prediction of endometriosis with serum and peritoneal fluid markers: a prospective controlled trial. Hum Reprod 2002;17:426–31.

188. Eyster KM, Boles AL, Brannian JD et al. DNA microarray analysis of gene expression markers of endometriosis. Fertil Steril 2002;77:38.

189. Taylor RN, Lundeen SG, Giudice LC. Emerging role of genomics in endometriosis research. Fertil Steril 2002;78:694–8.

190. Kao LC, Germeyer A, Tulac S et al. Expression profiling of endometrium from women with endometriosis reveals candidate genes for disease-based implantation failure and infertility. Endocrinology 2003;144:2870–81.

191. Lebovic DI, Baldocchi RA, Mueller MD et al. Altered expression of a cell-cycle suppressor gene, Tob-1, in endometriotic cells by cDNA array analyses. Fertil Steril 2002;78:849–54.

6. Endometriosis is an Inflammatory Disease

Neal G. Mahutte, Umit Kayisli and Aydin Arici

Endometriosis is associated with changes in both cell-mediated and humoral immunity. Although the peritoneal fluid of women with endometriosis contains increased numbers of immune cells, their function appears to be altered from an inhibitory to a facilitatory role. Leukocytes that would normally clear endometrial cells from the peritoneal cavity instead appear to allow their proliferation via an assortment of growth factors and cytokines.

Whether these immunologic alterations induce endometriosis or are a direct consequence of its presence is unclear. So far it has proved difficult to separate 'the chicken from the egg'. Nevertheless, the breadth and depth of immunologic alterations appear to play an important role in allowing endometriosis implants to persist and progress at all stages of the disease.

The inflammatory changes found in women with endometriosis may also contribute to the symptomatology of pain and infertility. Accumulations of inflammatory cells increase the release of prostaglandins, further induce tissue damage and may result in scarring. As a result, dysmenorrhea may progress to dyspareunia and chronic pelvic pain. Additionally, scar tissue may alter fallopian tube integrity, and the inflammatory environment may impair folliculogenesis, fertilization, and embryo implantation.

For all of these reasons, endometriosis is an inflammatory disease. It is almost impossible to isolate the effects of endometriotic implants from their associated immunologic alterations, yet to unravel the pathogenesis of endometriosis and to develop new therapies for its treatment requires a comprehensive understanding of the immune alterations intrinsic to its existence.

IMMUNE ALTERATIONS IN ENDOMETRIOSIS

The major immune alterations identified in endometriosis are outlined in Table 6.1. They

---

Table 6.1 Immune alterations in endometriosis

Increased macrophage number and activity
- Increased angiogenic factors (VEGF, MIF, IL-8, IL-6 TGF-β, TNF-α)
- Increased endometrial growth factors (PDGF, TGF-β, MDGF, EGF, IL-8)
- Increased chemotactic factors (MCP-1, RANTES, IL-8, GROα)

Increased cytokine production
- Source: leukocytes, endometriosis implants and mesothelial cells
- TNF-α, MCP-1, INF-γ, IL-1, IL-2, IL6, IL-8, GROα

Increased humoral immune responses
- Increased B-cell activity
- Increased immunoglobulins and complement proteins

Decreased cell-mediated immunity
- Decreased natural killer cell responsiveness to ectopic endometrial cells
- Decreased T-cell responsiveness to ectopic endometrial cells

VEGF = vascular endothelial growth factor; MIF = macrophage migration inhibitory factor; IL = interleukin; TGF = transforming growth factor; TNF = tumor necrosis factor; PDGF = platelet-derived growth factor; MDGF = macrophage-derived growth factor; EGF = epidermal growth factor; MCP = monocyte chemoattractant protein; RANTES = regulated on activation, normal T-cell expressed and secreted; GRO = growth-regulated; INF = interferon

---

include increases in activated macrophages, humoral immune responses, and inflammatory cytokines in the peritoneal fluid. Concomitantly, there is a decline in cell-mediated immunity, manifested by decreased natural killer (NK) cell activity and possibly decreased T-cell responsiveness.

Macrophages are the most abundant nucleated cells found in peritoneal fluid. Although their numbers vary during the menstrual cycle, they are most elevated in the proliferative phase after menstruation. Macrophages play a key role in first-line host defense mechanisms. Macrophages may directly phagocytose and destroy invading microorganisms, or indirectly contribute to their demise by the secretion of substances including proinflammatory cytokines, reactive oxygen species, prostaglandins, growth factors, and complement.[1] Indeed, cell-mediated immune responses are believed to play a critical role in clearing ectopic endometrial cells from the peritoneal cavity.[2]

One of the most consistent changes in the peritoneal fluid of women with endometriosis is the significantly increased concentration of activated macrophages.[3-5] Macrophages are also abundant in and around endometriosis implants themselves (Figure 6.1). Although peritoneal macrophages from normal fertile women suppress endometrial cell proliferation, those from women with endometriosis have the opposite effect. Indeed, it has been shown that these macrophages stimulate endometrial cell proliferation and induce angiogenesis. Both of these functions are controlled by the synthesis and secretion of prostaglandins and cytokines. Such factors, derived from activated peritoneal macrophages, also modulate other immune responses that contribute to the survival and persistence of endometriosis implants.

In women with endometriosis there also appear to be other signs of decreased cell-mediated surveillance, recognition, and destruction of exfoliated endometrial cells. Although NK cells are more abundant in the peritoneal fluid of women with endometriosis, they demonstrate decreased cytotoxicity.[5,6] Both peripheral and peritoneal NK cells from women with endometriosis are less cytotoxic to endometrial cells.[7,8] Moreover, NK-cell cytotoxicity has been inversely correlated with the stage of endometriosis.[9] Although the cause of decreased NK-cell cytotoxicity is unknown, byproducts of macrophages are a likely source of this suppression. Indeed, both sera and peritoneal fluid from women with endometriosis have been shown to reduce NK-cell cytotoxicity.[10,11]

Women with endometriosis also have increased numbers of T lymphocytes in the peritoneal fluid, especially T-helper (Th) cells.[5] Indeed, the ratio of T-helper to T-suppressor cells is elevated in the peritoneal fluid of women with endometriosis compared to normal controls.[2] The same finding has also been reported when comparing endometriotic tissue to eutopic endometrium.[12]

Endometriosis has also been associated with polyclonal B-cell activation and increased autoantibodies.[13] In particular, elevated IgG and IgA have been identified in the peritoneal fluid of women with endometriosis.[14] Other components of the humoral immunity pathway that may be elevated in women with endometriosis include complement component 3 (C3).[15]

PATHOGENESIS OF ENDOMETRIOSIS

Retrograde menstruation is a universal phenomenon, and implantation of exfoliated endometrial cells is the most widely accepted theory for the development of endometriosis. Why endometriosis develops in some women but not others is unknown. Nevertheless, one of the critical factors believed to determine the outcome of retrograde menstrual tissue is the host immune response.

Five critical steps have been postulated to explain the development of endometriosis lesions (Table 6.2). The two initial steps are attachment of endometrial cells to the peritoneal surface, and invasion of these cells into the mesothelium. After these steps, angiogenesis around the nascent implant, endometrial cellular proliferation, and recruitment of inflammatory cells subservient to the implant become important. Although the endometriotic tissue influences each of these steps, they are also highly influenced by immune cells and inflammatory cytokines (Table 6.3).

ATTACHMENT OF ENDOMETRIAL CELLS TO MESOTHELIAL CELLS

Endometrial tissue is endowed with the capability of adhering to peritoneal tissue.[16] This process is probably mediated by integrins at the peritoneal surface.[17] Endometrial adhesion to mesothelial cells is also fostered by inflammatory cytokines such as IL-8.

IL-8 concentrations are elevated in the peritoneal fluid of women with endometriosis, particularly in the most active stages of the disease.[18,19] IL-8 can be produced by a variety of cell types, including macrophages, endometrial cells, mesothelial cells, endothelial cells, and fibro-

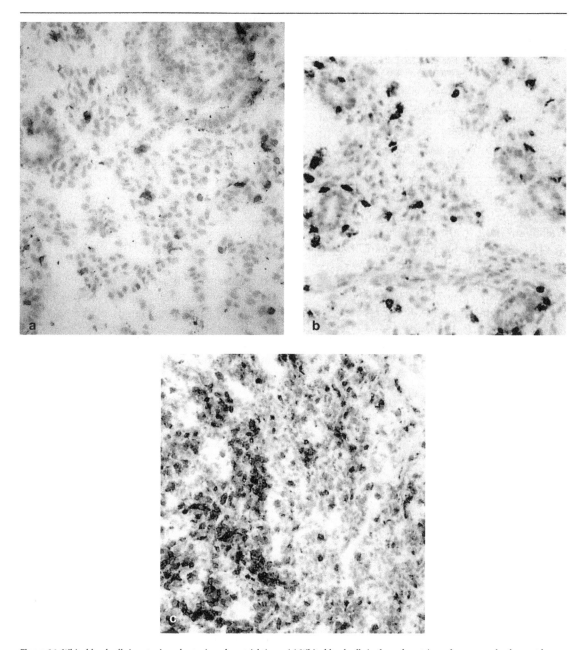

Figure 6.1 White blood cells in eutopic and ectopic endometrial tissue. (a) White blood cells in the endometrium of a woman who does not have endometriosis. (b) White blood cells in the eutopic endometrium of a woman with endometriosis. (c) White blood cells surrounding ectopic endometrial tissue in a woman with endometriosis. Note the marked increase in staining. The predominant cell type accounting for the increase is the macrophage.

blasts. Endometriosis lesions themselves can also produce IL-8. Indeed, IL-8 is markedly expressed in vivo by both endometrial glands and stromal cells (Figure 6.2).[20] In vitro production of IL-8 may be induced by IL-1β. Not only is IL-1β up-regulated by estradiol, but IL-1β is present in

Table 6.2 Critical factors in the pathogenesis of endometriosis

Attachment of endometrial cells to mesothelial cells

Invasion of endometrial cells into the mesothelium

Angiogenesis near nascent endometriosis implants

Proliferation of ectopic endometrial cells

Recruitment of inflammatory cells that support persistence of the implants

significantly increased concentrations in women with endometriosis.[21] Also, tumor necrosis factor-α (TNF-α) induces the production of IL-8 by neutrophils, and TNF-α is elevated in the peritoneal fluid of women with endometriosis.

IL-8 is believed to play a key role in the pathogenesis of endometriosis. IL-8 expression by endometrial cells is highest in the late secretory and early proliferative phase, the time when retrograde menstruation occurs.[22] It has been shown that IL-8 stimulates the adhesion of endometrial stromal cells to fibronectin in a concentration-dependent manner.[23] Thus, IL-8 may play an important role in the initial attachment of endometrial cells to the peritoneal surface. Interestingly, it has also been shown that in vitro attachment of endometrial stromal cells to extracellular matrix upregulates IL-8 gene expression.[24]

INVASION OF ENDOMETRIAL CELLS INTO THE MESOTHELIUM

After the initial attachment of endometrial cells to the mesothelium early endometriosis lesions invade the extracellular matrix of the peri-

Table 6.3 Cytokines elevated in the peritoneal fluid of women with endometriosis

Cytokine	Source	Function
RANTES	Endometrial stromal cells Hematopoietic cells	Chemoattractant for: • monocytes • memory T cells
IL-1	Endometriosis implants Activated macrophages	Induces endometriotic stromal cells to secrete VEGF and IL-6 Increases IL-8 Increases MCP-1 Increases sICAM-1 Activates T-lymphocytes Differentiates B-lymphocytes
IL-8	Macrophages Endometrial cells Mesothelial cells Fibroblasts and endothelial cells	Stimulates adhesion of endometrial cells to fibronectin Stimulates angiogenesis Stimulates endometrial cell proliferation Chemoattractant and antiapoptotic factor for neutrophils
TNF-α	Leukocytes: • Macrophages • Neutrophils • Activated lymphocytes • NK cells Endometrial epithelial cells (greatest in secretory phase) Endometrial stromal cells (greatest in proliferative phase)	Promotes adherence of cultured stromal cells to mesothelial cells Increases endometrial epithelial cell prostaglandin production Initiates cytokine cascade and the inflammatory response Kills certain cell lines
VEGF	Endometriotic implants Activated macrophages	Stimulates angiogenesis
MCP-1	Macrophages Endometrial cells	Recruits and activates macrophages

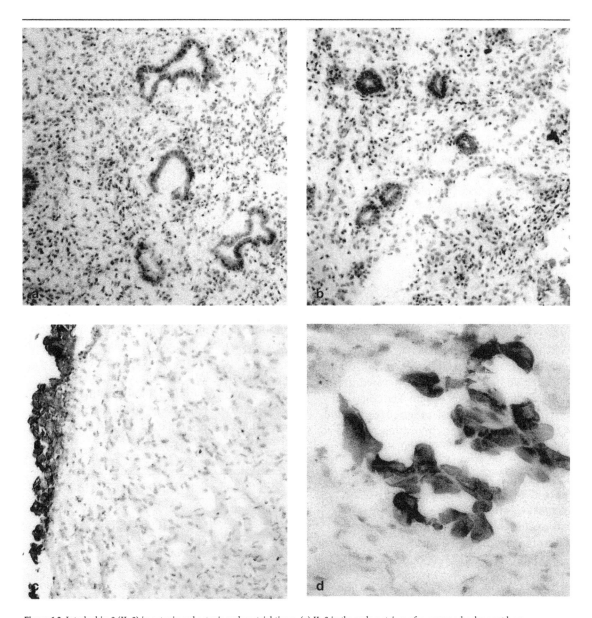

Figure 6.2 Interleukin-8 (IL-8) in eutopic and ectopic endometrial tissue. (a) IL-8 in the endometrium of a woman who does not have endometriosis. (b) IL-8 in the eutopic endometrium from a woman with endometriosis. (c) Strong staining of IL-8 within an endometriosis implant. Note the absence of staining in the surrounding peritoneal tissue. (d) Close-up of IL-8 staining in an endometriosis implant.

toneum.[25] Secretion of metalloproteinases plays a key role in endometrial cell invasion of the extracellular matrix.

IL-8 facilitates endometrial cell invasion of the peritoneal surface. In vitro metalloproteinases activity is upregulated when endometrial cells are exposed to IL-8, especially when those cells are also grown in the presence of extracellular matrix proteins.[26] Thus, IL-8-stimulated attachment of endometrial cells to extracellular matrix may induce further IL-8 expression via a positive feedback mechanism, and simultaneously facilitate endometrial cell invasion.

ANGIOGENESIS NEAR NASCENT ENDOMETRIOSIS IMPLANTS

A key condition for the survival and growth of ectopic endometrial tissue following successful adhesion is the establishment of a new blood supply. Active endometriosis implants are markedly vascularized. The ability to induce angiogenesis derives both as a byproduct of leukocyte recruitment and directly from the endometrial glands and stroma (Table 6.4). Important mediators of local angiogenesis include vascular endothelial growth factor (VEGF), macrophage migration inhibitory factor (MIF), IL-8, interferon-γ, fibroblast growth factor, and platelet-derived growth factor (PDGF).[26–28]

VEGF is a potent angiogenic factor expressed by activated macrophages, neutrophils, and endometriotic implants. VEGF is elevated in the peritoneal fluid of women with endometriosis, and its expression is most pronounced around red lesions rather than the more inactive black powder-burn implants.[27,29] Endometriosis is an estrogen-sensitive disease, and it has been clearly shown that estradiol upregulates VEGF gene transcription in endometrial stromal cells.[30] Estradiol has also been shown to promote VEGF production by peritoneal macrophages.[31] Moreover, the endogenous expression of aromatase within endometriosis implants augments local estradiol concentrations, and hence VEGF production.[32] Finally, hypoxia stimulates VEGF expression, and this may play a significant stimulatory role in the initial stages of exfoliated endometrial cell survival.

Another important angiogenic factor is the multifunctional cytokine MIF.[33] MIF is produced by ectopic endometrial cells (both glandular and stromal) as well as inflammatory cells such as macrophages and lymphocytes, and is a potent mitogenic factor for endothelial cells. It also has the ability to activate and inhibit macrophage migration. Thus, in addition to directly inducing angiogenesis it also helps retain macrophages in the area of the implant, thereby augmenting the release of other growth factors and angiogenic factors. Finally, endothelial cells actually produce MIF, thus potentially further amplifying neovascularization by paracrine and autocrine mechanisms.

Table 6.4 Inflammatory cytokines mediating angiogenesis, endometrial cell proliferation and recruitment of inflammatory cells

Angiogenesis near nascent endometriosis implants
• IL-8, VEGF, MIF, interferon-γ, FGF, PDGF

Proliferation of endometrial cells
• IL-8, PDGF, MDGF, EGF, TGF-β

Recruitment of inflammatory cells that support persistence of the implants
• IL-8, MCP-1, MIF, RANTES

IL = interleukin; VEGF = vascular endothelial growth factor; MIF = macrophage migration inhibitory factor; FGF = fibroblast growth factor; PDGF = platelet-derived growth factor; MDGF = macrophage-derived growth factor; EGF = epidermal growth factor; TGF-β = transforming factor-β; MCP-1 = monocyte chemoattractant protein-1; RANTES = regulated on activation, normal T-cell expressed and secreted

---

PROLIFERATION OF ENDOMETRIAL CELLS

Endometrial cell proliferation is enhanced by peripheral blood monocytes from patients with endometriosis.[34] In contrast, monocytes from fertile women significantly suppress endometrial cell proliferation. A variety of monocyte-derived endometrial cell growth factors have been identified. These include IL-8, PDGF, macrophage-derived growth factor (MDGF), epidermal growth factor (EGF), and transforming growth factor-β (TGF-β).[35]

IL-8 induces proliferation of endometrial cells via an autocrine mechanism. In vitro, IL-8 increases endometrial stromal cell proliferation in a concentration-dependent manner, and anti-IL-8 antibody inhibits endometrial stromal proliferation.[22]

PDGF is a substance released by activated macrophages. It is elevated in the peritoneal fluid of women with endometriosis. PDGF induces endometrial stromal cell proliferation in a dose-dependent manner.[36,37] PDGF and TGF-β also induce upregulation of Fas ligand on endometrial stromal cells. When Fas ligand-bearing endometrial cells come in contact with Fas-bearing immune cells, the interaction may trigger immune cell death. Thus, not only may PDGF and TGF-β stimulate endometrial cell proliferation, they may also help these cells escape immune surveillance.[38]

RECRUITMENT OF INFLAMMATORY CELLS THAT SUPPORT PERSISTENCE OF THE IMPLANTS

Numerous factors contribute to the recruitment and activation of leukocytes in women with endometriosis (Table 6.4). These include monocyte chemotactic protein-1 (MCP-1), IL-8, MIF, and regulated on activation, normal T-cell expressed and secreted (RANTES). Endometriotic lesions themselves express these cytokines. However, they are also secreted by other cell types. For example, mesothelial cells produce MCP-1, as well as macrophages themselves, especially in the proliferative phase of women with endometriosis.[39,40] Indeed, MCP-1 concentrations in the peritoneal fluid of women with endometriosis are markedly elevated over controls.[41]

RANTES is a chemoattractant for monocytes and memory T cells secreted by hematopoietic cells and endometrial stromal cells. Increased concentrations of RANTES have been identified in the peritoneal fluid of women with moderate to severe endometriosis. In vitro production of RANTES by endometrial stromal cells is induced by TNF-α and IFN-γ. The production of RANTES by endometrial stromal cells may also be up-regulated by IL-1β, a pleiotrophic macrophage-derived cytokine.[42] It has been hypothesized that this provides a feedforward inflammatory loop where IL-1β from activated macrophages stimulates RANTES production, which in turn induces monocyte chemotaxis and further IL-1β.[43]

IL-8 is another cytokine with important chemotactic properties. It exerts chemotactic activity on neutrophils and macrophages and also inhibits neutrophil apoptosis, even in the presence of Fas engagement.[44]

IMPACT OF INFLAMMATORY MILIEU ON FERTILITY

The inflammatory milieu in endometriosis has the potential to compromise fertility via a variety of mechanisms (Table 6.5). Folliculogenesis may be impaired, especially in advanced-stage endometriosis. Higher rates of apoptosis have been documented in granulosa cells obtained from women with endometriosis undergoing in vitro fertilization (IVF) compared with patients with tubal factor, male factor, or idiopathic infertility.[45] Granulosa cell apoptotic bodies have been shown to predict oocyte quality, and the incidence of apoptotic bodies increases with the severity of endometriosis.[46,47]

Alterations in the follicular fluid of women with endometriosis may also compromise oocyte quality (Table 6.6). In natural cycles IL-6 levels are elevated, whereas follicular fluid VEGF levels are decreased.[48] Additionally, granulosa cell production of inflammatory cytokines, such as IL-1β, IL-8 and tumor necrosis factor-α (TNF-α), may be increased in women with endometriosis.[49] Follicular fluid TNF-α levels have been

---

Table 6.5 Inflammatory changes contributing to endometriosis-associated infertility

Compromised oocyte quality
- Increased granulosa cell apoptosis
- Altered follicular fluid

Impaired fertilization
- Decreased sperm motility
- Increased sperm phagocytosis

Implantation defects
- Decreased integrin $\alpha v\beta 3$ and LIF
- Increased embryotoxicity

LIF = leukemia inhibitory factor

Table 6.6 Alterations in the follicular fluid of women with endometriosis

Increased
- IL-1β, IL-6, IL-8
- TNF-α
- MCP-1
- Endothelin-1
- Natural killer cells, B lymphocytes, monocytes

Decreased
- VEGF

IL = interleukin; TNF = tumor necrosis factor; MCP = monocyte chemotactic protein; VEGF = vascular endothelial growth factor

correlated with poor-quality oocytes, and it has been speculated that the cytokine-induced proinflammatory milieu may disturb oocyte fertilization.[50]

In natural cycles, endometriosis has been associated with reduced fertilization rates.[51] Spermatozoa incubated with follicular fluid from women with endometriosis demonstrate significantly lower zona binding than do spermatozoa incubated in follicular fluid samples from women with tubal factor infertility. Additionally, sperm mixed with peritoneal fluid from women with endometriosis perform poorly on zona-free hamster egg–sperm penetration assays.[52] Antibodies to transferrin and α_2-HS inhibit sperm motility in vitro and are commonly found in the peritoneal fluid of women with endometriosis.[53,54] In addition, peritoneal macrophages in women with endometriosis demonstrate higher sperm phagocytic activity than do peritoneal macrophages in women without the disease.[55]

Impairments of implantation have also been documented in women with endometriosis. In murine models peritoneal fluid from infertile women with endometriosis decreases implantation rates and markers of endometrial receptivity such as leukemia inhibitory factor (LIF) and integrin $\alpha v\beta 3$.[56] In humans it has been reported that implantation window-specific integrins, such as $\alpha v\beta 3$, are absent in women with endometriosis.[57] Moreover, aberrant expression of HOX-A10 and HOX-A11, homeobox genes essential for implan-

tation, has been documented in midluteal phase endometrium from women with endometriosis.[58] Finally, it has been reported that serum and peritoneal fluid samples from infertile women with endometriosis are embryotoxic to two-cell mouse embryos.[59]

RELATIONSHIP OF INFLAMMATORY MILIEU TO PELVIC PAIN

Activated immune responses and accumulations of inflammatory cells may also contribute to pelvic pain. The prolonged survival and activation of macrophages and neutrophils results in chronic inflammation, and may contribute to tissue damage and scarring. Such effects directly trigger sensory neurons, or indirectly lead to pain via the formation of adhesions.

Pelvic adhesions are a significant cause of morbidity, being found in 30–50% of women operated as for chronic pelvic pain. Adhesion formation classically involves three components: an acute inflammatory response, fibrinolysis, and metalloproteinases. Thus far, three important proinflammatory cytokines have been identified in adhesion formation/reformation: IL-1, TNF-α, and IL-6.[60] All three may be elevated in the peritoneal fluid of women with endometriosis.

The relationship between prostaglandins and pelvic pain is less clear. There is a significant increase in the release of prostaglandins E_2 and $F_{2\alpha}$ from peritoneal macrophages in women with endometriosis.[61] Although some investigators have correlated dysmenorrhea with prostaglandin production, this has not been a consistent finding.[62,63]

CONCLUSION

Immunologic changes play a role in the development and progression of endometriosis. The major alterations include elevated macrophages, decreased NK-cell cytotoxicity, and increases in inflammatory cytokines. Although leukocytes perpetuate the immune response via autocrine and paracrine mechanisms, endometriosis implants themselves also provide a major source of proinflammatory mediators. In addition to sustaining the endometriotic lesions, these factors may also contribute to the major clinical manifestations of endometriosis, i.e. pain and infertility.

REFERENCES

1. Halme J, White C, Kauma S, Estes J, Haskill S. Peritoneal macrophages from patients with endometriosis release growth factor activity in vitro. J Clin Endocrinol Metab 1988;66:1044–9.

2. Dmowski WP, Gebel HM, Braun DP. The role of cell-mediated immunity in pathogenesis of endometriosis. Acta Obstet Gynecol Scand 1994;159(Suppl):7–14.

3. Halme J, Becker S, Hammond MG, Raj MH, Raj S. Increased activation of pelvic macrophages in infertile women with mild endometriosis. Am J Obstet Gynecol 1983;145:333–7.

4. Zeller JM, Henig I, Radwanska E, Dmowski WP. Enhancement of human monocyte and peritoneal macrophage chemiluminescence activities in women with endometriosis. Am J Reprod Immunol Microbiol 1987;13:78–82.

5. Hill JA, Faris HM, Schiff I, Anderson DJ. Characterization of leukocyte subpopulations in the peritoneal fluid of women with endometriosis. Fertil Steril 1988;50:216–22.

6. Oosterlynck DJ, Meuleman C, Waer M, Vandeputte M, Koninckx PR. The natural killer activity of peritoneal fluid lymphocytes is decreased in women with endometriosis. Fertil Steril 1992;58:290–5.

7. Oosterlynck DJ, Cornillie FJ, Waer M, Vandeputte M, Koninckx PR. Women with endometriosis show a defect in natural killer activity resulting in a decreased cytotoxicity to autologous endometrium. Fertil Steril 1991;56:45–51.

8. Wilson TJ, Hertzog PJ, Angus D et al. Decreased natural killer cell activity in endometriosis patients: relationship to disease pathogenesis. Fertil Steril 1994;62:1086–8.

9. Ho HN, Chao KH, Chen HF et al. Peritoneal natural killer cytotoxicity and CD25+ CD3+ lymphocyte subpopulation are decreased in women with stage III–IV endometriosis. Hum Reprod 1995;10:2671–5.

10. Oosterlynck DJ, Meuleman C, Waer M, Koninckx PR, Vandeputte M. Immunosuppressive activity of peritoneal fluid in women with endometriosis. Obstet Gynecol 1993;82:206–12.

11. Kanzaki H, Wang HS, Kariya M, Mori T. Suppression of natural killer cell activity by sera from patients with endometriosis. Am J Obstet Gynecol 1992;167:257–61.

12. Witz CA, Montoya IA, Dey TD, Schenken RS. Characterization of lymphocyte subpopulations and T cell activation in endometriosis. Am J Reprod Immunol 1994;32:173–9.

13. Nothnick WB. Treating endometriosis as an autoimmune disease. Fertil Steril 2001;76:223–31.

14. Badawy SZ, Cuenca V, Kaufman L, Stitzel A, Thompson M. The regulation of immunoglobulin production by B cells in patients with endometriosis. Fertil Steril 1989;51:770–3.

15. Isaacson KB, Coutifaris C, Garcia CR, Lyttle CR. Production and secretion of complement component 3 by endometriotic tissue. J Clin Endocrinol Metab 1989;69:1003–9.

16. Witz CA, Dechaud H, Montoya-Rodriguez IA et al. An in vitro model to study the pathogenesis of the early endometriosis lesion. Ann NY Acad Sci 2002;955:296–307.

17. Witz CA, Takahashi A, Montoya-Rodriguez IA, Cho S, Schenken RS. Expression of the alpha2beta1 and alpha3beta1 integrins at the surface of mesothelial cells: a potential attachment site of endometrial cells. Fertil Steril 2000;74:579–84.

18. Ryan IP, Tseng JF, Schriock ED et al. Interleukin-8 concentrations are elevated in peritoneal fluid of women with endometriosis. Fertil Steril 1995;63:929–32.

19. Arici A, Tazuke SI, Attar E, Kliman HJ, Olive DL. Interleukin-8 concentration in peritoneal fluid of patients with endometriosis and modulation of interleukin-8 expression in human mesothelial cells. Mol Hum Reprod 1996;2:40–5.

20. Akoum A, Lawson C, McColl S, Villeneuve M. Ectopic endometrial cells express high concentrations of interleukin (IL)-8 in vivo regardless of the menstrual cycle phase and respond to oestradiol by up-regulating IL-1-induced IL-8 expression in vitro. Mol Hum Reprod 2001;7:859–66.

21. Fakih H, Baggett B, Holtz G et al. Interleukin-1: a possible role in the infertility associated with endometriosis. Fertil Steril 1987;47:213–17.

22. Arici A, Seli E, Zeyneloglu HB et al. Interleukin-8 induces proliferation of endometrial stromal cells: a potential autocrine growth factor. J Clin Endocrinol Metab 1998;83:1201–5.

23. Garcia-Velasco JA, Arici A. Interleukin-8 stimulates the adhesion of endometrial stromal cells to fibronectin. Fertil Steril 1999;72:336–40.

24. Garcia-Velasco JA, Arici A. Interleukin-8 expression in endometrial stromal cells is regulated by integrin-dependent cell adhesion. Mol Hum Reprod 1999;5:1135–40.

25. Spuijbroek MD, Dunselman GA, Menheere PP, Evers JL. Early endometriosis invades the extracellular matrix. Fertil Steril 1992;58:929–33.

26. Arici A. Local cytokines in endometrial tissue: the role of interleukin-8 in the pathogenesis of endometriosis. Ann NY Acad Sci 2002;955:101–9.

27. Donnez J, Smoes P, Gillerot S, Casanas-Roux F, Nisolle M. Vascular endothelial growth factor (VEGF) in endometriosis. Hum Reprod 1998;13:1686–90.

28. Taylor RN, Lebovic DI, Mueller MD. Angiogenic factors in endometriosis. Ann NY Acad Sci 2002;955:89–100.

29. McLaren J, Prentice A, Charnock-Jones DS, Smith SK. Vascular endothelial growth factor (VEGF) concentrations are elevated in peritoneal fluid of women with endometriosis. Hum Reprod 1996;11:220–3.

30. Shifren JL, Tseng JF, Zaloudek CJ et al. Ovarian steroid regulation of vascular endothelial growth factor in the human endometrium: implications for angiogenesis during the menstrual cycle and in the pathogenesis of endometriosis. J Clin Endocrinol Metab 1996;81:3112–18.

31. McLaren J, Prentice A, Charnock-Jones DS et al. Vascular endothelial growth factor is produced by peritoneal fluid macrophages in endometriosis and is regulated by ovarian steroids. J Clin Invest 1996;98:482–9.

32. Noble LS, Simpson ER, Johns A, Bulun SE. Aromatase expression in endometriosis. J Clin Endocrinol Metab 1996;81:174–9.

33. Kats R, Metz CN, Akoum A. Macrophage migration inhibitory factor is markedly expressed in active and early-stage endometriotic lesions. J Clin Endocrinol Metab 2002;87:883–9.

34. Braun DP, Muriana A, Gebel H et al. Monocyte-mediated enhancement of endometrial cell proliferation in women with endometriosis. Fertil Steril 1994;61:78–84.

35. Hammond MG, Oh ST, Anners J, Surrey ES, Halme J. The effect of growth factors on the proliferation of human endometrial stromal cells in culture. Am J Obstet Gynecol 1993;168:1131–6.

36. Surrey ES, Halme J. Effect of platelet-derived growth factor on endometrial stromal cell proliferation in vitro: a model for endometriosis? Fertil Steril 1991;56:672–9.

37. Munson L, Upadhyaya NB, Van Meter S. Platelet-derived growth factor promotes endometrial epithelial cell proliferation. Am J Obstet Gynecol 1995;173:1820–5.

38. Garcia-Velasco JA, Arici A, Zreik T, Naftolin F, Mor G. Macrophage derived growth factors modulate Fas ligand expression in cultured endometrial stromal cells: a role in endometriosis. Mol Hum Reprod 1999;5:642–50.

39. Arici A, Oral E, Attar E, Tazuke SI, Olive DL. Monocyte chemotactic protein-1 concentration in peritoneal fluid of women with endometriosis and its modulation of expression in mesothelial cells. Fertil Steril 1997;67:1065–72.

40. Akoum A, Kong J, Metz C, Beaumont MC. Spontaneous and stimulated secretion of monocyte chemotactic protein-1 and macrophage migration inhibitory factor by peritoneal macrophages in women with and without endometriosis. Fertil Steril 2002;77:989–94.

41. Akoum A, Lemay A, McColl S, Turcot-Lemay L, Maheux R. Elevated concentration and biologic activity of monocyte chemotactic protein-1 in the peritoneal fluid of patients with endometriosis. Fertil Steril 1996;66:17–23.

42. Lebovic DI, Chao VA, Martini JF, Taylor RN. IL-1beta induction of RANTES (regulated upon activation, normal T cell expressed and secreted) chemokine gene expression in endometriotic stromal cells depends on a nuclear factor-kappaB site in the proximal promoter. J Clin Endocrinol Metab 2001;86:4759–64.

43. Lebovic DI, Mueller MD, Taylor RN. Immunobiology of endometriosis. Fertil Steril 2001;75:1–10.

44. Kwak JY, Park SW, Kim KH, Na YJ, Lee KS. Modulation of neutrophil apoptosis by plasma and peritoneal fluid from patients with advanced endometriosis. Hum Reprod 2002;17:595–600.

45. Toya M, Saito H, Ohta N et al. Moderate and severe endometriosis is associated with alterations in the cell cycle of granulosa cells in patients undergoing in vitro fertilization and embryo transfer. Fertil Steril 2000;73:344–50.

46. Nakahara K, Saito H, Saito T et al. The incidence of apoptotic bodies in membrana granulosa can predict prognosis of ova from patients participating in in vitro fertilization programs. Fertil Steril 1997;68:312–17.

47. Nakahara K, Saito H, Saito T et al. Ovarian fecundity in patients with endometriosis can be estimated by the incidence of apoptotic bodies. Fertil Steril 1998;69:931–5.

48. Pellicer A, Albert C, Mercader A et al. The follicular and endocrine environment in women with endometriosis: local and systemic cytokine production. Fertil Steril 1998;70:425–31.

49. Carlberg M, Nejaty J, Froysa B et al. Elevated expression of tumour necrosis factor alpha in cultured granulosa cells from women with endometriosis. Hum Reprod 2000;15:1250–5.

50. Lee KS, Joo BS, Na YJ et al. Relationships between concentrations of tumor necrosis factor-alpha and nitric oxide in follicular fluid and oocyte quality. J Assist Reprod Genet 2000;17:222–8.

51. Cahill DJ, Wardle PG, Maile LA, Harlow CR, Hull MG. Ovarian dysfunction in endometriosis-associated and unexplained infertility. J Assist Reprod Genet 1997;14:554–7.

52. Aeby TC, Huang T, Nakayama RT. The effect of peritoneal fluid from patients with endometriosis on human sperm function in vitro. Am J Obstet Gynecol 1996;174:1779–83.

53. Mathur SP. Autoimmunity in endometriosis: relevance to infertility. Am J Reprod Immunol 2000;44:89–95.

54. Pillai S, Rust PF, Howard L. Effects of antibodies to transferrin and alpha 2-HS glycoprotein on in vitro sperm motion: implications in infertility associated with endometriosis. Am J Reprod Immunol 1998;39:235–42.

55. Jha P, Farooq A, Agarwal N, Buckshee K. In vitro sperm phagocytosis by human peritoneal macrophages in endometriosis-associated infertility. Am J Reprod Immunol 1996;36:235–7.

56. Illera MJ, Juan L, Stewart CL et al. Effect of peritoneal fluid from women with endometriosis on implantation in the mouse model. Fertil Steril 2000;74:41–8.

57. Lessey BA, Castelbaum AJ, Sawin SW et al. Aberrant integrin expression in the endometrium of women with endometriosis. J Clin Endocrinol Metab 1994;79:643–9.

58. Taylor HS, Bagot C, Kardana A, Olive D, Arici A. HOX gene expression is altered in the endometrium of women with endometriosis. Hum Reprod 1999;14:1328–31.

59. Martinez-Roman S, Balasch J, Creus M, et al. Immunological factors in endometriosis-associated reproductive failure: studies in fertile and infertile women with and without endometriosis. Hum Reprod 1997;12:1794–9.

60. Cheong YC, Shelton JB, Laird SM et al. IL-1, IL-6 and TNF-alpha concentrations in the peritoneal fluid of women with pelvic adhesions. Hum Reprod 2002;17:69–75.

61. Karck U, Reister F, Schafer W, Zahradnik HP, Breckwoldt M. PGE2 and PGF2 alpha release by human peritoneal macrophages in endometriosis. Prostaglandins 1996;51:49–60.

62. Koike H, Egawa H, Ohtsuka T et al. Correlation between dysmenorrheic severity and prostaglandin production in women with endometriosis. Prostaglandins Leuk Essent Fatty Acids 1992;46:133–7.

63. Rapkin A, Bhattacherjee P. Peritoneal fluid eicosanoids in chronic pelvic pain. Prostaglandins 1989;38:447–52.

7. Cytokine Regulation

Daniela Hornung

Cytokines are important mediators of intercellular communication within the immune system. They target a variety of cells and show proliferative, chemoattractant, differentiative, or cytostatic effects. Most cytokines are coupled to intracellular signaling and second-messenger pathways with the help of high-affinity receptors on target cell membranes.[1-4]

Immune system mediators such as cytokines and chemokines have important roles in the pathogenesis of endometriosis, which is associated with an inflammatory peritoneal environment. Macrophages, at 85% (between 0.4 and 1.6×10^6 cells/mL), constitute the majority of cells within the peritoneal cavity[5,6] (Figure 7.1). Others include eosinophils, mast cells, lymphocytes, and mesothelial cells. Endometriosis patients have increased numbers of activated macrophages compared to healthy controls.[7] These cells secret various local products, such as growth factors and cytokines. The following cytokines and growth factors are important inflammatory mediators in the peritoneal fluid of patients with endometriosis:interleukins IL-1, IL-4, IL-5, IL-6, IL-8, IL-10, IL-12, IL-13, RANTES (regulated upon activation, normal T cell-expressed and secreted), eotaxin, TNF-α (tumor necrosis factor-α), IFN-γ (interferon-γ), ENA-78 (epithelial neutrophil-activating protein-78), MCP-1 (monocyte chemotactic protein), EGF (epidermal growth factor), IGF (insulin-like growth factor), TGF-β (transforming growth factor-β), CSF (colony-stimulating factor), PDGF (platelet-derived growth factor), and VEGF (vascular endothelial growth factor). Usually, levels correlate with the severity of the disease, with the highest amounts of cytokines being present in advanced stages of endometriosis. Other cytokines are not different between endometriosis and control patients without disease; some are decreased in endometriosis patients[8-38] (Table 7.1). Cytokines are produced not only by immune cells, but also by endometriotic implants themselves. Supposedly, they play a role in the development and progression of endometriosis as well as in endometriosis-associated infertility.[39] Oocyte maturation, sperm mobility, sperm–egg interaction, embryo development, and implantation might be compromised by an imbalance of cytokines and growth factors.[40-46] Cytokines are paracrine mediators for steroid hormone actions. They have to be very precisely regulated within the tissue microenvironment owing to their potency in relatively low concentrations (high pM concentrations).[47]

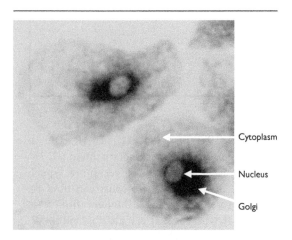

Cytoplasm

Nucleus

Golgi

Figure 7.1 Peritoneal macrophages are the majority of cells within the peritoneal cavity of patients with endometriosis and healthy controls. Immunohistochemistry confirmed the presence of peritoneal macrophages and demonstrated the morphology of these cells. CD68, an oxidized LDL scavenger receptor, stained mainly the Golgi, with sparing of the nucleus, and showed only very weak staining of the cytoplasm.

INTERLEUKIN-1

IL-1 has a molecular weight of 17 kDa. It is secreted mainly by activated macrophages and monocytes and can activate T lymphocytes and

Table 7.1 Cytokine and growth factor concentrations in the peritoneal fluid (PF) of patients with endometriosis compared to patients without endometriosis

Cytokine/growth factor	Increased concentrations in PF of endometriosis patients compared to controls without endometriosis	Unchanged concentrations in PF of endometriosis patients compared to controls without endometriosis	Decreased concentrations in PF of endometriosis patients compared to controls without endometriosis
IL-1	8, 9	10, 11	
IL-4	12	13, 14	
IL-5		11, 13	
IL-6	11, 13, 15, 16		
IL-8	17, 18		
IL-10		19	
IL-12		20	
IL-13			19
RANTES	21		
Eotaxin	22		
TNF-α	15, 23, 24	10, 25	
IFN-γ		17, 18, 21, 23, 25, 26	
ENA-78	Mueller et al., pers. comm.		
MCP-1	27		
EGF		28, 29	
IGF	30, 31		
TGF-β	32, 33		
CSF	34	13	
PDGF	35, 36		
VEGF	37, 38		

differentiate B lymphocytes and other progenitor cells. IL-1 is an important factor for inflammation and the immune response.[48] The possibility of stimulating fibroblast proliferation might be an important factor of IL-1 to provoke adhesion formation and implant proliferation in endometriosis patients.[49,50] IL-1 can stimulate the secretion of other cytokines and prostaglandins, and is embryotoxic.

The IL-1 system has two receptors, two ligands, and one soluble antagonist. The IL-1 receptor family consists of several proteins with low amino acid homology. The three known receptors of IL are IL-1R type I (80 kDa), IL-1R type II (68 kDa) and the IL-1R accessory protein (IL-1R AcP). Many cells express both receptors type I and II, and all three IL-1 isoforms can bind to both receptors. IL-1β has a higher affinity to IL-1R type II, whereas IL-1 can act only via IL-1R type I to transfer signals. The IL-1 receptor type II is known to bind to IL-1 and to inhibit its biological effects.[48,51] In situ hybridization and RT-PCR have shown that IL-1RII mRNA expression was significantly decreased in endometriosis, mainly in the early stages of disease (stages I and II). The reduced levels of IL-1RII mRNA in endometrium from endometriosis patients showed a profound defect in IL-1RII gene expression and, consequently, a reduced capability of endometrial tissue to downregulate IL-1 activity.[52]

The two receptor agonists IL-1α and IL-1β are synthesized as 31 kDa precursors and must be cleaved before they can act as mature forms of IL-1 (17 kDa). Both agonists are encoded by different genes and share only about 20% amino acid homology, but they have similar biologic activities and bind to the same receptors. The soluble IL-1 receptor antagonist is called IL-1ra. This antagonist can inhibit the binding of IL-1α and IL-1β to the IL-1 receptor type I. The intracellular form (icIL-1ra) is described mainly in epithelial cells; sIL-1ra is the secreted form of this IL antagonist.[53] Serum concentrations of sIL-1RII were significantly lower in women with stage I and II endometriosis than in control women. The serum of women with endometriosis induced higher secretion of MCP-1 by U937 cells than that of control women, and recombinant IL-1RII significantly blocked that secretion. Kharfi and Akoum concluded that sIL-1RII might be a key factor involved in the pathogenesis of endometriosis, as these patients have a deficiency in the mechanisms involved in the downregulation of IL-1.[54]

In different studies, IL-1 was elevated in the peritoneal fluid of endometriosis patients,[8,9] whereas in other studies no elevated levels of IL-1 were reported.[10,11] IL-1β mRNA was increased in peritoneal macrophages from patients with mild endometriosis, whereas patients with moderate and severe endometriosis had increased levels of IL-1ra mRNA in their peritoneal macrophages.[55] The authors concluded that a switch in gene expression must take place with disease progression.

Transcription of RANTES mRNA is upregulated by IL-1β via a nuclear-κ B response element in the proximal RANTES gene promoter. These results demonstrate a feedforward regulatory loop in the pathogenesis of endometriosis: IL-1β, secreted from activated peritoneal macrophages, can lead to additional macrophage recruitment via RANTES production from endometriotic stromal cells.[56] IL-1β promotes the growth of endometriotic lesions through inhibition of Tob-1. These findings associate IL-1β with an alteration of cell-cycle gene expression in cells derived from endometriotic implants.[57] Estradiol and IL-1β exert a synergistic stimulatory action on RANTES expression by endometriotic stromal cells. These findings reveal a new regulatory mechanism by which IL-1β produced by activated macrophages can, together with ovarian and locally (by aromatase) produced estradiol, enhance macrophage and T-cell recruitment, leading to an exacerbation of the local immuno-inflammatory milieu.[58]

Together with IL-6 and TNF-α, IL-1 is involved in adhesion formation. In patients with severe endometriosis and adhesions, Cheong et al.[50] were able to show increased levels of IL-1 in the peritoneal fluid. Sillem et al[49] could demonstrate that treatment of endometriosis cell cultures with IL-1 would increase the adhesion of these cells to laminin and fibronectin. They concluded that inflammatory cytokines such as IL-1 and TNF-α may facilitate the adhesion of retrogradely menstruated endometrial fragments.

The intercellular adhesion molecule-1 (ICAM-1) is an important mediator between the immune and the endometrial systems. ICAM mRNA is significantly higher in endometriosis cells than in endometrium cells from the same patient. IL-1β was able to increase sICAM-1 (the soluble form of ICAM) shedding from endometrial cells in a concentration-dependent manner. The IL-1β-mediated induction could be slightly enhanced by co-treatment with estradiol. Vigano et al[59] concluded that the release of higher concentrations of sICAM-1 might be one of the mechanisms by which ectopic endometrial cells escape immunosurveillance.

INTERLEUKIN-4

IL-4 is a cytokine with both stimulatory and inhibitory effects on the inflammatory system, such as macrophage inhibition and T-cell activation. It is expressed in T helper cells type 2 (Th2), can inhibit cytokine synthesis of IL-1, IL-6 and TNF-α, and enhance IL-8 production. Gazvani and colleagues[14] did not see any difference in IL-4 concentration in the peritoneal fluid of patients with endometriosis compared to healthy controls, whereas Hsu et al[12] described higher levels of IL-4 mRNA and protein in peritoneal cells and peripheral blood monocytes of affected women.

INTERLEUKIN-5

IL-5 is an eosinophil chemoattractant and can be demonstrated by immunohistochemistry in endometriosis tissue samples. Degranulating eosinophils are present in the majority of endometriosis implants, as shown by immunohistochemistry and Western blotting of eosinophil peroxidase, but only in a few of the secretory-phase and in none of the proliferative-phase normal endometrium samples.[60] IL-5 levels in the peritoneal fluid of endometriosis patients tends to be higher than in PF of normal controls.[11]

INTERLEUKIN-6

IL-6 is a 23–26 kDa phosphoglycoprotein produced by a variety of different cell types, including macrophages, monocytes, endothelial cells, fibroblasts, and endometrial stromal and epithelial cells. It represents an autocrine or paracrine activator of monocyte/macrophage differentiation. IL-6 can enhance the secretion of other cytokines and enzymes of estrogen synthesis. Owing to a higher rate of differentiation from monocytes to macrophages, IL-6 might be responsible for a greater accumulation of peritoneal macrophages in patients with moderate or severe endometriosis. IL-6 was found at elevated levels in peritoneal fluid from patients with advanced and active stages of endometriosis.[15] In other studies the variance was high, so that no statistically significant differences could be noted between controls and patients with endometriosis.[16] IL-6 is an inhibitor of endometrial stromal cell proliferation. Because decreased levels of soluble IL-6

receptor were found in the peritoneal fluid of patients with endometriosis, Rier and colleagues[61] suggested that endometriotic stromal cells might escape the growth inhibitory effects of IL-6.

INTERLEUKIN-8

IL-8 is a cytokine with angiogenic and neutrophil chemotactic activity. This 8 kDa peptide is produced by monocytes, lymphocytes, fibroblasts, and epithelial and endothelial cells. It can be stimulated by different proinflammatory substances, such as LPS, TNF-α, or IL-1. Its angiogenic characteristics might be responsible for the neovascularization and proliferation of endometriosis implants. IL-8 belongs to the α- or C-X-C chemokine family with four conserved cysteine residues, where the first cysteine residues are separated by a variable amino acid. IL-8 is responsible for neutrophil and T-lymphocyte recruitment. It might also be an important factor for the attachment of endometrial fragments to the peritoneal surface, as it can induce the expression of several adhesion molecules. IL-8 is elevated in the peritoneal fluid of patients with endometriosis, and the concentrations correlate with the severity of disease.[17,18] IL-8 may play a role in the growth and maintenance of ectopic implants, as it can stimulate endometrial cell proliferation both directly and indirectly by stimulating leukocytes to secret other cytokines and growth factors. Gazvani et al[62] showed that IL-8 had a dose-dependent stimulatory effect on the survival of endometrial cells, whereas anti-IL-8 significantly inhibited the survival of endometrial cells from women with endometriosis compared to cells from women without endometriosis. These effects varied according to disease stage and the concentration of cytokines.

INTERLEUKIN-10

Interleukin 10 is an important immunomodulatory cytokine, produced by Th2 cells and inhibiting macrophages. IL-10 concentrations were not elevated in the peritoneal fluid of patients with endometriosis compared to healthy controls.[19] IL-10 downregulated Tob-1, a cell-cycle suppressor gene, in endometriotic stromal cells, but had no significant effect on normal endometrial stromal cells.[57] Concentrations of peritoneal IL-10 were significantly elevated in women with early-stage endometriosis, and this may lead to a decrease in activated peritoneal CD4+ Th1 cells.[63]

INTERLEUKIN-12

IL-12 is a key immunomodulatory, heterodimeric cytokine composed of p40 and p35 chains and produced by macrophages and monocytes. It can induce the proliferation and cytotoxicity of natural killer cells and T cells. In several studies, concentrations of IL-12 are detectable in low concentrations in the peritoneal fluid, but they are not significantly affected by the presence or absence of endometriosis implants.[20,64] In contrast, significantly higher levels of the free p40 chains of IL-12 were detected in the peritoneal fluid of women with endometriosis compared to women without the disease. In addition, the IL-12 plus free p40/IL-12 ratio was increased in women with severe endometriosis. When NK (natural killer) cells were pretreated with heterodimeric IL-12 they exhibited an enhanced cytotoxic response toward endometrial fragments. This IL-12-induced cytotoxicity could be inhibited by the p40 subunit in a dose-dependent manner. The inhibitory effect of the p40 subunit was mediated by the downregulation of IL-12 high-affinity binding sites on NK cells, as measured by a decrease in IL-12 binding capacity and inhibition of surface IL-12 receptor β_1-chain expression and inhibition of phosphorylation of STAT4 protein. STAT4 is a signal transducer and activator of transcription. The excess of p40 in the peritoneal fluid of patients with endometriosis could be related to the NK cell defect associated with endometriosis.[65]

The intraperitoneal injection of IL-12 into the peritoneal cavity of C57BL/6 and BALB/c mice was able to reduce the weight and surface area of endometriotic implants. This in vivo mouse model demonstrated that IL-12 is able to significantly reduce the implantation and proliferation of endometriosis.[66] IL-12 could possibly be a specific agent to correct the p40-induced NK cell defect and an immune system stimulator as new therapy for the treatment of endometriosis.

INTERLEUKIN-13

IL-13 is produced by Th2 cells and can inhibit the secretion of proinflammatory cytokines by activated macrophages. IL-13 is significantly reduced in the peritoneal fluid of patients with endometriosis compared with women without this disease.[19] The immunolocalization of IL-13 was noted in isolated peritoneal fluid cells, and in the stromal and glandular compartments of endometrium and endometriosis implants. No cycle-dependent differences were seen in the immunolocalization or peritoneal fluid concentration of IL-13. McLaren and colleagues speculated that the lack of suppression of macrophage activation by reduced amounts of IL-13 might be one factor in the pathogenesis of endometriosis. Odukoya et al[67] could find no significant difference in the expression of IL-13 mRNA in ovarian endometrioma compared to healthy ovarian tissue.

RANTES

RANTES (regulated upon activation, normal T cell-expressed and secreted) belongs to the β- or C-C chemokine family with two cystein residues adjacent to each other. The size of RANTES is 8 kDa and it is a chemoattractant for monocytes, memory T cells, and eosinophils. These cells are the predominant leukocytes in the peritoneal fluid of women with endometriosis.[68] RANTES protein was identified immunohistochemically[69] (Figure 7.2) and RANTES mRNA was confined by in situ hybridization[70] (Figure 7.3) in stromal cells of normal endometrium and ectopic implants. In histological serial sections, CD68-positive macrophages were in the same regions where prominent RANTES mRNA was seen by

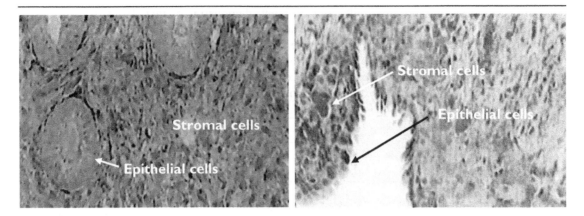

Figure 7.2 Immunohistochemical localization of RANTES (regulated upon activation, normal T cell-expressed and secreted) protein in human endometrium and ovarian endometrioma. A section of normal midproliferative endometrium was stained with RANTES antibodies and counterstained with hematoxylin. Positive staining of stromal cells with sparing of epithelial cells in the glands could be detected (left). A similar staining pattern occured in the ovarian endometrioma: positive immunostaining of the stromal cells with sparing of the cyst epithelium. Unaffected ovary also showed only very weak staining for RANTES (right).

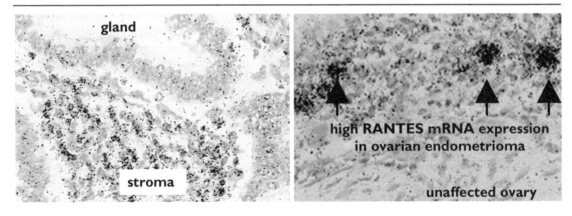

Figure 7.3 In situ hybridization of RANTES mRNA in normal midproliferative endometrium (left) and ovarian endometrioma (right). RANTES gene expression could be detected in the stromal compartment between glands, but not in the glands themselves. Ovarian endometrioma showed a similar staining pattern: intense spots of RANTES mRNA within the stromal cells (black arrows), but no positive signals in the epithelial layer or in the unaffected ovary.

in situ hybridization[70] (Figure 7.4). These macrophages might be recruited to areas of stromal RANTES expression. In vitro, RANTES is only actively synthesized by stromal cells derived from normal endometrium and endometriosis implants, if these cells are treated with proinflammatory cytokines, for example with TNF-α, IFN-γ or IL-1β. RANTES mRNA was identified by in situ hybridization in not more than 10–20%

of the stimulated endometriosis stromal cells, the other 80–90% being free of RANTES mRNA[70] (Figure 7.5). This observation suggests that only a subpopulation of endometriotic stromal cells is responsible for RANTES mRNA expression. Subconfluent monolayers of endometriotic epithelial cells did not show evidence of RANTES mRNA expression, either at baseline or after 48 hours of cytokine stimulation (Figure 7.6). The

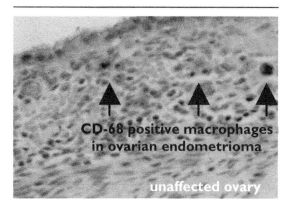

Figure 7.4 Immunohistochemistry demonstrated CD-68-positive macrophages in the stromal compartment of an adjacent section of ovarian endometrioma (Figure 7.3), where large amounts of RANTES mRNA could be demonstrated by in situ hybridization. These macrophages are possibly recruited to areas of intense RANTES expression.

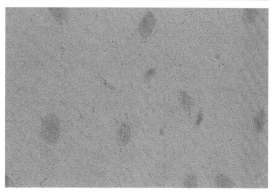

Figure 7.6 In situ hybridization demonstrated that endometrial epithelial cells did not contain RANTES mRNA, even when cells were cultured with 100 ng/mL TNF-α for 48 hours.

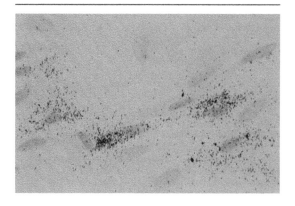

Figure 7.5 In situ hybridization demonstrated RANTES mRNA in a subpopulation of some isolated endometriotic stromal cells (about 10–20%), when cells were cultured with 100 ng/mL TNF-α for 48 hours.

difference between expression of basal RANTES in vivo and in vitro, with the necessity for exogenous cytokine stimulation for RANTES expression in cultured cells, suggests that paracrine or juxtacrine cytokines are important mediators of this inflammatory loop. It was proposed that epithelial–stromal interactions are essential steps for the pathophysiology of endometriosis. Epithelial cells themselves do not synthesize RANTES transcripts or protein basally or under

cytokine stimulation, but they can secret TNF-α, which in turn stimulates stromal cells to secret RANTES.[71] The ability of stromal cells within endometriosis implants to produce this potent chemokine may be a factor in the recruitment of inflammatory cells into the peritoneal cavity. The chemotactic activity of RANTES was tested on U937 cells, a human monocytic cell line, in Boyden chamber assays[72] (Figure 7.7). Similar to human peritoneal macrophages these cells expressed the human RANTES receptors CCR-1 and CCR-5. Both receptors are G protein-coupled receptors with high affinity for RANTES (CCR-1 >CCR-5). Expression of CCR-1 can be upregulated in U937 cells and peritoneal macrophages by 48 hours' stimulation with the cytokines IFN-γ and TNF-α[72] (Figure 7.8). Over a range of 0–1000 pg/mL recombinant human RANTES had a linear, direct effect on monocyte migration (Figure 7.9). Peritoneal fluid and conditioned media induced dose-dependent effects on monocyte migration that were correlated with the concentrations of immunoreactive RANTES, as measured by ELISA. The addition of antihuman RANTES antibodies to peritoneal fluid or conditioned media neutralized the chemoattractant effects by 70–75%, and heat denaturation neutralized the chemoattractant effects by more than 95% (Figure 7.10), indicating that the chemoattractant factors are proteinaceous in nature.

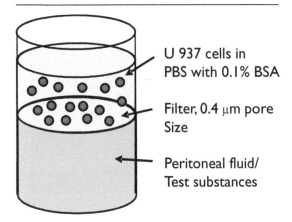

Figure 7.7 Model of a Boyden chamber. The upper chamber is separated from the lower chamber by a permeable 0.4 μm pore size polyethylene terphthalene (PET) track-etched membrane. U937 cells, a human histiocytic cell line, were induced to display monocytic differentiation and chemotactic responsiveness after treatment with 1 mmol/L 8-bromo-cAMP. Peritoneal fluid and/or test substances were placed in the bottom wells (600 μL/well), 500 000 activated U937 cells in 200 μL PBS with 0.1% BSA added to the top compartment. After 2 hours' incubation filters were washed, migrated cells were fixed to the underside of the membrane, stained with crystal violet, and the optical absorption measured at 570 nm.

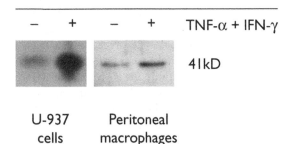

Figure 7.8 Western blot demonstration of CCR-1, the highest-affinity human RANTES receptor (41 kDa), in U937 cells and primary peritoneal macrophages. Cells were stimulated by 100 ng/mL TNF-α and IFN-γ for 48 hours (+) or not stimulated (−). A substantial increase of CCR-1 protein was seen in both cell types after cytokine stimulation.

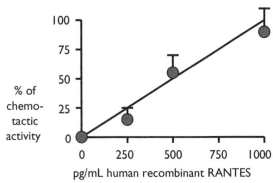

Figure 7.9 Monocyte migration across Boyden chamber. Recombinant human RANTES had a direct linear effect on migration of U937 cells in the range between 0 and 1000 pg/mL.

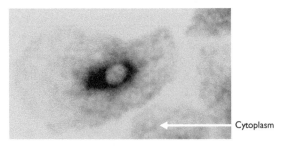

Figure 7.10 A pool of 16 peritoneal fluids was tested for monocyte chemotaxis in Boyden chambers and the results normalized to 100%. The same pool was tested after incubation to 95°C for 5 minutes and showed a reduction of chemotaxis of more than 95%. Specific monoclonal human RANTES antibodies inhibited the chemotactic activity of the peritoneal fluid pool by 70%.

Receptor neutralizing antibodies to CCR-1 and CCR-5 inhibited monocyte chemotaxis by 80–85%.[72]

Thioglycollate medium, a non-specific irritant, has been shown to promote a monocytic peri-toneal exudate in rodent models. As in human endometriosis, RANTES appears to play a critical role in the inflammation induced by thiogly-collate in the mouse. Co-treatment with neutral-izing anti-RANTES antibodies dramatically inhibited the action of thioglycollate to induce cellular accumulation and cytokine secretion. Hence, although the RANTES pathway appears to predominate, other inflammatory mediators also contribute to the macrophage accumulation stimulated by thioglycollate. This result also indicates that RANTES acts downstream of the thioglycollate effect and supports the impor-

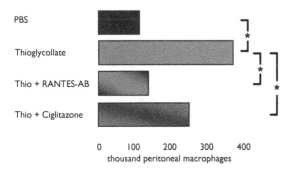

PBS

Thioglycollate

Thio + RANTES-AB

Thio + Ciglitazone

0   100   200   300   400
thousand peritoneal macrophages

Figure 7.11 Effect of RANTES antibodies and ciglitazone on peritoneal macrophage number. Peritoneal cells from mice in the control (PBS) group were counted directly after collection. The number of cells recovered from mice treated with thioglycollate was increased threefold compared to the control PBS group. Treatment with thioglycollate (Thio) plus neutralizing RANTES antibodies significantly reduced macrophage numbers by 60%. Mice treated with thioglycollate plus ciglitazone showed a 32% reduction in cell numbers relative to thioglycollate alone. * indicates statistical significance ($P<0.05$).

tance of this chemokine pathway in peritoneal inflammation.[73]

RANTES antibodies are very expensive, are not orally bioavailable, and long-term treatment may lead to the production of anti-idiotypic or neutralizing antibodies. In contrast, TZDs (thiazolidinediones), activators of PPAR-γ (peroxisome proliferator activated receptor gamma) are affordable non-peptide compounds with anti-inflammatory effects that would counter RANTES activity. Ciglitazone, a TZD, significantly reduced leukocyte infiltration in the mouse model (Figure 7.11). TZD were first used as orally bioavailable insulin-sensitizing agents. They are currently under investigation in the treatment of inflammatory diseases, including arthritis and colitis. Although in these experiments an intraperitoneal route of administration was chosen, this drug has high oral bioavailability.[73]

Other studies suggest that TZD ligands of PPAR-γ could exert anti-inflammatory effects by interfering with cytokine production in endothelial or T cells. On the basis of these preclinical experiments it was proposed that this class of pharmaceutical agents be evaluated as a potential adjunct to the treatment of human endometriosis.

EOTAXIN

Eotaxin is an α- or C-C chemokine of 8.4 kDa whose major biological activity is the chemoattraction of eosinophils. However, recent studies indicate that it may dictate a broader scope of activities on myeloid cells both during development and in pathological states. The detection of immunoreactive eotaxin protein in the luminal epithelium of normal endometrium, and more intense staining in the glandular epithelium of endometriosis biopsies, indicates that these tissues have the potential to accumulate this chemokine[6] (Figure 7.12). The distribution of eotaxin staining is similar to observations of the related C-C monocyte chemokine MCP-1. The accumulation of immune cell activator proteins in human endometrium and endometriosis is cell specific. Epithelial cells isolated from endometriomas could be induced to secrete eotaxin if they were treated with IFN-γ, TNF-α, estradiol, and medroxyprogesterone acetate. Isolated stromal cells from normal endometrium and endometriosis lesions failed to secrete eotaxin under basal, cytokine, and/or steroid hormone-stimulated conditions.[6] The human eotaxin receptor CCR-3 is expressed by eosinophils and by endometrial epithelial cells,[74] so it is possible that eotaxin can increase its secretion on the same epithelial cells where it is produced by coupling on CCR-3 receptors (autocrine activity). Pelvic fluid concentrations of eotaxin were statistically elevated in women with advanced stages of active disease[6] (Figure 7.13). This supports the proposal that active endometriosis lesions secrete eotaxin and other cytokines into the peritoneal environment. Endometriotic epithelial cells have a preferential ability to synthesize and secrete eotaxin. The production of eotaxin seems to be under endocrine and paracrine control, with enhanced secretion under conditions that mimic the secretory phase of the menstrual cycle. Eotaxin, together with other cytokines and immune cells, contributes to an inflammatory milieu in the reproductive tract and might lead to endometriosis-associated infertility. The precise role of this

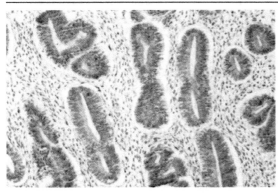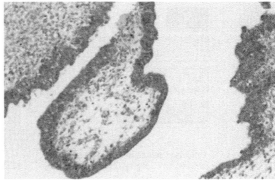

Figure 7.12 Immunohistochemical localization of eotaxin protein in human endometrium and ovarian endometrioma. A section of normal secretory endometrium was stained with eotaxin antibodies and counterstained with hematoxylin. Predominantly epithelial staining could be seen (left). A similar staining pattern occured in the ovarian endometrioma: positive immunostaining of the epithelial layer of the ovarian endometrioma (right).

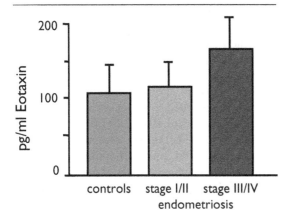

Figure 7.13 Peritoneal fluid concentrations of eotaxin were measured using an ELISA. Patients with moderate and severe endometriosis had significant higher levels of eotaxin than control subjects without endometriosis or patients with minimal and mild endometriosis.

chemokine remains unknown; however, these findings suggest that allergic and autoinflammatory phenomena associated with this syndrome may be linked to the recruitment of eosinophils and other myeloid cells into the peritoneal cavity.

TUMOR NECROSIS FACTOR-α

Tumor necrosis factor-α (TNF-α) is a pleiotropic cytokine of 17 kDa produced mainly by activated macrophages, neutrophils, activated lymphocytes, NK cells, and some non-hematopoietic cells. Its primary function is to serve as an initiator of a cascade of cytokines and other inflammatory factors. TNF-α was first described as a killer of several cell lines, especially tumor cell lines. It is also embryotoxic.[75]

TNF-α is localized in normal endometrium and in endometriosis implants. The strongest protein staining in normal endometrium is seen in epithelial cells of the secretory phase. Some staining can also be seen in stromal cells of the proliferative phase. This different pattern of distribution suggests a different hormonal and local regulation of TNF-α.[76,77]

In endometriosis implants TNF-α is localized more to the epithelial than to the stromal compartment, with very weak staining of the unaffected ovarian tissue[70] (Figure 7.14). Cell cultures of endometrial and endometriosis epithelial cells are able to produce immunoreactive TNF-α. In mixed epithelial and stromal cell cultures of endometriosis implants, Zhao and colleagues reported a RANTES secretion without exogenous added cytokines. This stromal cell-derived cytokine must have been stimulated by TNF-α from surrounding epithelial cells.[71]

In peritoneal fluid from patients with endometriosis TNF-α is increased compared to

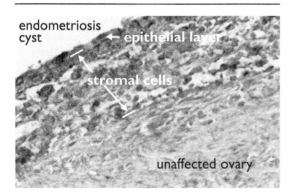

Figure 7.14 Immunohistochemical localization of TNF-α protein in human ovarian endometrioma. Strong positive staining of epithelial cells and also positive staining of stromal cells is demonstrated. Unaffected ovary showed only very weak staining for TNF-α.

healthy controls. The concentrations correlate with the severity of the disease and might be responsible for infertility.[21,22] One of the mechanisms for the reduction of fertility by TNF-α is decreased sperm motility.[78]

Recombinant human TNF-binding protein-1 (r-hTBP-1), the soluble form of TNF-α receptor type 1, inhibits the development of endometriosis in baboons, as shown by d'Hooghe et al.[79] In a rat model r-hTBP-1 was also able to inhibit the development of experimentally induced endometriosis.[80] Both groups could demonstrate the potential effectiveness of r-hTBP-1 for the treatment of endometriosis and the important role of TNF-α for the development of this disease.

Peritoneal fluid from women with endometriosis or recombinant TNF-α was able to enhance the proliferation of endometrial cell cultures from women with endometriosis. The soluble TNF-receptor etanercept blocked this enhanced proliferation. Braun et al[81] suggest a therapy for endometriosis with agents that block the effects of TNF-α.

IFN-γ

Interferon-γ is a 17 kDa proinflammatory cytokine with a variety of cytotoxic and immuno-modulatory effects. This potent inducer of cell-mediated immunity is produced by Th1 cells and can activate macrophages and inhibit endometrial proliferation. The IFN-γ receptor is expressed on the surface of most cell types, apart from erythrocytes. The concentration of IFN-γ did not differ between healthy controls and endometriosis patients,[26] so it seems that IFN-γ is not one of the most important cytokines for the pathogenesis of endometriosis. Together with other cytokines, for example TNF-α, however, it has additive effects for an inflammatory environment. Also, IFN-γ is an embryotoxic agent and can inhibit sperm motility.[78] In leukocytes from endometriosis implants, mRNA levels of IFN-γ are significantly greater than in leukocytes from normal endometrium.[82] Levels of IFN-γ in eutopic endometrium of women with adenomyosis were also significantly increased compared to those of controls. Mononuclear cells of these affected patients produced higher levels of IFN-γ when cultured for 24 hours.[83]

ENA-78 (EPITHELIAL-CELL DERIVED NEUTROPHIL ACTIVATING PROTEIN-78)

ENA-78 is an α- or C-X-C chemokine with angiogenic activity. It has a molecular weight of 8 kDa and a size of 78 amino acids, and acts on the CXCR2 receptor. Neutrophils attracted by ENA-78 can produce VEGF, which promotes neovascularization of endometriotic implants. ENA-78 was detected in 56% of women with endometriosis but in only 13% of unaffected women (a statistically significant difference).[84]

MCP-1 (MONOCYTE CHEMOTACTIC PROTEIN-1)

Monocyte chemotactic protein-1 belongs to a superfamily of small molecular weight cytokines (8.7 kDa) and is a member of the C-C or β chemokines. MCP-1 receptors (CCR2) are expressed mainly by monocytes. MCP-1 can induce leukocyte chemotaxis with different degrees of cellular specificity, and is responsible for monocyte infiltration into tissue and tumors.

MCP-1 is secreted by endometrial cells. This secretion is upregulated in patients with endometriosis. It is also secreted by activated peritoneal macrophages, and as endometriosis patients have an increased number of activated macrophages this might be one of the mechanisms by which levels of MCP-1 are increased in the peritoneal fluid of such patients.

MCP-1 production by endometriotic cells can be stimulated with IL-1 and TNF-α.[27]

In stages I and II of endometriosis the chemotactic activity of peritoneal fluid was increased compared to that of healthy controls; 40–53% of this chemotactic activity was inhibited if polyclonal rabbit anti-MCP-1 antibodies were added to the peritoneal fluid.[85]

MCP-1 might be one important factor for the recruitment and activation of peritoneal macrophages in endometriosis. These macrophages and their cytokine secretions are part of a pelvic inflammation with reduced fertility, as many of these cytokines (e.g. IL-1 and TNF-α) disturb sperm motion and sperm–egg penetration, or have embryotoxic properties. On the other hand, they produce growth factors that promote endometriotic implant growth and proliferation.

EGF (EPIDERMAL GROWTH FACTOR)

Epidermal growth factor is synthesized as a 160 kDa precursor. The mature soluble peptides have a size of 6 kDa after proteolytic cleavage. TGF-α, heparin-binding EGF, and amphiregulin are the three members of the EGF family. EGF is mitogenic for mesenchymal and epithelial cells, and TGF-α has angiogenic activity as well. The EGF receptor is a 170 kDa transmembrane tyrosin kinase receptor which is responsible for the transduction of mitogenic EGF signals. EGF receptors could be detected in normal endometrium and in endometriosis implants.[86] Peritoneal fluid concentrations of EGF were not different in patients with or without endometriosis.[28,29]

IGF (INSULIN-LIKE GROWTH FACTOR)

Insulin-like growth factors are non-glycosylated peptides of 7 kDa. IGF type 1 receptor is a heterotetrameric transmembrane complex similar to the classic insulin receptor. It binds IGF-I and II ligands and acts via tyrosine kinase domains in its β subunits. IGF type II receptor is a single membrane-spanning protein. Six forms of human IGF-binding proteins are described with a molecular weight between 24 and 45 kDa. These proteins are not only IGF transporters, they also exert bioactivity and are modulated by serine proteases.

Plasma IGF-1 levels are higher in cases of severe endometriosis, whereas levels locally in the endometrium are reduced, which might explain infertility, as IGF facilitates the implantation of the human embryo.[87] IGF-1 levels were significantly higher in the peritoneal fluid of patients with endometriosis, whereas IGFBP-2 and IGFBP-3 levels were lower in the peritoneal fluid of affected women.[88] Akoum et al[89] demonstrated increased IGFBP-3 in endometriosis implants and in the endometrium of patients with endometriosis.

TGF-β (TRANSFORMING GROWTH FACTOR-β)

Transforming growth factor-β is a macrophage and T cell-derived pleiotropic cytokine of 25 kDa with three different isoforms. It is a potent chemoattractant for monocytes, an inhibitor of T, B and NK cell activity, and an inducer of angiogenesis.

TGF-β receptors are expressed on many cell types with three different subunits, I, II, and III, which are not fully described. TGF-β can stimulate the growth of some cells and inhibit the growth of others. It is an important factor for tissue development and morphological changes, for example for cyclic changes to the endometrium.

TGF-β is increased in patients with endometriosis compared to healthy controls or infertile women without endometriosis. Oosterlynck and colleagues[32] proposed that TGF-β could exert mitogenic activity for endometriosis implants.

CSF (COLONY-STIMULATING FACTOR)

Colony stimulating factors are able to stimulate in vitro the colony formation of hematopoietic progenitor cells. In vivo they are responsible for the generation, proliferation, activation, and migration of macrophages (M-CSF), granulocytes (G-CSF), and both granulocytes and macrophages (GM-CSF). M-CSF are homodimeric glycosylated proteins of 40–90 kDa. The receptor is a cell surface protein with high affinity encoded by the proto-oncogene c-*fms*. In the peritoneal fluid of endometriosis patients, M-CSF is elevated in positive correlation with the severity of disease.[34]

GM-CSF is a glycoprotein of 18–22 kDa that binds to two cell surface receptors, a high-affinity receptor, with α and β subunits, and a low-affinity complex. GM-CSF is expressed in the glandular epithelium of endometrium and endometriosis implants, with most prominent staining in the secretory phase of the cycle.[90] GM-CSF is not elevated in patients with endometriosis.[13]

PDGF (PLATELET-DERIVED GROWTH FACTOR)

Platelet-derived growth factor is a cationic glycoprotein of 32 kDa with chemotactic and mitogenic activity for mesenchymal and stromal cells. It is secreted not only by platelets, but also by macrophages and other cells. In the pelvic fluid, PDGF is significantly elevated in patients with endometriosis compared to controls.[36] PDGF promotes endometrial epithelial cell proliferation.[91] Pelvic fluid and purified PDGF could stimulate the incorporation of thymidine into DNA from human endometrial stromal cell cultures, suggesting an important role of PDGF in the growth and progression of the disease.[92] PDGF induced a dose-dependent upregulation of FAST expression (Fas-Fas ligand), which signals Fas-mediated cell death of activated immune cells.[36] This could be a mechanism by which endometrial

cells escape immune surveillance following implantation and growth.

VEGF (VASCULAR ENDOTHELIAL GROWTH FACTOR)

Vascular endothelial growth factor is a very potent and specific angiogenic factor. VEGF receptors Flt-1 (fms-like tyrosine kinase) and KDR (kinase domain receptor) are tyrosine kinase receptors. Binding of VEGF to its receptors leads to dimer formation, autophosphorylation, and activation of mitogen-activated protein kinases. Four mRNA species of VEGF are described, and the 165 and 121 amino acid residues form glycosylated homodimers of 45 and 35 kDa, respectively. The 189 and 206 amino acid species are not actively secreted into the extracellular space. Release of bioactive VEGF fragments can be induced by hypoxia, IL-1β, PDGF, TGF-β, EGF, PGE_2, plasmin cleavage, or heparin. In normal endometrium, VEGF protein is localized to endometrial glands with focal immunostaining at the apical surface[93] (Figure 7.15), whereas stromal cells are diffusely and weakly positive for VEGF. The physiological roles of VEGF in endometrium are neovascularization after menstrual shedding, and facilitating the implantation of the embryo by causing local

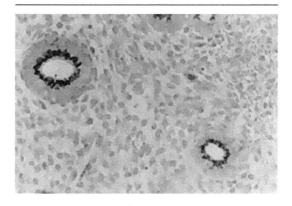

Figure 7.15 Immunohistochemistry of normal midproliferative endometrium localized VEGF protein to endometrial glands with focal concentration at the apical surface of the gland.

edema. In patients with endometriosis, VEGF is produced by endometriotic implants and peritoneal macrophages, causing increased VEGF levels in the peritoneal fluid, with positive correlation to the stage of endometriosis.[35,36] Antiangiogenic therapy may be a possible new approach in the treatment of endometriosis. Dabrosin et al,[94] in a mouse model of endometriosis, suggested the use of gene therapy with transient overexpression of the gene for the natural angiogenesis inhibitor angiostatin, delivered to the peritoneum by a replication-deficient adenovirus vector (AdAngiostatin). They were able to eradicate experimentally induced endometriosis in all 14 treated mice, and propose local or target delivery of the gene to avoid prolonged systemic effects and impaired ovarian function.

REFERENCES

1. Lebovic DI, Mueller MD, Taylor RN. Immunobiology of endometriosis. Fertil Steril 2001;75:1–10.
2. Ryan IP, Taylor RN. Endometriosis and infertility: new concepts. Obstet Gynecol Surv 1997;52:365–71.
3. Giudice LC, Tazuke SI, Swierz L. Status of current research on endometriosis. J Reprod Med 1998;43:252–62.
4. Ryan IP, Moore ES, Taylor RN. Cytokines in endometriosis. In: Hill JH, ed. Cytokines in Human Reproduction. New York: Wiley-Liss, 2000;259–85.
5. Syrop CH, Halme J. Peritoneal fluid environment and infertility. Fertil Steril 1987;48:1–9.
6. Hornung D, Waite LL, Ricke EA et al. Nuclear peroxisome proliferator-activated receptors alpha and gamma have opposing effects on monocyte chemotaxis in endometriosis. J Clin Endocrinol Metab 2001;86:3108–14.
7. Olive D, Weinberg JB, Haney AF. Peritoneal macrophages and infertility: the association between cell number and pelvic pathology. Fertil Steril 1985;44:772–7.
8. Fakih H, Baggett B, Holtz G et al. Interleukin-1: a possible role in the infertility associated with endometriosis. Fertil Steril 1987;47:213–17.
9. Mori H, Sawairi M, Nakagawa M et al. Peritoneal fluid interleukin-1β and tumor necrosis factor in patients with benign gynecologic disease. Am J Reprod Immunol 1991;26:62–7.
10. Keenan JA, Chent TT, Chadwell NL et al. IL-1β, TNF-α and IL-2 in peritoneal fluid and macrophage-conditioned media of women with endometriosis. Am J Reprod Immunol 1995;34:381–5.
11. Koyama N, Matsuura K, Okamura H. Cytokines in the peritoneal fluid of patients with endometriosis. J Reprod Med 1993;43:45–50.
12. Hsu CC, Yang BC, Wu MH et al. Enhanced interleukin-4 expression in patients with endometriosis. Fertil Steril 1997;67:1059–64.
13. Punnonen J, Teisala K, Ranta H et al. Increased levels of interleukin-6 and interleukin-10 in the peritoneal fluid of patients with endometriosis. Am J Obstet Gynecol 1996;174:1522–6.
14. Gazvani MR, Bates MD, Vince GS et al. Peritoneal fluid concentrations of interleukin-4 in relation to the presence of

endometriosis, its stage and the phase of the menstrual cycle. Acta Obstet Gynecol Scand 2001;80:361–3.
15. Harada T, Yoshioka H, Yoshida S et al. Increased interleukin-6 levels in peritoneal fluid of infertile patients with active endometriosis. Am J Obstet Gynecol 1997;176:593–7.
16. Tseng JF, Ryan IP, Milam TD et al. Interleukin-6 secretion in vitro is upregulated in ectopic and eutopic endometrial stromal cells from women with endometriosis. J Clin Endocrinol Metab 1996;81:1118–22.
17. Ryan IP, Tseng JF, Schriock ED et al. Interleukin-8 concentrations are elevated in peritoneal fluid of patients with endometriosis. Fertil Steril 1995;63:929–32.
18. Arici A, Tazuke SI, Attar E et al. Interleukin-8 concentrations in peritoneal fluid of patients with endometriosis and modulation of interleukin-8 expression in human mesothelial cells. Mol Hum Reprod 1996;2:40–5.
19. McLaren J, Dealtry G, Prentice A et al. Decreased levels of the potent regulator of monocyte/macrophage activation, interleukin-13, in the peritoneal fluid of patients with endometriosis. Hum Reprod 1997;12:1307–10.
20. Zeyneloglu HB, Senturk LM, Seli E et al. The peritoneal fluid levels of interleukin-12 in women with endometriosis. Am J Reprod Immunol 1998;39:152–6.
21. Khorram O, Taylor RN, Ryan IP et al. Peritoneal fluid concentrations of the cytokine RANTES correlate with the severity of endometriosis. Am J Obstet Gynecol 1993;169:1545–9.
22. Hornung D, Dohrn K, Sotlar K et al. Localization in tissues and secretion of eotaxin by cells from normal endometrium and endometriosis. J Clin Endocrinol Metab 2000;85:2604–8.
23. Eisermann J, Gast MJ, Pineda J et al. Tumor necrosis factor in peritoneal fluid of women undergoing laparoscopic surgery. Fertil Steril 1988;50:573–9.
24. Hill JA, Anderson DJ. Lymphocyte activity in the presence of peritoneal fluid from fertile women and infertile women with and without endometriosis. Am J Obstet Gynecol 1989;161:861–4.
25. Vercellini P, Benedetti FD, Rossi E et al. Tumor necrosis factor in plasma and peritoneal fluid of women with and without endometriosis. Gynecol Obstet Invest 1993;36:39–41.
26. Keenan JA, Chen TT, Chadwell NL et al. Interferon–gamma (IFN-γ) and interleukin-6 (IL-6) in peritoneal fluid and macrophage-conditioned media of women with endometriosis. Am J Reprod Immunol 1994;32:180–3.
27. Arici A, Oral E, Attar E et al. Monocyte chemotactic protein-1 concentration in peritoneal fluid of women with endometriosis and its modulation of expression in mesothelial cells. Fertil Steril 1997;67:1065–72.
28. De Leon FD, Vijayakumar R, Brown M et al. Peritoneal fluid volume, estrogen, progesterone, prostaglandin, and epidermal growth factor concentrations in patients with and without endometriosis. Obstet Gynecol 1986;68:189–94.
29. Huang JC, Papasakelariou C, Dawood MY. Epidermal growth factor and basic fibroblast growth factor in peritoneal fluid of women with endometriosis. Fertil Steril 1996;65:931–4.
30. Giudice LC, Dsupin BA, Gargosy SE et al. The insulin-like growth factor system in human peritoneal fluid: its effect on endometrial stromal cells and its potential relevance to endometriosis. J Clin Endocrinol Metab 1994;79:1284–93.
31. Sbracia M, Zupi E, Alo P et al. Differential expression of IGF-I and IGF-II in eutopic and ectopic endometria of women with endometriosis and in women without endometriosis. Am J Reprod Immunol 1997;37:326–9.
32. Oosterlynck DJ, Meuleman C, Waer M et al. Transforming growth factor-beta activity is increased in peritoneal fluid from women with endometriosis. Obstet Gynecol 1994;83:287–92.

33. Pizzo A, Salmeri FM, Ardita FV et al. Behaviour of cytokine levels in serum and peritoneal fluid of women with endometriosis. Gynecol Obstet Invest 2002;54:82–7.

34. Fukaya T, Sugawara J, Yoshida H et al. The role of macrophage colony stimulating factor in the peritoneal fluid in infertile patients with endometriosis. Tohoku J Exp Med 1994;172:221–6.

35. Halme J, White C, Kauma S et al. Peritoneal macrophages from patients with endometriosis release growth factor activity in vitro. J Clin Endocrinol Metab 1988;66:1044–9.

36. Garcia-Velasco JA, Arici A, Zreik T et al. Macrophage derived growth factors modulate Fas ligand expression in cultured endometrial stromal cells:a role in endometriosis. Mol Hum Reprod 1999;5:642–50.

37. Shifren JL, Tseng JF, Zaloudek CJ et al. Ovarian steroid regulation of vascular endothelial growth factor in the human endometrium: implications for angiogenesis during the menstrual cycle and in the pathogenesis of endometriosis. J Clin Endocrinol Metab 1996;81:3112–18.

38. McLaren J, Prentice A, Charnock-Jones DS et al. Vascular endothelial growth factor is produced by peritoneal fluid macrophages in endometriosis and is regulated by ovarian steroids. J Clin Invest 1996;98:482–9.

39. Iwabe T, Harada T, Terakawa N. Role of cytokines in endometriosis-associated infertility. Gynecol Obstet Invest 2002;53:19–25.

40. Curtis P, Jackson AE. Adverse effects on sperm movement characteristics in women with minimal and mild endometriosis. Br J Obstet Gynaecol 1993;100:165–9.

41. Drudy L, Lewis SEM, Kinsella CB et al. The influence of peritoneal fluid from patients with minimal stage or treated endometriosis on sperm motility parameters using computer-assisted semen analysis. Hum Reprod 1994;9:2418–23.

42. Arumugam K. Endometriosis and infertility: raised iron concentration in the peritoneal fluid and its effect on the acrosome reaction. Hum Reprod 1994;9:1153–7.

43. Coddington CS, Oehninger S, Cunningham DS et al. Peritoneal fluid from patients with endometriosis decreases sperm binding to the zona pellucida in the hemizona assay: a preliminary report. Fertil Steril 1992;57:783–6.

44. Marcos RN, Gibbons WE, Findley WE. Effect of peritoneal fluid on in vitro cleavage of 2-cell mouse embryos: possible role in infertility associated with endometriosis. Fertil Steril 1985;44:678–83.

45. Taketani Y, Kuo TM, Mizuno M. Comparison of cytokine levels and embryo toxicity in peritoneal fluid from infertile women with untreated or treated endometriosis. Am J Obstet Gynecol 1992;167:265–70.

46. Gomez-Torres MJ, Acien P, Campos A et al. Embryotoxicity of peritoneal fluid in women with endometriosis. Its relation with cytokines and lymphocyte populations. Hum Reprod 2002;17:777–81.

47. Taylor RN, Ryan IP, Moore ES et al. Angiogenesis and macrophage activation in endometriosis. Ann NY Acad Sci 1997;828:194–207.

48. Bankers-Fulbright J, Kalli K, McKean D. Interleukin-1 signal transduction. Life Sci 1996;59:61–83.

49. Sillem M, Prifti S, Monga B et al. Integrin-mediated adhesion of uterine endometrial cells from endometriosis patients to extracellular matrix proteins is enhanced by tumor necrosis factor alpha (TNF-alpha) and interleukin-1 (IL-1). Eur J Obstet Gynecol Reprod Biol 1999;87:123–7.

50. Cheong YC, Shelton JB, Laird SM et al. IL-1, IL-6 and TNF-alpha concentrations in the peritoneal fluid of women with pelvic adhesions. Hum Reprod 2002;17:69–75.

51. Haskill S, Martin G, Van Le L et al. cDNA cloning of an intracellular form of the human interleukin 1 receptor antagonist associated with epithelium. Proc Natl Acad Sci USA 1991;88:3681–5.

52. Kharfi A, Akoum A. Correlation between decreased type-II interleukin-1 receptor and increased monocyte chemotactic protein-1 expression in the endometrium of women with endometriosis. Am J Reprod Immunol 2001;45:193–9.

53. Simon C, Frances A, Piquette G et al. The immune mediator interleukin-1 receptor antagonist (IL-1ra) prevents embryo implantation. Endocrinology 1994;134:521–8.

54. Kharfi A, Akoum A. Soluble interleukin-1 receptor type II blocks monocyte chemotactic protein-1 secretion by U937 cells in response to peripheral blood serum of women with endometriosis. Fertil Steril 2002;78:836–42.

55. Mori H, Sawairi M, Nakagawa M et al. Expression of interleukin-1 (IL-1) beta messenger ribonucleic acid (mRNA) and IL-1 receptor antagonist mRNA in peritoneal macrophages from patients with endometriosis. Fertil Steril 1992;57:535–42.

56. Lebovic DI, Chao VA, Martini JF et al. IL-1beta induction of RANTES (regulated upon activation, normal T cell expressed and secreted) chemokine gene expression in endometriotic stromal cells depends on a nuclear factor–kappaB site in the proximal promoter. J Clin Endocrinol Metab 2001;86:4759–64.

57. Lebovic DI, Baldocchi RA, Mueller MD et al. Altered expression of a cell-cycle suppressor gene, Tob-1, in endometriotic cells by cDNA array analyses. Fertil Steril 2002;78:849–54.

58. Akoum A, Lemay A, Maheux R. Estradiol and interleukin-1beta exert a synergistic stimulatory effect on the expression of the chemokine regulated upon activation, normal T cell expressed, and secreted in endometriotic cells. J Clin Endocrinol Metab 2002;87:5785–92.

59. Vigano P, Gaffuri B, Somigliana E et al. Expression of intercellular adhesion molecule (ICAM)-1 mRNA and protein is enhanced in endometriosis versus endometrial stromal cells in culture. Mol Hum Reprod 1998;4:1150–16.

60. Blumenthal RD, Samoszuk M, Taylor AP et al. Degranulating eosinophils in human endometriosis. Am J Pathol 2000;156:1581–8.

61. Rier SE, Zarmakoupis PN, Hu X et al. Dysregulation of interleukin-6 responses in ectopic endometrial stromal cells: correlation with decreased soluble receptor levels in peritoneal fluid of women with endometriosis. J Clin Endocrinol Metab 1995;80:1431–7.

62. Gazvani R, Smith L, Fowler PA. Effect of interleukin-8 (IL-8), anti-IL-8, and IL-12 on endometrial cell survival in combined endometrial gland and stromal cell cultures derived from women with and without endometriosis. Fertil Steril 2002;77:62–7.

63. Ho HN, Wu MY, Chao KH et al. Peritoneal interleukin-10 increases with decrease in activated (CD4+) T lymphocytes in women with endometriosis. Hum Reprod 1997;12:2528–33.

64. Gazvani R, Bates M, Vince G et al. Concentration of interleukin-12 in the peritoneal fluid is not influenced by the presence of endometriosis, its stage or the phase of the menstrual cycle. Acta Obstet Gynecol Scand 2001;80:175–8.

65. Mazzeo D, Vigano P, Di Blasio AM et al. Interleukin-12 and its free p40 subunit regulate immune recognition of endometrial cells: potential role in endometriosis. J Clin Endocrinol Metab 1998;83:911–16.

66. Somigliana E, Vigano P, Rossi G et al. Endometrial ability to implant in ectopic sites can be prevented by interleukin-12 in a murine model of endometriosis. Hum Reprod 1999;14:2944–50.

67. Odukoya OA, Ajjan R, Lim K et al. The pattern of cytokine mRNA expression in ovarian endometriomata. Mol Hum Reprod 1997;3:393–7.

68. Halme J, Becker S, Haskill S. Altered maturation and function of peritoneal macrophages: possible role in pathogenesis of endometriosis. Am J Obstet Gynecol 1987;156:783–9.

69. Hornung D, Ryan IP, Chao VA et al. Immunolocalization and regulation of the chemokine RANTES in human endometrial and

endometriosis tissues and cells. J Clin Endocrinol Metab 1997;82:1621–8.

70. Hornung D, Klingel K, Dohrn K et al. Regulated on activation, normal T-cell-expressed and -secreted mRNA expression in normal endometrium and endometriotic implants: assessment of autocrine/paracrine regulation by in situ hybridization. Am J Pathol 2001;158:1949–54.

71. Zhao D, Pritts EA, Hornung D et al. Epithelial–stromal interactions induce RANTES expression in endometriosis. Fertil Steril 2002;77:O75.

72. Hornung D, Bentzien F, Wallwiener D et al. Chemokine bioactivity of RANTES in endometriotic and normal endometrial stromal cells and peritoneal fluid. Mol Hum Reprod 2001;7:163–8.

73. Hornung D, Chao VA, Vigne JL et al. Thiazolidinedione (TZD) inhibition of peritoneal inflammation. J Gynecol Obstet Invest 2003;55:20–4.

74. Zhang J, Lathbury LJ, Salamonsen LA. Expression of the chemokine eotaxin and its receptor, CCR3, in human endometrium. Biol Reprod 2000;62:404–11.

75. Nedwin G, Naylor S, Sakaguchi A et al. Human lymphotoxin and tumor necrosis factor genes: structure, homology and chromosomal localization. Nucleic Acids Res 1985;13:6361–73.

76. Tabibzadeh S. Ubiquitous expression of TNF-alpha/cachectin immunoreactivity in human endometrium. Am J Reprod Immunol 1991;26:1–4.

77. Hunt J, Chen H, Hu X et al. Tumor necrosis factor-alpha messenger ribonucleic acid and protein in human endometrium. Biol Reprod 1992;47:141–7.

78. Estrada LS, Champion HC, Wang R et al. Effect of tumour necrosis factor-alpha (TNF-alpha) and interferon-gamma (IFN-gamma) on human sperm motility, viability and motion parameters. Int J Androl 1997;20:237–42.

79. D'Hooghe TM, Cuneo S, Nugent N et al. Recombinant human TNF binding protein-1 (r-hTBP-1) inhibits the development of endometriosis in baboons: a prospective, randomized, placebo- and drug-controlled study. Fertil Steril 2001;76:O2, Suppl.3.

80. D'Antonio M, Martelli F, Peano S et al. Ability of recombinant human TNF binding protein-1 (r-hTBP-1) to inhibit the development of experimentally induced endometriosis in rats. J Reprod Immunol 2000;48:81–98.

81. Braun DP. Peritoneal fluid-mediated enhancement of eutopic and ectopic endometrial cell proliferation is dependent on tumor necrosis factor-alpha in women with endometriosis. Fertil Steril 2002;78:727–32.

82. Klein NA, Pergola GM, Tekmal RR et al. Cytokine regulation of cellular proliferation in endometriosis. Ann NY Acad Sci 1994;734:322–32.

83. Sotnikova N, Antsiferova I, Malyshkina A. Cytokine network of eutopic and ectopic endometrium in women with adenomyosis. Am J Reprod Immunol 2002;47:251–5.

84. Mueller MD, Mazzucchelli L, Buri C, Lebovic DI, Dreher E, Taylor RN. Epithelial neutrophil-activating peptide 78 concentrations are elevated in the peritoneal fluid of women with endometriosis. Fertil Steril 2003;79:815–20.

85. Akoum A, Lemay A, McColl SR et al. Elevated concentration and biologic activity of monocyte chemotactic protein-1 in the peritoneal fluid of patients with endometriosis. Fertil Steril 1996;66:17–23.

86. Prentice A, Thomas EJ, Weddell A et al. Epidermal growth factor receptor expression in normal endometrium and endometriosis: an immunohistochemical study. Br J Obstet Gynaecol 1992;99:395–8.

87. Druckmann R, Rohr DU. IGF-1 in gynaecology and obstetrics: update 2002. Maturitas 2002;41(Suppl 1):65–83.

88. Kim JG, Suh CS, Kim SH et al. Insulin-like growth factors (IGFs), IGF-binding proteins (IGFBPs), and IGFBP-3 protease activity in the peritoneal fluid of patients with and without endometriosis. Fertil Steril 2000;73:996–1000.

89. Akoum A, Lemay A, Lajeuness Y et al. Immunohistochemical localization of insulin-like growth factor-binding protein-3 in eutopic and ectopic endometrial tissues. Fertil Steril 1999;72:1085–92.

90. Sharpe-Timms KL, Bruno PL, Penney LL et al. Immunohistochemical localization of granulocyte–macrophage colony-stimulating factor in matched endometriosis and endometrial tissues. Am J Obstet Gynecol 1994;171:740–5.

91. Munson L, Upadhyaya NB, Van Meter S. Platelet-derived growth factor promotes endometrial epithelial cell proliferation. Am J Obstet Gynecol 1995;173:1820–5.

92. Surrey ES, Halme J. Effect of platelet-derived growth factor on endometrial stromal cell proliferation in vitro: a model for endometriosis? Fertil Steril 1991;56:672–9.

93. Hornung D, Lebovic DI, Shifren JL et al. Vectorial secretion of vascular endothelial growth factor by polarized human endometrial epithelial cells. Fertil Steril 1998;69:909–15.

94. Dabrosin C, Gyorffy S, Margetts P et al. Therapeutic effect of angiostatin gene transfer in a murine model of endometriosis. Am J Pathol 2002;161:909–18.

8. Matrix Metalloproteinases and Endometriosis

Kevin G. Osteen and Kaylon L. Bruner-Tran

FUNCTIONAL ENDOMETRIAL BIOLOGY AND THE ETIOLOGY OF ENDOMETRIOSIS

The basic biology of the human endometrium is intimately linked to cyclic ovarian steroid production, creating a unique endometrial architecture which supports and controls the highly invasive events of implantation and placentation. During a woman's reproductive life the endometrium consists of morphologically and functionally distinct layers: the stratum basalis, which lies adjacent to the myometrium, the stratum spongiosum or intermediate layer, and the stratum compactum. It is from the stratum basalis that the surface of the endometrium regenerates after each episode of cyclic tissue shedding, whereas the two uppermost layers, referred to jointly as the stratum functionalis, undergo coordinated histologic and cytologic changes in preparation for pregnancy.[1] In the absence of nidation, steroids drive the reassembly of the endometrial stratum functionalis by coordinating distinct patterns of cell–cell communication across each phase of the menstrual cycle. Although rare among adult tissues, extensive tissue restructuring is a hallmark of the human reproductive cycle and numerous matrix metalloproteinases (MMPs), as well as their natural inhibitors (TIMPs), exhibit cell-specific and cycle-dependent expression in both the ovary and the endometrium.[2]

Recent research has suggested that steroid-mediated MMP expression may provide a critical link between normal endometrial remodeling and the invasive mechanisms required for the establishment of ectopic endometrial growth. Clinically, endometriosis is more common in women whose menstrual flow is excessive or of long duration,[3] and viable endometrial tissue has been identified in the peritoneum of women at the time of menstruation.[4] In early research stud-

ies, primates were found to develop endometriosis following surgically induced peritoneal menstruation,[5] and Ridley and Edwards[6] successfully induced endometriosis in two of 15 women who voluntarily allowed peritoneal injection of their own menstrual tissue. Although the opportunity for ectopic growth of endometrial tissue is clearly provided by physical displacement during retrograde menstruation, the local paracrine environment, coupled with an altered pattern of MMP expression and activity, probably dictates the incidence of endometriotic tissue growth at various sites within the peritoneal cavity. Certainly, the peritoneal fluid is a rich source of steroids, growth factors, and cytokines, many of which can promote or inhibit the selective expression and activation of members of the MMP family.[7]

MMP EXPRESSION PATTERNS DURING THE MENSTRUAL CYCLE

In order to appreciate the potential role of members of the MMP family on the pathophysiology of endometriosis, it is necessary to first consider the role of these enzymes in normal endometrial physiology. Following menstruation, repair of the broken epithelium covering the luminal surface is among the initial events required to re-establish local tissue integrity. Expression of MMP-7 mRNA can be localized to the epithelium during early postmenstrual repair, as well as focally during estrogen-stimulated cell growth and tissue remodeling during the proliferative phase.[8] MMP-9 has also recently been reported to be expressed by the epithelium and may be the only MMP expressed in both endometrial epithelium and stroma.[8,9] Although epithelial cell expression of MMPs is rather limited, the endometrial stroma exhibits a more complex cellular architecture and MMP-1, MMP-2, MMP-3, MMP-8, MMP-9,

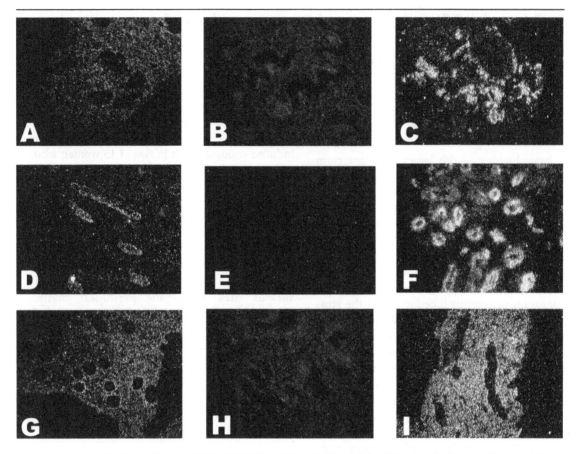

Figure 8.1 In situ hybridization localization of MMP-3 (A-C), MMP-7 (D-F), and MMP-11 (G-I) mRNA in formalin-fixed, paraffin-embedded normal endometrium removed during the proliferative (A, D, G), secretory (B, E, H) or menstrual phases (C, F, I). Magnification 200×.

MMP-10, MMP-11, and MT1-MMP are variably expressed by fibroblasts, immune cells, and vascular cells during the menstrual cycle.[2,10–15] Among endometrial cell types specialized stromal fibroblasts appear to be most sensitive to steroids, often directing the growth and differentiation of adjacent cells, including the expression of MMPs. Differential regulation of specific members of the MMP family is common: for example, MMP-11 mRNA is often observed to be more highly expressed among stromal cells than is MMP-3, which is often expressed focally near the stromal–glandular interface (Figure 8.1). In contrast to periods of endometrial growth in response to estrogen, most MMPs are not expressed during the progesterone-dominated secretory phase,[2,8,10,16] although MMP-2 mRNA is constitutively expressed throughout the cycle.[10] The cell-specific expression of MMP-3 and MMP-7 has been examined in primate endometrium during experimental menstrual cycles, and the cell-specific expression of these MMPs appears to follow a similar cyclic pattern as reported in humans.[17,18] However, in contrast to human studies, focal expression of MMP-3 and MMP-7 has been reported to disappear during the late proliferative phase in the macaque endometrium, prior to the postovulatory rise in progesterone.[19]

TIMP EXPRESSION PATTERNS DURING THE MENSTRUAL CYCLE

The expression of specific MMPs among various cell types within the endometrium allows for controlled remodeling of this unique organ system. However, the endometrium is highly vascular and overall tissue integrity must be maintained to prevent bleeding as matrix breakdown and regrowth progresses. To achieve appropriate tissue stability during the dynamics of menstrual cycle remodeling, natural inhibitors of MMPs, called TIMPs, are generally coexpressed with MMPs. Rodgers et al[10] were among the first to demonstrate the specific expression of TIMP-1 mRNA in the human endometrium, in both epithelial and stromal cells across each phase of the menstrual cycle, with relative levels increasing in the stromal compartment during the late secretory phase. The greatest intensity of hybridization signal of TIMP-1 was found in early premenstrual tissues.[10] Zhang and Salamonsen have reported immunoreactive TIMP-1 protein in all tissue compartments of the human endometrium throughout the cycle, with the most intense staining localized to luminal epithelium.[20] Although TIMP-1 can be found in uterine flushings at the end of the menstrual cycle,[21] the TIMPs are clearly involved in stabilization of the uterine vasculature throughout the cycle and are abundantly expressed in vascular cells of the secretory endometrium.[10] In the primate endometrium TIMP-1 expression demonstrates a shift to the stratum basalis following the breakdown and bleeding events in the upper functionalis region, further suggesting a role of TIMP in tissue repair and stabilization after menstruation.[19] If pregnancy is established, continued progesterone production prevents menstruation by promoting continued endometrial stability during the extensive tissue remodeling that occurs at the maternal–fetal interface. Not surprisingly, investigators have reported increasing levels of all four TIMP proteins in various cell types during endometrial maturation and during pregnancy.[2] For example, TIMP-1, TIMP-2, and TIMP-3 proteins increase during progesterone-mediated in vitro decidualization of human stromal cells,[20] and TIMP-4 has been reported to be present in term decidua in vivo.[22] In the absence of pregnancy steroid support to the endometrium decreases, promoting the expression of numerous MMPs and TIMPs within an inflammatory-like local tissue environment. In contrast to the steroid-mediated regulation of members of the MMP system during the proliferative and secretory phases, the loss of steroid support at the end of the cycle results in broad expression of MMP and TIMP in association with menstrual breakdown. Although human and primate studies have linked retrograde menstruation to the pathophysiology of endometriosis, the specific role of members of the MMP family in this disease remains to be fully established. Exploring the expression of members of the MMP family during menstruation may provide insight into the invasive potential of endometrial fragments entering the peritoneal cavity, a requirement for the establishment of endometriosis.

MMP AND TIMP EXPRESSION PATTERNS DURING MENSTRUATION

As detailed above, the expression pattern of MMP and TIMP changes dramatically across the menstrual cycle, reflecting the unique biological requirements for cell-specific growth and differentiation, menstrual breakdown, and tissue repair. Compared to MMP expression, TIMP expression levels fluctuate less during the proliferative and secretory phases of the cycle, whereas menstruation is associated with increases in both MMP and TIMP expression.[8,10,16,23–25] The coexpression of numerous members of the MMP family allows for the zone-specific breakdown of the upper functionalis region of the endometrial surface while preserving the capacity for rapid tissue regrowth from the basalis. A variety of vascular changes have been classically associated with the earliest events initiating menstruation (reviewed by Bulletti et al[26]). However, the expression of members of the MMP family by the many cell types within the endometrium can also be implicated in the initiation and progression of menstruation.[2,27] As steroid levels fall just prior to menstrual breakdown, focal expression of MMP-7 mRNA can be observed in epithelial cells.[8] As menstruation progresses, MMP-1, MMP-3, MMP-7, MMP-9, and MMP-11, MT1-MMP, and MT2-MMP mRNA become broadly expressed among epithelial, stromal, immune, and vascular components.[8,14,16,28,29] Importantly, MMP activation is necessary for enzyme activity, regardless of mRNA expression patterns. In this regard, both estrogen and progesterone appear necessary for maintaining overall tissue integrity in the endometrium, as organ cultures of endometrial tissue react to steroid withdrawal by releasing numerous MMPs, which can be readily measured by zymography.[16,25] In addition, MMP-1, MMP-3, MMP-7, and MMP-9 have each been shown to be both expressed and activated during the menstrual phase.[30]

The regulatory mechanisms by which declining levels of steroids induce MMP and TIMP expression at the time of menstruation has not been determined, although Salamonsen et al[16] have suggested that because of the focal nature of menstruation-associated MMP expression, progesterone withdrawal alone is unlikely to be the primary regulatory factor. In contrast, recent studies indicate that proinflammatory cytokines play a pivotal role in stimulating MMP expression, as both estrogen and progesterone levels fall prior to menstruation.[12,27,31-33] Periods of dramatic tissue

breakdown, repair, growth-associated remodeling, and pregnancy-associated differentiation are essential components of normal endometrial biology and are clearly associated with specific expression patterns of members of the MMP family. Although these processes are linked to the role of the endometrium to support successful pregnancy, the steroid-mediated expression of MMPs during the menstrual cycle appears also to provide a mechanism for the invasive processes that contribute to the pathophysiology of endometriosis. Extensive clinical and experimental evidence indicates that a woman's estrogen exposure contributes to her overall risk for endometriosis, whereas progesterone exposure during pregnancy or therapeutically may prevent or regress disease in some women.[34-36] In an experimental model of endometriosis, steroid-mediated regulation of endometrial MMP expression and action has been linked to the ability of human endometrial fragments to establish viable ectopic lesions in the peritoneum of nude mice.[37] As shown in Figure 8.2, ectopic lesions in this experimental model resemble human endometriosis both grossly and histologically, and demonstrate the expression of MMP mRNA.

THE MMP SYSTEM AND ENDOMETRIOSIS

The epidemiology and natural history of endometriosis are complex and lack consensus, and

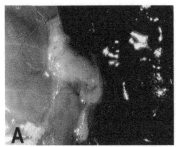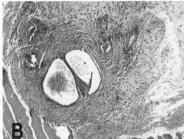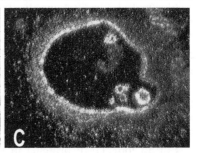

Figure 8.2 Human endometrium growing as experimental endometriosis in nude mice. (A) Gross appearance (magnification 15×); (B) microscopic appearance of a formalin-fixed paraffin-embedded lesion stained with hematoxlyin and eosin (magnification 200×); (C) in situ hybridization localization of MMP-7 mRNA in a human lesion removed from a nude mouse (magnification 200×).

hence numerous theories have been offered to explain the development of the disease.[34] Nevertheless, the mechanical distribution of endometrial tissue through retrograde menstruation represents a plausible explanation for the development of most cases of endometriosis in women, as originally described by Sampson.[38] The retrograde menstruation theory proposes that endometriosis develops from the implantation of menstrual tissue refluxed through the fallopian tubes into the peritoneal space. The most common intraperitoneal locations for the disease, in descending order of incidence, are the ovaries, the uterus, the posterior cul-de-sac, and the fallopian tubes.[34] Superficial or surface implant sites of endometriosis retain the most resemblance to normal endometrium, especially locations on the ovary, suggesting an importance of the local environment on disease etiology. Nevertheless, the discriminating factor(s) in determining the development of active endometriosis only in certain individuals probably involves a complex array of potentially interactive influences, including steroid exposure, immunologic disturbances, genetic predisposition, and perhaps environmental toxin exposure.

The precise role(s) of MMPs or TIMPs in the development and progression of endometriosis remains speculative, although several laboratories have implicated protease activity in the establishment and progression of endometriosis in patients with the disease,[39–41] as well as in experimental models.[37,42] A number of studies indicate that altered regulation of MMPs may be a component of the pathophysiology of endometriosis. Normally, the postovulatory rise in serum progesterone levels leads to a suppression of endometrial MMPs while initiating a gradual increase in TIMP-1 and TIMP-3 expression.[2,27] The suppression of MMPs during the secretory phase of the menstrual cycle occurs within an increasingly proinflammatory environment which gradually develops in the endometrium prior to the beginning of menstruation.[27,43] The broadest expression of MMPs and TIMPs in the normal endometrium appears to occur as progesterone levels fall and the influence of proinflammatory cytokines

becomes more pronounced.[2] Both MMPs and TIMPs have been reported to increase in menstrual tissue and menstrual fluid,[2,30] and numerous proinflammatory cytokines may further influence expression of the MMP family within the peritoneum.[39] Experimental models of endometriosis support the theory that decreased progesterone action and increased exposure to proinflammatory cytokines can lead to increased ectopic growth.[37,44,45] Additionally, at ectopic growth sites endometrial tissue may exhibit a reduced sensitivity to progesterone, an increased local production of estrogen, and an altered ability to metabolize steroids,[46–50] conditions that appear to promote local proinflammatory cytokine action.[51] A proinflammatory peritoneal environment coupled with the altered steroid sensitivity of endometriotic implants may significantly alter their expression of MMPs and TIMPs compared to normal endometrium. Indeed, in the natural human disease MMP-1 and MMP-2 protein are more highly expressed, whereas TIMP-1 and TIMP-2 are significantly reduced in endometriotic tissues compared to normal endometrium.[52] Szamatowicz et al[53] also found that levels of MMP-9 protein are higher and TIMP-1 protein levels are lower in the peritoneal fluid of women with endometriosis than in disease-free women. Recent studies would indicate that the expression of the MMP family is also altered in the eutopic endometrium of women with endometriosis. Chung et al[54] have demonstrated lower levels of TIMP-3 mRNA expression in both eutopic endometrium and endometriotic lesions compared to disease-free women, although MMP-9 mRNA was increased at the ectopic sites. In women with endometriosis, we have found the cell-specific mRNA expression of MMP-3, MMP-7, and MMP-11 to be elevated in the eutopic endometrium during the progesterone-dominated secretory phase of the cycle (Figure 8.3), and these enzymes fail to respond to progesterone suppression in vitro.[55,56] Differential display analysis of eutopic endometrium obtained from endometriosis patients compared to autologous endometriotic lesions found no alterations among MMP genes during the proliferative

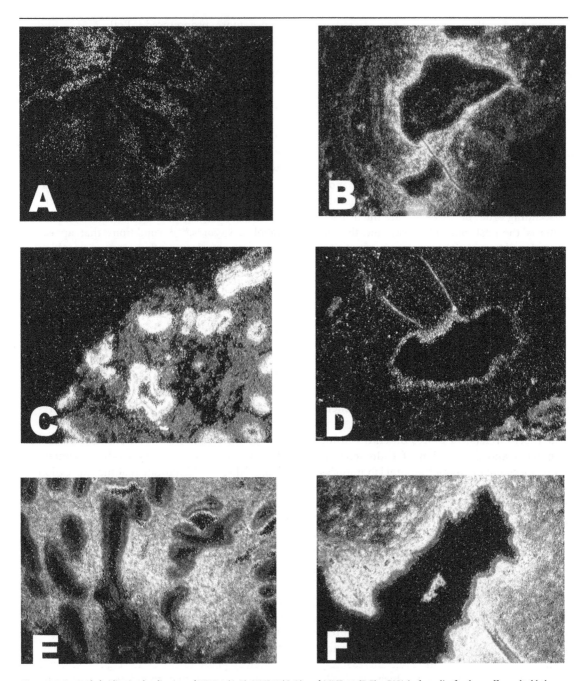

Figure 8.3 In situ hybridization localization of MMP-3 (A-B), MMP-7 (C-D), and MMP-11 (E-F) mRNA in formalin-fixed, paraffin-embedded endometrium (A, C, E) or endometriosis (B, D, F) removed during the secretory phase from women with endometriosis.

phase.[57] However, an analysis of progesterone-responsive genes in women with endometriosis versus disease-free controls identified aberrant

expression of MMPs and numerous other genes during the secretory phase of the cycle.[58] The above studies would suggest that dysregulation of

MMP and TIMP family members can occur at both eutopic and ectopic sites of endometrial growth in women with endometriosis. However, the altered regulation of MMP family members in eutopic tissues of women with endometriosis may represent a key mechanistic link to the selective establishment of this disease only in certain women. More studies are needed to determine the cellular and molecular pathways of MMP regulation that may become altered in association with the disease process of endometriosis. Identifying these pathways may allow for the design of more effective diagnostic and therapeutic regimens for this complex and persistent disease.

ACKNOWLEDGEMENTS

These studies were supported by The Special Cooperative Centers Program in Reproduction Research (NIH# U54 HD37321), EPA# GR 826300 (KGO) and The Endometriosis Association (KGO, KB-T).

REFERENCES

1. Noyes RA, Hertig AT, Rick J. Dating the endometrial biopsy. Fertil Steril 1950;1:3–25.
2. Curry TE Jr, Osteen KG. Cyclic changes in the matrix metalloproteinase system in the ovary and uterus. Biol Reprod 2001;64:1285–96.
3. Cramer DW, Wilson E, Stillman RJ et al. The relationship of endometriosis to menstrual characteristics, smoking and exercise. JAMA 1986;255:1904–8.
4. Lui DTY. Endometriosis: its association with retrograde menstruation, dysmenorrhea and tubal pathology. Br J Obstet Gynaecol 1986;93:859–64.
5. TeLinde RW, Scott RB. Experimental endometriosis. Am J Obstet Gynecol 1950;60:1147–73.
6. Ridley JH, Edwards IK. Experimental endometriosis in the human. Am J Obstet Gynecol 1958;76:783–90.
7. Osteen KG, Bruner-Tran KL, Ong D, Eisenberg E. Paracrine mediators of endometrial matrix metalloproteinase expression: potential targets for progestin-based treatment of endometriosis. Ann NY Acad Sci 2002;955:139–46.
8. Rodgers WH, Osteen KG, Matrisian LM, Navre M, Gorstein F. Expression and localization of matrilysin, a matrix metalloproteinase, in the human endometrium. Am J Obstet Gynecol 1993;168:253–60.
9. Skinner JL, Riley SC, Gebbie AE, Glasier AF, Critchley HO. Regulation of matrix metalloproteinase-9 in endometrium during the menstrual cycle and following administration of intrauterine levonorgestrel. Hum Reprod 1999;14:793–9.
10. Rodgers WH, Matrisian LM, Giudice LC et al. Patterns of matrix metalloproteinase expression in cycling endometrium imply differential functions and regulation by steroids. J Clin Invest 1994;94:946–53.
11. Vincent AJ, Malakooti N, Zhang J et al. Endometrial breakdown in women using Norplant is associated with migratory cells expressing matrix metalloproteinase-9 (gelatinase B). Hum Reprod 1999;14:807–15.
12. Singer CF, Marbaix E, Lemoine P, Courtoy PJ, Eeckhout Y. Local cytokines induce differential expression of matrix metalloproteinases but not their tissue inhibitors in human endometrial fibroblasts. Eur J Biochem 1999;259:40–5.
13. Vincent AJ, Salamonsen LA. The role of matrix metalloproteinases and leukocytes in abnormal uterine bleeding associated with progestin-only contraceptives. Hum Reprod 2000;15:135–43.
14. Zhang J, Hampton AL, Nie G, Salamonsen LA. Progesterone inhibits activation of latent matrix metalloproteinase (MMP)-2 by membrane-type 1 MMP: enzymes coordinately expressed in human endometrium. Biol Reprod 2000;62:85–94.
15. Maatta M, Soini Y, Liakka A, Autio-Harmainen H. Localization of MT1-MMP, TIMP-1, TIMP-2, and TIMP-3 messenger RNA in normal, hyperplastic, and neoplastic endometrium. Enhanced expression by endometrial adenocarcinomas is associated with low differentiation. Am J Clin Pathol 2000;114:402–11.
16. Salamonsen LA, Butt AR, Hammond FR, Garcia S, Zhang J. Production of endometrial matrix metalloproteinases, but not their tissue inhibitors, is modulated by progesterone withdrawal in an in vitro model for menstruation. J Clin Endocrinol Metab 1997;82:1409–15.
17. Brenner RM, Rudolph L, Matrisian L, Slayden OD. Non-human primate models: artificial menstrual cycles, endometrial matrix metalloproteinases and s.c. endometrial grafts. Hum Reprod 1996;11:150–64.
18. Cox KE, Sharpe-Timms KL, Kamiya N et al. Differential regulation of stromelysin-1 (matrix metalloproteinase-3) and matrilysin (matrix metalloproteinase-7) in baboon endometrium. J Soc Gynecol Invest 2000;7:242–8.
19. Rudolph-Owen LA, Slayden OD, Matrisian LM, Brenner RM. Matrix metalloproteinase expression in *Macaca mulatta* endometrium: evidence for zone-specific regulatory tissue gradients. Biol Reprod 1998;59:1349–59.
20. Zhang J, Salamonsen LA. Tissue inhibitor of metalloproteinases (TIMP)-1,-2 and -3 in human endometrium during the menstrual cycle. Mol Hum Reprod. 1997 3:735-41.
21. Laird SM, Dalton CF, Okon MA et al. Metalloproteinases and tissue inhibitor of metalloproteinase 1 (TIMP-1) in endometrial flushings from pre- and post-menopausal women and from women with endometrial adenocarcinoma. J Reprod Fertil 1999;115:225–32.
22. Riley SC, Leask R, Denison FC et al. Secretion of tissue inhibitors of matrix metalloproteinases by human fetal membranes, decidua and placenta at parturition. J Endocrinol 1999;162:351–9.
23. Tabibzadeh S. Signals and molecular pathways involved in apoptosis, with special emphasis on human endometrium. Hum Reprod Update 1995;1:303–23.
24. Kokorine I, Marbaix E, Henriet P et al. Focal cellular origin and regulation of interstitial collagenase (matrix metalloproteinase-1) are related to menstrual breakdown in the human endometrium. J Cell Sci 1996;109:2151–60.
25. Salamonsen LA, Woolley DE. Matrix metalloproteinases in normal menstruation. Hum Reprod 1996;11:124–33.
26. Bulletti C, De Ziegler D, Albonetti A, Flamigni C. Paracrine regulation of menstruation. J Reprod Immunol 1998;39:89–104.
27. Salamonsen LA, Woolley DE. Menstruation: induction by matrix metalloproteinases and inflammatory cells. J Reprod Immunol 1999;44:1–27.

28. Marbaix E, Donnez J, Courtoy PJ, Eeckhout Y. Progesterone regulates the activity of collagenase and related gelatinases A and B in human endometrial explants. Proc Natl Acad Sci USA. 1992;89:11789–93.

29. Nayak NR, Critchley HO, Slayden OD et al. Progesterone withdrawal up-regulates vascular endothelial growth factor receptor type 2 in the superficial zone stroma of the human and macaque endometrium: potential relevance to menstruation. J Clin Endocrinol Metab 2000;85:3442–52.

30. Koks CA, Groothuis PG, Slaats P et al. Matrix metalloproteinases and their tissue inhibitors in antegradely shed menstruum and peritoneal fluid. Fertil Steril 2000;73:604–12.

31. Lockwood CJ, Krikun G, Hausknecht VA, Papp C, Schatz F. Matrix metalloproteinase and matrix metalloproteinase inhibitor expression in endometrial stromal cells during progestin-initiated decidualization and menstruation-related progestin withdrawal. Endocrinology 1998;139:4607–13.

32. Schatz F, Krikun G, Runic R et al. Implications of decidualization-associated protease expression in implantation and menstruation. Semin Reprod Endocrinol 1999;17:3–12.

33. Keller NR, Sierra-Rivera E, Eisenberg E, Osteen KG. Progesterone exposure prevents matrix metalloproteinase-3 (MMP-3) stimulation by interleukin-1α in human endometrial stromal cells. J Clin Endocrin Metab 2000;85:1611–19.

34. Halme J, Stovall D. Endometriosis and its medical management. In: Wallach EE, Zacur HA, eds. Reproductive medicine and surgery. St Louis: Mosby, 1995; 695–710.

35. Olive DL. Medical treatment: alternatives to danazol. In: Schenken RS, ed. Endometriosis: Contempory Concepts and Clinical Management. Philadelphia: JB Lippincott, 1989;192.

36. Ramzy I. Pathology. In: Schenken RS, ed. Endometriosis: Contemporary Concepts and Clinical Management. Philadelphia: JB Lippincott, 1989; 60.

37. Bruner KL, Matrisian LM, Rodgers WH, Gorstein F, Osteen KG. Suppression of matrix metalloproteinases inhibits establishment of ectopic lesions by human tissue in nude mice. J Clin Invest 1997;99:2851–7.

38. Sampson JA. Peritoneal endometriosis due to menstrual dissemination of endometrial tissues into the peritoneal cavity. Am J Obstet Gynecol 1927;14:422–69.

39. Osteen KG, Bruner KL, Sharpe-Timms KL. Steroid and growth factor regulation of matrix metalloproteinase expression and endometriosis. Semin Reprod Endocrinol 1996;14:247– 55.

40. Saito T, Mizumoto H, Kuroki K et al. Expression of MMP-3 and TIMP-1 in endometriosis and the influence of Danazol. Acta Obstet Gynecol Jpn 1995;47:495–6.

41. Sharpe-Timms Kl, Keisler LW, McIntush EW, Keisler DH. Tissue inhibitor of metalloproteinase-1 concentrations are attenuated in peritoneal fluid and sera of women with endometriosis and restored in sera by gonadotropin-releasing hormone agonist therapy. Fertil Steril 1998;69:1128–34.

42. Sillem M, Hahn U, Coddington CC III et al. Ectopic growth of endometrium depends on its structural integrity and proteolytic activity in the cynomolgus monkey (*Macaca fascicularis*) model of endometriosis. Fertil Steril 1996;66:468–73.

43. Osteen KG, Bruner-Tran KL, Keller NR, Eisenberg E. Progesterone-mediated endometrial maturation limits matrix metalloproteinase (MMP) expression in an inflammatory-like environment: a regulatory system altered in endometriosis. Ann NY Acad Sci 2002;955:37–47.

44. Bruner KL, Keller NK, Osteen KG. Interleukin-1 "opposes suppression of human endometrial matrix metalloproteinases by progesterone in a model of experimental endometriosis. In: Lemay A, Maheux R, eds. Understanding and Managing Endometriosis: Advances in Research and Practice. New York: Parthenon Publishing, 1999.

45. Maas JW, Groothuis PG, Dunselman GA et al. Development of endometriosis-like lesions after transplantation of human endometrial fragments onto the chick embryo chorioallantoic membrane. Hum Reprod 2001;16:627–31.

46. Lessey BA, Metzger DA, Haney AF, McCarty KS Jr. Immunohistochemical analysis of estrogen and progesterone receptors in endometriosis: comparison with normal endometrium during the menstrual cycle and the effect of medical therapy. Fertil Steril 1989;49:229–35.

47. Bergqvist A, Ferno M. Oestrogen and progesterone receptors in endometriotic tissue and endometrium: comparison of different cycle phases and ages. Hum Reprod 1993; 8:2211–17.

48. Misao R, Iwagaki S, Fujimoto J, Sun W, Tamaya T. Dominant expression of progesterone receptor isoform B mRNA in ovarian endometriosis. Horm Res 1999;52:30–34.

49. Noble LS, Simpson ER, Johns A, Bulun SE. Aromatase expression in endometriosis. J Clin Endocrin Metab 1996;81:174–9.

50. Zeitoun K, Takayama K, Sasano H et al. Deficient 17-a-hydroxysteroid dehydrogenase type 2 expression in endometriosis: failure to metabolize 17-a-estradiol. J Clin Endocrin Metab 1998;83:4474–80.

51. Tseng JF, Ryan IP, Milam TD et al. Interleukin-6 secretion in vitro is up-regulated in ectopic and eutopic endometrial stromal cells from women with endometriosis. J Clin Endocrinol Metab 1996;81:1118–22.

52. Wenzl RJ, Heinzl H. Localization of matrix metalloproteinase-2 in uterine endometrium and ectopic implants. Gynecol Obstet Invest 1998;45:253–57.

53. Szamatowicz J, Laudanski P, Tomaszewska I. Matrix metalloproteinase-9 and tissue inhibitor of matrix metalloproteinase-1: a possible role in the pathogenesis of endometriosis. Hum Reprod 2002;17:284–8.

54. Chung HW, Wen Y, Chun SH et al. Matrix metalloproteinase-9 and tissue inhibitor of metalloproteinase-3 mRNA expression in ectopic and eutopic endometrium in women with endometriosis: a rationale for endometriotic invasiveness. Fertil Steril 2001;75:152–9.

55. Bruner-Tran KL, Webster-Clair D, Osteen KG. Experimental endometriosis: the nude mouse as a xenographic host. Ann NY Acad Sci 2002;955:328–39.

56. Bruner-Tran KL, Eisenberg E, Yeaman G et al. Steroid and cytokine regulation of matrix metalloproteinase expression in endometriosis and the establishment of experimental endometriosis in nude mice. J Clin Endocrinol Metab 2002;87:4782–91.

57. Eyster KM, Boles AL, Brannian JD, Hansen KA. DNA microarray analysis of gene expression markers of endometriosis. Fertil Steril 2002;77:38–42.

58. Kao LC, Tulac S, Imani B et al. Expression profile comparisons in eutopic endometrium between women with and without endometriosis during the window of implantation. Fertil Steril 2002;77:S27–8.

9. The Biology of Endometriosis: Aromatase and Endometriosis

Serdar E. Bulun, Zongjuan Fang, Gonca Imir, Bilgin Gurates, Mitsutoshi Tamura, Bertan Yilmaz, David Langoi, Sanober Amin, Sijun Yang and Santanu Deb

INTRODUCTION

Endometriosis is one of the most prominent public health problems in the US.[1,2] It is characterized by the presence of endometrial glands and stroma within the pelvic peritoneum and other extrauterine sites, and is linked to pelvic pain and infertility. It is estimated to affect 5% of women of reproductive age.[1,2] Endometriosis is a polygenically inherited disease of complex multifactorial etiology.[3] Sampson's theory of transplantation of endometrial tissue on the pelvic peritoneum via retrograde menstruation is the most widely accepted explanation for the development of pelvic endometriosis because of convincing circumstantial and experimental evidence.[4] Because retrograde menstruation is observed in almost all cycling women, endometriosis is postulated to develop as a result of the coexistence of a defect in clearance of the menstrual efflux from pelvic peritoneal surfaces, possibly involving the immune system.[5] Alternatively, intrinsic molecular aberrations in pelvic endometriotic implants have been proposed to significantly contribute to the development of endometriosis. Aberrant expression of aromatase, certain cytokines and tissue metalloproteinases, deficiency of 17β-hydroxysteroid dehydrogenase (17β-HSD) type 2, and resistance to the protective action of progesterone are some of these molecular abnormalities.[6–12] Because endometriosis is an estrogen-dependent disorder, aromatase expression and 17β-HSD type 2 deficiency are of paramount importance in its pathophysiology. Aromatase causes the accumulation of the biologically active estrogen estradiol (E_2) in this tissue. 17β-HSD type 2, which metabolizes E_2 to estrone (E_1), is deficient in endometriosis. The combination of these two abnormalities serves to maintain high levels of E_2 in endometriotic tissue.

MECHANISMS OF ESTROGEN BIOSYNTHESIS IN HUMAN TISSUES

The enzyme aromatase catalyzes the conversion of androstenedione and testosterone to estrone and estradiol. The gene that encodes this enzyme is expressed in a number of human tissues and cells, such as ovarian granulosa cells, placental syncytiotrophoblasts, adipose tissue and skin fibroblasts, and the brain. In women of reproductive age the ovary is the most important site of estrogen biosynthesis, and this takes place in a cyclic fashion. Upon binding of follicle-stimulating hormone (FSH) to its G protein-coupled receptor in the granulosa cell membrane, intracellular cAMP levels rise and enhance the binding of two critical transcription factors, steroidogenic factor-1 (SF-1) and cAMP response element-binding protein (CREB), to the classically located proximal promoter II of the aromatase gene.[13,14] This, in turn, activates aromatase expression and consequently estrogen secretion from the preovulatory follicle.[14,15]

On the other hand, in postmenopausal women estrogen formation takes place in extraglandular tissues such as the adipose tissue and skin[16–18] (Figure 9.1). In contrast to cAMP regulation of aromatase expression in the ovary, this is controlled primarily by cytokines (IL-6, IL-11, TNF-α) and glucocorticoids via the alternative use of promoter I.4 in adipose tissue and skin fibroblasts.[15] The major substrate for aromatase in adipose tissue and skin is androstenedione of adrenal origin. In postmenopausal women approximately 2% of circulating androstenedione

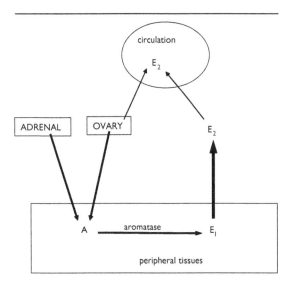

Figure 9.1 Mechanisms of estrogen production. Estradiol (E_2) is either directly secreted by the ovary or produced in peripheral sites (adipose tissue and skin). The principal substrate for extraglandular aromatase activity in ovulatory women is androstenedione (A) of adrenal and ovarian origin. In women receiving GnRH agonists or postmenopausal women, however, the adrenal remains the primary source of androstenedione. Androstenedione is converted by aromatase to estrone (E_1) in adipose tissue and skin fibroblasts. Estrone is further converted to estradiol by 17β-HSD (reductase) activity in these peripheral tissues. Thus, peripheral aromatization is the major source for circulating estradiol in the postmenopausal period or during ovarian suppression.

is converted to estrone, which is further converted to estradiol in these peripheral tissues. This may give rise to significant serum levels of estradiol capable of causing endometrial hyperplasia or even carcinoma.[17,18]

AROMATASE IN ENDOMETRIOSIS

Endometrium and myometrium contain extremely high levels of estrogen receptors and thus are prime targets for estrogen. Until recently, estrogen action has been classically seen as occurring only via an 'endocrine' mechanism: in other words, it was thought that only circulating estradiol, whether secreted by the ovary or formed in the adipose tissue, could exert an estrogenic effect after delivery to target tissues via the bloodstream. Studies on aromatase expression in breast cancer demonstrated that paracrine mechanisms play an important role in estrogen action in this tissue.[19] Estrogen produced by aromatase activity in breast adipose tissue fibroblasts was demonstrated to promote the growth of adjacent malignant breast epithelial cells.[20] Finally, we demonstrated an 'intracrine' effect of estrogen in uterine leiomyomas and endometriosis: estrogen produced by aromatase activity in the cytoplasm of leiomyoma smooth muscle cells or endometriotic stromal cells can exert its effects by readily binding to its nuclear receptor within the same cell.[6,21,22] Disease-free endometrium and myometrium, on the other hand, lack aromatase expression.[21,22]

Among estrogen-responsive pelvic disorders, aromatase expression was studied in the greatest detail in endometriosis.[6,7,22,23] First, extremely high levels of aromatase mRNA were found in extraovarian endometriotic implants and endometriomas. Secondly, endometriosis-derived stromal cells in culture incubated with a cAMP analog displayed extraordinarily high levels of aromatase activity comparable to that in placental syncytiotrophoblasts.[22] These exciting findings led us to test a battery of growth factors, cytokines, and other substances that might induce aromatase activity via a cAMP-dependent pathway in endometriosis. PGE_2 was found to be the most potent known inducer of aromatase activity in endometriotic stromal cells.[22] In fact, this PGE_2 effect was found to be mediated via the cAMP-inducing EP_2 receptor subtype (our unpublished observations). Moreover, estrogen was reported to increase PGE_2 formation by stimulating cyclooxygenase type-2 (COX-2) enzyme in endometrial stromal cells in culture.[24] Thus, a positive feedback loop for continuous local productions of estrogen and PG is established, favoring the proliferative and inflammatory characteristics of endometriosis (Figure 9.2). In addition, aromatase mRNA was also detected in the eutopic endometrial samples of women with moderate to severe endometriosis (but not in those of disease-free women), albeit in much smaller quantities than from endometriotic implants.[6] This may be suggestive of a genetic defect in women with

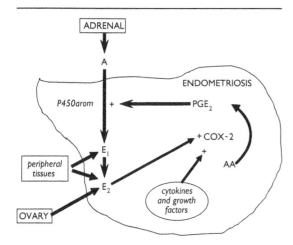

Figure 9.2 A positive feedback cycle for estrogen and prostaglandin formation. Estradiol (E_2) in an endometriotic lesion arises from several body sites. In an ovulatory woman, estradiol is secreted directly from the ovary in a cyclic fashion. In the early follicular phase and after menopause, peripheral tissues (adipose and skin) are the most important sources to account for the circulating estradiol. Estradiol is also produced locally in the endometriotic implant itself in both ovulatory and postmenopausal women. The most important precursor, androstenedione (A) of adrenal origin, becomes converted to estrone (E_1), which in turn is reduced to estradiol in the peripheral tissues and endometriotic implants. We demonstrated significant levels of 17β-hydroxysteroid dehydrogenase type 1 (reductase) expression in endometriosis, which catalyzes the conversion of estrone to estradiol.[12] Estradiol both directly and indirectly (through cytokines) induces cyclooxygenase-2 (COX-2), which gives rise to elevated concentrations of prostaglandin E_2 (PGE_2) in endometriosis.[24] PGE_2 in turn is the most potent known stimulator of aromatase in endometriotic stromal cells.[22] This establishes a positive feedback loop in favor of continuous estrogen formation in endometriosis.

endometriosis, which is manifested by this subtle finding in the eutopic endometrium. We propose that when defective endometrium with low levels of aberrant aromatase expression reaches the pelvic peritoneum by retrograde menstruation, it causes an inflammatory reaction that exponentially increases local aromatase activity – i.e. estrogen formation – induced directly or indirectly by PG and cytokines.[22]

It would be rather naive to propose that aberrant aromatase expression is the only important molecular mechanism in the development and growth of pelvic endometriosis, as there may be many other molecular mechanisms that favor its development: abnormal expression of proteinase-type enzymes that remodel tissues or their inhibitors (matrix metalloproteinases, tissue inhibitor of metalloproteinase-1), certain cytokines (IL-6, RANTES), and growth factors (EGF) are some of these.[8-11] Alternatively, a defective immune system that fails to clear peritoneal surfaces of the retrograde menstrual efflux has been proposed in the development of endometriosis.[5,25] The development of endometriosis in an individual woman probably requires the coexistence of a threshold number of these aberrations. None the less, the clinical importance of aromatase expression pertains, as we were able to treat endometriosis using aromatase inhibitors.[26,27]

REGULATION OF AROMATASE EXPRESSION IN ENDOMETRIOTIC STROMAL CELLS

PGE_2 induces aromatase activity strikingly by increasing cAMP levels in endometriotic stromal cells.[22] On the other hand, neither cAMP analogs nor PGE_2 was capable of stimulating any detectable aromatase activity in eutopic endometrial stromal cells in culture. The obvious question was: what are the molecular differences that give rise to aromatase expression in endometriosis and its inhibition in eutopic endometrium? To address this, we first determined that the cAMP-inducible promoter II was used for in vivo aromatase expression in endometriotic tissue.[7] Then, a stimulatory transcription factor, SF-1, and an inhibitory factor, chicken ovalbumin upstream promoter transcription factor (COUP-TF), were found to compete for the same binding site in aromatase promoter II. COUP-TF was ubiquitously expressed in both eutopic endometrium and endometriosis, whereas SF-1 was expressed specifically in endometriosis but not in eutopic endometrium, and binds to aromatase promoter more avidly than COUP-TF.[7] Thus, SF-1 and other transcription factors (e.g. CREB) activate transcription in endometriosis, whereas COUP-TF, which occupies the same DNA site in eutopic endometrium, inhibits this process[7] (Figure 9.3). In summary, one of the molecular alterations leading to local aromatase expression

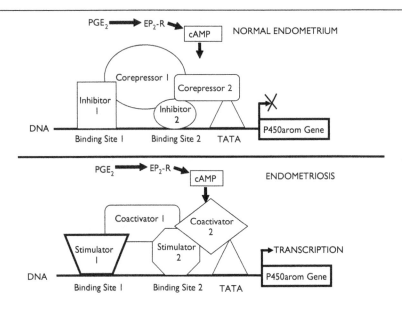

Figure 9.3 Molecular mechanism of aberrant aromatase expression in endometriosis. Normally, aromatase is not expressed in endometrium. Thus, there is no local estrogen formation. This is maintained by inhibitory proteins that bind to DNA in the promoter region of the *P450arom* gene. These inhibitory factors may directly bind to DNA in the promoter region (inhibitors 1 and 2), or may bind to transcription factors and repress their activities through protein–protein interactions (co-repressors 1 and 2). In endometriosis, however, the inhibitors and co-repressors are decreased or absent. Instead, they are replaced by aberrantly present proteins that bind to the *P450arom* promoter and activate its transcription. Again, these proteins either directly bind to DNA as classic transcription factors (stimulators 1 and 2) or interact with DNA-binding proteins and enhance their transcriptional activity (coactivators 1 and 2). PGE$_2$, prostaglandin E$_2$; EP$_2$-R, type 2 receptor for PGE$_2$; cAMP, cyclic adenosine monophosphate; P450arom, aromatase P450.

in endometriosis but not in normal endometrium is the aberrant production of SF-1 in endometriotic stromal cells, which overcomes the protective inhibition maintained normally by COUP-TF in the eutopic endometrium.

RATIONALE FOR TREATMENT OF ENDOMETRIOSIS WITH AROMATASE INHIBITORS

Endometriosis is successfully suppressed by estrogen deprivation with GnRH analogs or the induction of surgical menopause. Control of pelvic pain with GnRH agonists is usually successful during and immediately after the treatment, whereas pain associated with endometriosis returns in up to 75% of cases.[28,29] There may be many reasons for the failure of GnRH agonist treatment. One likely explanation is the presence of significant estradiol production that continues

in the adipose tissue, skin, and endometriotic implant per se during the GnRH agonist treatment (Figure 9.4). Therefore, blockage of aromatase activity in these extraovarian sites with an aromatase inhibitor may keep larger numbers of patients in remission for longer periods of time. The most striking evidence for the significance of extraovarian estrogen production is the recurrence of endometriosis after successfully completed hysterectomy and bilateral salpingo-oophorectomy in a number of women.[26,30] Endometriotic tissue in one such aggressive case was found to express much higher levels of aromatase mRNA than did premenopausal endometriosis.[26] We reported the treatment of a 57-year-old overweight woman who had recurrence of severe endometriosis after hysterectomy and bilateral salpingo-oophorectomy. Two additional laparotomies were performed owing to persistent severe pelvic pain and bilateral ureter-

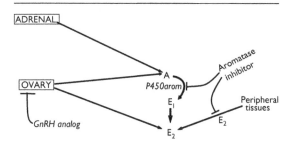

Figure 9.4 The role of aromatase inhibition in the treatment of endometriosis. Estrogen formation takes place via various mechanisms in endometriosis patients: (a) delivery from the ovary and peripheral tissues via circulation, and (b) local biosynthesis in endometriosis. GnRH analogs will eliminate estradiol secreted by the ovary by downregulating the hypothalamic–pituitary unit. In cases resistant to treatment with GnRH agonists or in postmenopausal endometriosis, the use of aromatase inhibitors to block estrogen formation in the peripheral tissues as well as in endometriotic stromal cells may be critical in controlling the growth of endometriosis.

al obstruction leading to left renal atrophy and right hydronephrosis. Treatment with megestrol acetate was ineffective. A large (3 cm) vaginal endometriotic lesion contained unusually high levels of aromatase mRNA. The patient was given anastrozole (an aromatase inhibitor) for 9 months. Despite the addition of calcium and alendronate (a non-steroidal inhibitor of bone resorption), bone density in the lumbar spine decreased by 6.2%. The occurrence of significant bone loss in this particular case should be studied further. Dramatic relief of the pain and regression of the vaginal endometriotic lesion were observed within the first month of treatment. At the same time, circulating estradiol levels were reduced to 50% of the baseline value. Markedly high pretreatment levels of aromatase mRNA in the endometriotic tissue became undetectable in a repeat biopsy 6 months later, and the lesion had almost disappeared after 9 months of therapy. Two potential mechanisms may have accounted for this strikingly successful result. First, there was evidence of suppression of peripheral (i.e. skin and adipose tissue) aromatase activity, giving rise to a significant decrease in serum estradiol level. Second, unusually high levels of aromatase expression in the endometriotic lesion

disappeared after treatment with the aromatase inhibitor anastrozole. Besides the expected direct inhibition of aromatase activity in endometriosis by anastrozole, the disappearance of aromatase mRNA expression in the lesion may be explicable by the denial of estrogen that is known to stimulate local biosynthesis of PGE_2, which in turn stimulates aromatase expression (see Figure 9.2).

A recent publication now shows that premenopausal women with endometriosis can be treated with a combination of an aromatase inhibitor and norethindrone acetate. These women previously had not responded to the existing surgical or medical treatments, which is exemplified by multiple recurrences or persistence of pain during the treatment. After a 6-month treatment with letrozole and norethindrone acetate the majority of them had pain relief and decreased laparoscopically detectable endometriosis.[27]

In conclusion, aromatase inhibitors may represent a new generation of medications for the treatment of endometriosis in the near future. Larger clinical trials are needed to address this question.

AKNOWLEDGEMENTS

The preparation of this chapter was supported in part by NIH grants HD38691 and TW01339.

REFERENCES

1. Vessey MP, Villard-Mackintosh L, Painter R. Epidemiology of endometriosis in women attending family planning clinics. Br Med J 1993;306:182–4.
2. Kjerulff KH, Erickson BA, Langenberg PW. Chronic gynecological conditions reported by US women: findings from the National Health Information Survey, 1984 to 1992. Am J Public Health 1996;86:195–9.
3. Olive DL, Schwartz LB. Endometriosis. N Engl J Med 1993;328:1759–69.
4. Sampson JA. Peritoneal endometriosis due to the menstrual dissemination of endometrial tissue into the peritoneal cavity. Am J Obstet Gynecol 1927;14:422–5.
5. Halme J, White C, Kauma S et al. Peritoneal macrophages from patients with endometriosis release growth factor activity in vitro. J Clin Endocrinol Metab 1988;66:1044–9.
6. Noble LS, Simpson ER, Johns A et al. Aromatase expression in endometriosis. J Clin Endocrinol Metab 1996;81:174–9.
7. Zeitoun K, Takayama K, Michael MD et al. Stimulation of aromatase P450 promoter (II) activity in endometriosis and its

inhibition in endometrium are regulated by competitive binding of SF-1 and COUP-TF to the same cis-acting element. Mol Endocrinol 1999;13:239–53.

8. Khorram O, Taylor RN, Ryan IP et al. Peritoneal fluid concentrations of the cytokine RANTES correlate with the severity of endometriosis. Am J Obstet Gynecol 1993;169:1545–9.

9. Sharpe-Timms KL, Penney LL, Zimmer RL et al. Partial purification and amino acid sequence analysis of endometriosis protein-II (ENDO-II) reveals homology with tissue inhibitor of metalloproteinases-1 (TIMP-1). J Clin Endocrinol Metab 1995;80:3784–7.

10. Bruner KL, Matrisian LM, Rodgers WH et al. Suppression of matrix metalloproteinases inhibits establishment of ectopic lesions by human endometrium in nude mice. J Clin Invest 1997;99:2851–7.

11 Osteen KG, Bruner KL, Sharpe-Timms KL. Steroid and growth factor regulation of matrix metalloproteinase expression and endometriosis. Semin Reprod Endocrinol 1996;15:301–8.

12 Zeitoun K et al. Deficient 17β-hydroxysteroid dehydrogenase type 2 expression in endometriosis: failure to metabolize estradiol-17β. J Clin Endocrinol Metab 1998;83:4474–80.

13 Michael MD, Michael LF, Simpson ER. A CRE-like sequence that binds CREB and contributes to cAMP-dependent regulation of the proximal promoter of the human aromatase P450 (CYP19) gene. Mol Cell Endocrinol 1997;134:147–56.

14 Michael MD, Kilgore MW, Morohashi KI et al. Ad4BP/SF-1 regulates cyclic AMP-induced transcription from the proximal promoter (PII) of the human aromatase P450 (CYP19) gene in the ovary. J Biol Chem 1995;270:13561–6.

15 Simpson ER, Mahendroo MS, Means GD et al. Aromatase cytochrome P450, the enzyme responsible for estrogen biosynthesis. Endocrinol Rev 1994;15:342–55.

16 Ackerman GE, Smith ME, Mendelson CR et al. Aromatization of androstenedione by human adipose tissue stromal cells in monolayer culture. J Clin Endocrinol Metab 1981;53:412–17.

17 MacDonald PC, Rombaut RP, Siiteri PK. Plasma precursors of estrogen. I. Extent of conversion of plasma Δ⁴-androstenedione to estrone in normal males and non-pregnant normal, castrate and adrenalectomized females. J Clin Endocrinol Metab 1967;27:1103–11.

18 MacDonald PC, Edman CD, Hemsell DL et al. Effect of obesity on conversion of plasma androstenedione to estrone in post-menopausal women with and without endometrial cancer. Am J Obstet Gynecol 1978;130:448–55.

19 Bulun SE, Price TM, Mahendroo MS et al. A link between breast cancer and local estrogen biosynthesis suggested by quantification of breast adipose tissue aromatase cytochrome P450 transcripts using competitive polymerase chain reaction after reverse transcription. J Clin Endocrinol Metab 1993;77:1622–8.

20 Yue W, Wang JP, Hamilton CJ et al. In situ aromatization enhances breast tumor estradiol levels and cellular proliferation. Cancer Res 1998;58:927–32.

21 Bulun SE, Simpson ER, Word RA. Expression of the CYP19 gene and its product aromatase cytochrome P450 in human leiomyoma tissues and cells in culture. J Clin Endocrinol Metab 1994;78:736–43.

22 Noble LS, Takayama K, Zeitoun KM et al. Prostaglandin E$_2$ stimulates aromatase expression in endometriosis-derived stromal cells. J Clin Endocrinol Metab 1997;82:600–6.

23 Bulun SE, Mahendroo MS, Simpson ER. Polymerase chain reaction amplification fails to detect aromatase cytochrome P450 transcripts in normal human endometrium or deciduas. J Clin Endocrinol Metab 1993;76:1458–63.

24 Huang JC, Dawood MY, Wu KK. Regulation of cyclooxygenase-2 gene in cultured endometrial stromal cells by sex steroids. Proc Am Soc Reprod Med Meeting S5, 1996 [abstract].

25 Hill JA. Immunology and endometriosis. Fertil Steril 1992;58:262–4.

26 Takayama K, Zeitoun K, Gunby RT et al. Treatment of severe postmenopausal endometriosis with an aromatase inhibitor. Fertil Steril 1998;69:709–13.

27 Ailawadi RK, Jobanputra S, Kataria M et al. Treatment of endometriosis and chronic pelvic pain with letrozole and norethindrone acetate: a pilot study. Fertil Steril 2003;81:290–6.

28 Henzl MR, Corson SL, Moghissi K et al. Administration of nasal nafarelin as compared with oral danazol for endometriosis. N Engl J Med 1988;318:485–9.

29 Waller KG, Shaw RW. Gonadotropin-releasing hormone analogues for the treatment of endometriosis: long-term follow-up. Fertil Steril 1993;59:511–15.

30 Metzger DA, Lessey BA, Soper JT et al. Hormone-resistant endometriosis following total abdominal hysterectomy and bilateral salpingo-oophorectomy: correlation with histology and steroid receptor content. Obstet Gynecol 1991;78:946–50.

10. Animal Models

Henrik Falconer, Jason M. Mwenda and Thomas M. D'Hooghe

INTRODUCTION

Endometriosis has been well described and known for over 50 years, yet our current knowledge of its pathogenesis, the pathophysiology of related infertility, and spontaneous evolution is still unclear. Current treatments for endometriosis, including surgery and medical treatment, are neither curative nor without side effects. Medical treatment (i.e. hormonal treatment) affects the menstrual cycle and compromises fertility potential. Side effects that are caused by the hypoestrogenic condition associated with medical treatment can be annoying and unhealthy (vasomotor flushes, vaginal dryness, osteoporosis, etc.). These circumstances call for further research in endometriosis and for the development of new treatment and diagnostic tools.

Although endometriosis can be diagnosed by laparoscopy, there are several reasons why research in the field of endometriosis has not been as successful as one might expect. Two of the main reasons are poor study design, and the fact that at the time of diagnosis the duration of disease is unknown. The latter makes it particularly difficult to perform studies to determine the onset, etiology, or progression of the disease.[1] Study design is always a crucial matter in clinical research and in multifactorial diseases such as endometriosis, and adequate control groups are difficult to define. Finally, for ethical reasons it is difficult to carry out invasive studies in humans. For these reasons, alternative models for endometriosis research have been developed.

Both rodents and non-human primates have extensively been used in endometriosis research. It is obvious that a close phylogenetic relationship between animal and human is preferred. Even if it is possible to study certain aspects of a disease in rodents, it is not certain whether these findings can be transferred to humans. The use of primates has made it possible to induce endometriosis, with lesions similar to those seen in humans. This is important for research purposes, as spontaneous endometriosis in primates is most commonly minimal to mild. The ability to induce moderate to severe disease is crucial for the study of pathogenesis, endometriosis-associated subfertility, and drug effects. Endometriosis research in animal models has addressed most aspects of the disease, including pathogenesis, infertility, and the effects of new drugs.

SMALL ANIMALS

Several groups in endometriosis research have used rodent models (Table 10.1). The advantages of using rodents rather than primates are the low cost and ease of maintenance. However, these benefits probably do not make up for the disadvantages. The most important drawbacks are that rodents lack a menstrual cycle and do not have spontaneous endometriosis. The rat has spontaneous ovulation but its luteal phase is shorter than in humans, and the rabbit lacks a luteal phase. To study endometriosis in rodents, the disease must invariably be induced. Induced endometriosis in rodents differs significantly from the disease in humans, with rodents developing more cystic lesions that do not have the rich variations of appearance that can be seen in primates.

Rats, rabbits and hamsters have been used as models for induction of endometriosis. The disease has been induced using both auto- and xenotransplants. Autologous transplants have been performed in rabbits,[2] rats,[3] and hamsters[4] using uterine tissue removed at minilaparotomy. Syngenic mice have been used in the same fashion.[7]

Table 10.1 Rodents in endometriosis research (list not complete)

Rat	Hamster	Rabbit	Immunocompetent mice	Immunodeficient mice*
Jones 1984	Steinleitner et al. 1991	Jacobsen 1926	Cummings and Metcalf 1995	Zamah et al. 1984
Vernon and Wilson 1985		Weinstein et al. 1940	Rossi et al. 2000	Bergqvist et al. 1985
Golan et al. 1986		Levander and Norrman 1955		Bruner et al. 1997
Rajkumar et al. 1990		Merrill 1965		Awwad et al. 1999
Scharpe et al. 1991		Schenken and Asch1980		Nisolle et al. 2000
Barragan et al. 1992		Hahn et al. 1985		Somigliana et al. 200
Uchiide et al. 2002		Donnez et al. 1987		Fang et al. 2002
		Dunselman et al. 1989		Beliard et al. 2003
	Kaplan et al. 1989	Hull et al. 2003		

* Nude athymic mice or SCID mice

This non-physiological method of induction has caused several problems, such as adhesions interfering with fertility. The development of nude mice and SCID (severe combined immuno-deficiency) has made it possible to successfully implant human endometrium, thereby making it a more attractive model for the study of endo-metriosis. The endometrium can be obtained during surgery for benign conditions, or from simple uterine biopsies at any point of the men-strual cycle. The endometrium has then been implanted either at minilaparotomy,[5] subcuta-neously,[6] or after intraperitoneal inoculation.[7] Prior hormonal treatment of the implants may significantly increase the number of animals developing endometriosis according to some[8] (but not all[9,10]) investigators.

PATHOGENESIS

Among the more interesting studies in rodent models are the study of implantation of human endometrium and the progression of the disease in this model.[5] Studies of biopsied transplants in nude mice suggest that stromal cells are involved in the attachment process and that glandular cells contribute to the growth of endometriotic lesions. This was confirmed in the rat model,

showing infiltration of inflammatory cells in the stromal component of an autotransplant.[11] A study in normal immunocompetent mice demon-strated the dynamic aspects of endometriosis, with an initial decrease in endometriotic lesions followed by an increase.[12] The same authors reported that progression of the disease is dependent on intact ovarian function, whereas endometrial implantation on to the peritoneum is not. The cyclic expression of matrix metallo-proteinases (MMP) by human endometrium has been suggested to play a role in the invasive process necessary to establish endometriosis. In the SCID mouse model, suppression of steroid-regulated endometrial matrix metalloproteinases (MMP) inhibits the establishment of experimen-tal endometriosis.[13] Similar studies in nude mice showed that either eutopic or ectopic tissue from women with endometriosis exhibit patterns of altered MMP regulation in vivo.[14] In a nude mouse model, ectopic adhesion of endometrial cells to the peritoneum and the formation of endometriotic-like lesions were shown to involve the cooperation of epithelial and stromal cells through the secretion of growth factors, cytokines, and/or chemokines.[15] The progression of endometriosis is dependent on estrogen activ-ity, and the role of aromatase P450, the key enzyme for biosynthesis of estrogen, was investigated in transgenic mice. The authors concluded that an intact *P450arom* gene is essential for the growth of endometriotic lesions,[16] again supporting the crucial role of estrogen in the progression of endometriosis.

INFLAMMATORY RESPONSE AND IMMUNOLOGY

Recently, much of the attention in endometriosis research has been focused on the inflammatory response and immunology. Rock and Markham[17] hypothesized in 1992 that immunological factors may play an important role in pathogenesis. Several cytokines have been shown to be increased in women with endometriosis.[20] IL-8 and TNF-α from PF-derived macrophages promote endometrial cell proliferation, endometrial adhesion, and neoangiogenesis.[18–21] Furthermore, TNF-α and IL-1 from endometriotic lesions and mesothelial cells stimulates the production of IL-8 and RANTES, which in turn promote neoangiogenesis and the recruitment of macrophages, T cells, and eosinophils.[22–24] Other important pathogenic factors, such as turnover of MMP and neoangiogenesis, are also regulated by cytokines.[25]

Activation of the immune system in endometriosis has been demonstrated in rodents, both directly and indirectly through drugs modulating the immune system. Somigliana and coworkers used immunocompetent rats to demonstrate that interleukin-12 (IL-12) could reduce the total weight and surface area of experimentally induced endometriosis.[7] IL-12 is a proinflammatory cytokine that induces the production of interferon-γ and favors the differentiation of T-helper 1 (Th1) cells.[26] Transgenic mice offer the possibility of altering specific parts of the immune system by knocking out certain genes. β_2-Microglobulin (β_2M) is essential for the normal expression of major histocompatibility class I proteins, which are important for the maturation of T cells.[27] Using knockout mice deficient in either β_2M or IL-12, Somigliana et al reported reduced endo lesions in the former and increased

lesions in the latter.[28] The results from the IL-12-deficient group were not statistically significant but may support the previous study on IL-12 in endometriosis.[7] Furthermore, loxoribine, a powerful immunomodulatory drug that activates natural killer (NK) cells, was shown to reduce both epithelial and stromal components in rats with induced endometriosis.[29] Steinleitner et al assessed the effect of verapamil, a calcium channel-blocking agent known to inhibit macrophage activation, on reproduction in golden hamsters with autografted endometrium from the right uterine horn.[4] In treated animals the reproductive outcome was significantly better than in controls. Similar results were reported using the same model, but instead testing pentoxifylline,[30] a drug that affects the function of activated neutrophils and inhibits the synthesis of TNF-α.[31]

The role of cellular immunity, especially impaired NK-cell activity, is debated. Although studies in humans and non-human primates are somehow contradictory, studies in rodents seem to favor the hypothesis of decreased NK-cell activity in the pathogenesis of endometriosis. Using autograft splenocyte transplants, Ota and colleagues reported less NK-cell activity in experimentally induced endometriosis than in controls.[32] Interferon (IFN)-α_{2b}, used for the treatment of hepatitis C in humans, possesses both antiviral and immune-modifying properties, the latter by enhancing the activation of cytolytic T cells.[33] Rats with induced endometriosis were given IFN-α_{2b} either intraperitoneally or subcutaneously, with equal long-term results.[34] The drug was demonstrated to reduce the size of endometriotic lesions in the animals.

The results from these studies support the critical role of immunology in the pathogenesis of endometriosis, and future treatment could be directed against the immune system, although further studies are warranted in non-human primates and humans.

DRUG EFFECTS

The rodent model has been used extensively to study the efficacy of various drug treatments for endometriosis. All of the suppressing drugs in use, including GnRH analogs, danazol, and progesterone have been evaluated in rodents. In 1985, Hahn et al[35] reported that GnrRH analogs and danazol reduce the extent of endometriotic lesions in a rabbit model. However, recurrence was demonstrated in a rat model within 4[36] or 8 weeks after cessation of the drugs.[37] GnRH agonists reduced the extent of endometriosis, but merely acted as suppressive drugs without curative effect, a fact well known when treating endometriosis with GnRH agonists in women.

Only a few investigators have studied the treatment of endometriosis-associated infertility in rodents. Intraperitoneal injection of indomethacin in infertile rats with induced endometriosis has been reported to be more effective in restoring fertility and in reducing adhesions than have diathermy or danazol.[38] As mentioned previously, drugs that suppress macrophage activity (verapamil, pentoxifylline) may have a positive effect on endometriosis-associated subfertility.[4,17]

Promising new drugs in the treatment of endometriosis include antiprogestins such as onapristone, which has been reported to have antiproliferative properties on induced endometriosis in rats.[39] Recently, the anti-inflammatory agent TNF-α inhibitor has been demonstrated to reduce the extent of established endometriosis in rats.[40] Thiazolidimdiones (TZD), anti-inflammatory compounds currently under investigation for the treatment of inflammatory bowel disease and rheumatoid arthritis, can reduce macrophage activity in a mouse model.[41] Neoangiogenesis plays a crucial role in the implantation of ectopic endometrium to the peritoneum, and it has been reported recently that antiangiogenetic agents inhibited the growth of endometriotic lesions in nude mice xenografted with human endometrium.[42] The role of MMP has been discussed previously and an MMP inhibitor was found to reduce adenomyosis in a mouse model with experimentally induced endometriosis.[43] Most of these new immunomodulatory drugs, except for TNF-α blocking agents, have not yet been evaluated in non-human primates or women with endometriosis.

FERTILITY

In rabbits with induced endometriosis, impaired fertility has been reported by some[2,44–46] but not all investigators.[47–49] In 1980 Schenken and Asch[2] reported a 25% fertility rate in eight rabbits with induced endometriosis, which was lower than the 75% fertility rate in eight control animals. Minimal ovarian endometriosis induced in the rabbit[46] impaired ovulation, primarily through a mechanism related to periovarian adhesions. In contrast, other investigators have shown a 53% reduction in the fertility rate of rabbits with induced endometriosis, independent of adhesion formation.[44] Experiments with induced endometriosis in rabbits all suggest that adhesion formation may be a major factor interfering with fertility, although other factors are also likely to be involved. In a rabbit model with adhesion-free induced endometriosis[10] no differences were found between induction and control groups in the number of corpora lutea, the recovery rate of oocytes, the fertilization rate, the transport of fertilized ova,[47] the embryogenic cleavage stage 24 hours after mating, and the subsequent embryo development in vitro.[48,49] Although some investigators reported a normal fertility rate in rats with induced endometriosis,[50] others[3,38,51] demonstrated an impaired fecundity in these rodents. It cannot be excluded that, as in rabbits, surgically induced adhesions rather than ectopic endometrium may impair fertility in rats with experimental endometriosis. This also suggests that the induction of endometriosis in rodents introduces a major bias into the interpretation of study results.

CONCLUSION

Although several findings in human and non-human primate research have been supported in rodent models of endometriosis, it is still doubtful how representative these models are for the human disease.

Because of the lack of a menstrual cycle, the absence of spontaneous endometriosis, and the wide phylogenetic gap between rodents and humans, extrapolation of rodent data to the human situation remains difficult. Immuno-deficient mice (athymic, SCID) used for xeno-grafting human endometrium are likely to be a better model. However, detailed immunohisto-chemical analyses are required in order to rule out the bias caused by manipulation of the immune system in these mice. The multifactorial pathogenesis behind endometriosis demands a model more similar to humans than rodents.

NON-HUMAN PRIMATES

Non-human primate studies have been carried out using several species, including rhesus macaques, cynomolgus monkeys, and baboons (Table 10.2). The great apes (chimpanzee, gorilla, orang utang) are closest to humans in many anatomical and physiological aspects of repro-duction. However, as all of them are protected, endangered species in the wild, they cannot be used for endometriosis research.

Primates develop spontaneous disease and endometriosis has been reported in over 10 dif-ferent primate species. Not all of them are suitable as animal models for endometriosis research, and because of the specific demands, the baboon has been developed at the Institute of Primate Research, Nairobi, Kenya, as a model for

the study of endometriosis. The advantages of the baboon model will be addressed below.

GENETICS

As stated previously, the closer phylogenetic rela-tionship between non-human primates and humans makes them more attractive as models for endometriosis research than rodents. Many of the similarities among primate species are obvi-ous at the gross anatomical, physiological, and behavioral level, but only in recent decades has it become possible to quantify the underlying genetic basis of those similarities. Each of the 46 human chromosomes has a recognizable counterpart in the great apes, except for chromo-some 2. Baboons and rhesus monkeys have 42 diploid chromosomes, and their banding pat-terns reveal almost complete correspondence with those of human chromosomes.[52,53] Early works in immunogenetics[54] showed that non-human primates have a cluster of genes highly similar to the human major histocompatibility complex (MHC). MHC plays a central role in evoking the immune response to various types of antigen, making these similarities crucial when studying immunological response in non-human primates. Another example of the genetic similar-ities between humans and non-human primates is the fact that many proteins of non-human

---

Table 10.2 Non-human primates in endometriosis research (list not complete)

Rhesus monkey (*Macaca mulatta*)	Cynomolgus monkey (*Macaca fascicularis*)	Baboon (*Papio cynocephalus, Papio anubis*)
Jacobson 1926	DiZerega et al. 1980	D'Hoogeh et al. 1991
TeLinde and Scott 1950	Fanton and Hubbard 1983	Fazleabas et al. 2002
Dmowski et al. 1980	Schenken 1984	Dick et al. 2003
Werlin and Hodgen 1983		
Mann et al. 1986		
Hadfield et al. 1987		
Rier et al. 2001		
Zondervan et al. 2002		

primates have amino acid sequences that are 95–99% identical to sequences of homologous human proteins.[55] These genetic similarities contribute to the previously mentioned advantages of using non-human primates in endometriosis research. Moreover, it is possible to keep environmental factors constant and generate half-sibships in quite large numbers for some species.[56] These factors make it possible to study certain genetic aspects that cannot easily be studied in humans.

STUDIES IN NON-BABOON SPECIES

The prevalence of spontaneous endometriosis has recently been studied in rhesus monkeys from the Wisconsin National Primate Center. In a colony necropsied between 1981 and 2001, the prevalence was reported to be 31.4%.[57] Furthermore, increased prevalence with increasing age was demonstrated, as well as familial aggregation of endometriosis. Risk factors for the development of spontaneous endometriosis were studied in a case–control study using necropsy material from the same colony.[58] The authors reported that exposure to three or more estradiol implants or to one or two hysterotomies both significantly increased the risk of developing the disease. Exposure to one or more laparoscopies did not increase the risk for the development of endometriosis.[58]

Most endometriosis research in non-baboon species has been conducted in primates with induced disease. The first studies on inducing endometriosis in rhesus monkeys were carried out by Jacobson in 1926.[59] In this study, minced endometrial tissue was obtained after hysterotomy of the anterior uterine wall and was sown in the abdomen, or placed beneath the peritoneum in a few specific locations. This method resulted in implantation of endometrium on the surface of the uterus and adhesions in four animals, as documented by autopsy and pathological examination performed 9–12 months later. A new method for the induction of endometriosis was designed by Te Linde and Scott in 1950,[60] and involved the repositioning of the cervix into the abdominal cavity, thereby allowing intra-abdominal menstruation. This method was successful in five out of 10 rhesus monkeys, and endometriosis was evident 185–963 days after the induction. These results have been supported in several similar studies on the rhesus monkey. Endometriosis has also been successfully induced in the cynomolgus monkey.[61]

Several aspects of the disease have been studied in rhesus and cynomolgus monkeys. In the latter, the natural history of induced endometriosis was studied, and a tendency towards spontaneous disease progression was observed in non-pregnant monkeys.[61] After pregnancy, monkeys with minimal and mild disease had complete regression of macroscopic disease. Immunological aspects of the disease were studied in rhesus monkeys, and a reduced cellular immune response in vitro after intradermal injection of endometrial cells has been reported.[62] The influence of endometriosis on fertility was studied in cynomolgus monkeys with induced endometriosis; chemical and term pregnancy rates were lower in animals with moderate to severe disease compared to control animals.[63]

The impact of environmental effects on the pathogenesis has received attention during the last 10 years. Rier et al reported in 1993 that rhesus monkeys exposed to dioxins developed endometriosis, with incidence and severity being related to dose.[64] This study has been followed by three experiments in non-human primates, two using rhesus monkeys[65,66] and one using cynomolgus monkeys.[67] The relationship between dioxin exposure and endometriosis has not yet been accepted by the scientific research community, as some studies have failed to support the link.[65] The four studies in non-human primates, together with seven human epidemiological studies, have been extensively reviewed by Guo.[68] The value of the initial study by Rier et al[64] was considered to be limited with respect to power, study design, statistical analysis, and bias of confounding variables. As the material from this study was used again by Rier et al in 2001,[66] the same weaknesses apply to this study as well.[68] Arnold et al[65] could not reproduce the results of Rier et al, and the study by Yang et al[67] was not designed to examine the effects of dioxins as a causative factor in endometriosis. Epidemiological studies in humans seem to suffer from difficulties in defining cases and controls, and the odds ratio for the studies combined is likely to be close to 1.[68] In conclusion, there is very little in support of dioxins as causative agents of endometriosis.

Several studies on drug effects have been carried out in the primate model. GnRH agonists have been reported to be successful in reducing the degree of disease.[69,70] In monkeys treated with GnRH analogs and/or progesterone antagonists, all treatments reduced the extent of endometriosis but during antiprogestin treatment normal estradiol levels were maintained, suggesting that long-term treatment may be possible without the negative consequences of hypoestrogenism (i.e. reduced bone mass).[71] Still, antiprogestins remain a hormonal treatment with a considerable effect on the menstrual cycle and fertility potential.

THE BABOON AS A MODEL FOR ENDOMETRIOSIS RESEARCH

In the last 10–12 years the baboon has become the most widely used non-human primate model, and has been developed at the Institute of Primate Research, Nairobi, Kenya. The suitability of the baboon as a model in endometriosis research is due to a number of factors. First, baboons adapt well to captivity, with maintained menstrual cycling and fertility. Second, the menstrual cycle of the baboon is very similar to that of humans, generally given to be 31–34 days, with a range of between 20 and 50 days.[72] Third, the baboon shows a cyclic inflation and deflation of the perineal skin, enabling non-invasive follow-up of menstruation, follicular, and luteal phases. Fourth, adult female baboons weigh about 10–20 kg, a size that allows repeated blood sampling and the performance of complicated surgical procedures.[73] Fifth, transcervical curettage in the baboon does not differ significantly from the procedure in humans. The cervical channel of the baboon mimics that of the human, except for size.

The rhesus macaque, on the other hand, has a spiral-shaped channel, which makes it difficult to perform transcervical procedures. The endometriotic lesions in the baboon, both spontaneous and induced, mimic the lesions in humans, both in sense of shape and form as well as in location. This, together with the advantages shared with other non-human primates (genetics, spontaneous disease), makes the baboon the current gold standard for endometriosis research.

SPONTANEOUS AND INDUCED ENDOMETRIOSIS

In 1991, D'Hooghe et al,[74] in a pioneer experiment, observed spontaneous endometriotic lesions on the uterosacral ligaments and in the pouch of Douglas (46%), on the uterine peritoneum and the uterovesical fold (38%), and on uterine–omental adhesions (11%). The prevalence of endometriosis in baboons with proven fertility was reported to be 25%. Captivity has been reported to affect the development of spontaneous endometriosis,[75] although this could be subject to other factors apart from captivity per se (increased age, increased exposure to retrograde menstruation due to higher number of menstrual cycles uninterrupted by pregnancies). Ovarian involvement in the baboon has been found to be rare,[74,76] but has been reported in advanced disseminated endometriosis[77] and in one animal treated with high-dose azathioprine.[78] This fact has been considered one of the few disadvantages with the baboon model. The reason for the lack of ovarian endometriosis in baboons is unknown, but it has been speculated that the pathogenesis of ovarian endometriosis differs from that of the more common peritoneal disease. However, Dick et al[79] recently reported different data from the large baboon colony of Southwest National Regional Primate Research Center in San Antonio, USA. The authors reported 37% ovarian endometriosis in 43 baboons over a 14-year period, concluding that ovarian endometriosis was common in this particular colony. It was suggested that these high figures were due to genetic or husbandry differences between the colonies in USA and Kenya.

However, it is important to point out some of the differences with this study. First, Dick et al did not use laparoscopy to diagnose endometriosis, and all ovarian endometriosis was diagnosed at necropsy. Second, theirs was a retrospective study of pathology records, with some uncertainties regarding method of diagnosis. Third, the prevalence of endometriosis was remarkably low (43 cases out of 2926 reviewed records: 1.5%), suggesting that less advanced disease was undiagnosed. Fourth, almost half of the cases had disseminated disease, and only three cases of ovarian disease were found in localized endometriosis, a clinical entity not described by the authors. With this in mind, it is doubtful whether these results can be applied to the common presentation of endometriosis in baboons. Until further studies support Dick et al's findings, ovarian endometriosis should be considered rare in baboons.

The method of inducing endometriosis in baboons was described by D'Hooghe et al in 1995.[76] Endometrium was obtained either by transcervical curettage or at laparotomy (transfundal curettage). The endometrium was injected retroperitoneally or intraperitoneally, and the animals were followed using laparoscopy. The number, surface area, and volume of the endometriotic lesions and adhesions were measured to allow calculation of the rAFS score and stage according to the revised classification system of the American Society for Reproductive Medicine.[80] The authors concluded that intraperitoneal seeding of menstrual endometrium was more successful in inducing endometriotic lesions than retroperitoneal injection of either menstrual or luteal endometrium. The standard method of inducing endometriosis in the baboon is now to seed endometrial tissue, obtained through transcervical curettage, into the pelvic area using a transabdominal needle under laparoscopic vision.

PATHOGENESIS

Understanding the natural history of endometriosis is vital for further development in the field of endometriosis research. During repeated laparoscopies in baboons, D'Hooghe et al found that endometriosis is a dynamic process that undergoes periods of regression but which is ultimately progressive.[81] The remodeling, defined by the transition of lesions between typical, subtle, and suspicious implants, was observed in 23% of lesions. This work is important as it explains the clinical alterations that many patients experience, and also shows that endometriosis does not resolve spontaneously. A cornerstone in the pathogenesis of endometriosis is the Sampson theory of retrograde menstruation.[82] Thus, it has been considered highly important to present experimental data supporting the Sampson theory. Studies on retrograde menstruation in the baboon showed a prevalence of 83% in animals with endometriosis.[83] In humans, the prevalence has been found to be 76–90%.[84,85] Furthermore, retrograde menstruation was found to be more common in baboons with spontaneous endometriosis (83%) compared to animals with a normal pelvis (51%). In a series of experiments, the cervical channel in baboons was occluded using three different methods: insertion of silicone, electrocoagulation plus cervical suturing, and supracervical ligation.[86]

Endometriosis was found within 3 months in all baboons of the last group. These results, together with the experimental induction of endometriosis, support the Sampson theory of retrograde menstruation in the pathogenesis of endometriosis.

The effect of pregnancy on endometriosis is debated. Traditionally, endometriosis has been said to undergo regression during pregnancy. However, some investigators have reported the enlargement of endometriotic lesions during the first trimester and regression during the remainder of pregnancy.[87] More recent studies in baboons contradict these results, showing that pregnancy did not have significant effect on endometriosis during the first and second trimesters.[88]

In a recent study[89] the hypothesis that menstruation and the intrapelvic injection of endometrium affect inflammatory parameters in peritoneal fluid was tested in baboons. During menstruation, a significant increase occurred in the peritoneal fluid (PF) WBC concentration, the proportion of PF cells staining positive for TNF-α, TGF-β_1, and ICAM-1, and the PF concentration of TGF-β_1 and IL-6, compared to the follicular or luteal phase of the cycle. After intrapelvic injection of endometrium a significant increase was also found in PF WBC concentration, and in the proportion of PF cells staining positive for TNF-α, TGF-β_1, CD3, and HLA-DR. In summary, these data suggest that subclinical peritoneal inflammation occurs in baboons during menstruation and after the intrapelvic injection of endometrium. Recently, the phenomenon of subclinical peritoneal inflammation has also been described during menstruation in women.[90]

In women, endometrial expression of matrix metalloproteinases (MMP-3, MMP-7, and MMP-11) occurs during menstrual breakdown and during subsequent estrogen-mediated endometrial growth, but not during the secretory phase.[91] The cellular mechanisms required for the establishment of ectopic endometrial growth represent invasive events similar to those observed in cancer metastasis, and involve extensive degradation of the extracellular matrix.[92] In baboons with induced endometriosis, MMP-7 has been reported to regulate the invasion of endometrial tissue into the peritoneum.[93]

IMMUNOLOGY

Obviously, the Sampson theory is not sufficient to explain the full pathogenesis of endometriosis. As mentioned earlier, the prevalence of retrograde menstruation is higher than the prevalence of the disease. The role of the immune system was discussed in the rodent section, and in support of this, changes in white blood cell (WBC) population have been noted in women with endometriosis.[94-98] However, it is unclear whether these observations should be considered the cause or the consequence of endometriosis. This aspect is difficult to study in women, as most patients with pain, infertility, and endometriosis have had the disease for some time at the time of diagnosis.[1,99]

In baboons, the percentages of PB WBC subsets, determined by mouse antihuman monoclonal antibodies CD2, CD4, CD8, CD11B, CD20, and CD68, are comparable to those reported in humans, showing that WBC subsets in baboons can be analyzed with commercially available monoclonal antibodies.[100] In a previous study, the hypothesis was tested that PB and PF WBC populations are altered in baboons with spontaneous and induced endometriosis compared to animals without disease.[100] In peripheral blood, the percentage of CD4+ and IL-2 receptor-positive cells was increased in baboons with stages II–IV spontaneous or induced endometriosis, suggesting that alterations in PB WBC populations may be an effect of endometriosis. In PF the WBC concentration and percentages of CD68++ macrophages and CD8+ lymphocytes were only increased in baboons with spontaneous endometriosis and not in animals with induced disease, suggesting that alterations in PF WBC populations may lead to the development of endometriosis.[1,98,100]

The implantation of endometrial cells is dependent on several factors, such as neoangiogenesis and potentially decreased natural killer (NK) cell cytotoxicity.[101] D'Hooghe and colleagues[102] reported no difference in lymphocyte-mediated cytotoxicity and NK-cell activity between baboons with and without endometriosis, and the hypothesis of decreased clearance of endometrial cells due to reduced NK-cell activity was unsupported.

If endometriosis is a consequence of impaired function of the immune system, the use of immunosuppressive drugs would increase the size of lesions and possibly facilitate implantation. This was marginally demonstrated in baboons with spontaneous disease, treated with either methylprednisolone or azathioprine in high doses.[78] However, these findings did not apply to animals with induced disease, and therefore the hypothesis that endometriosis is caused by impaired immunity is not sufficiently supported by non-human primate data.

In summary, these two studies suggest that endometriosis may activate the immune/inflammatory system, but studies on the baboon model have not been able to support the theory[103] that endometriosis may result from decreased clearance of endometrial cells owing to reduced macrophage/natural killer cell activity.

DRUG EFFECTS

Considering the results emerging from studies in the baboon model, the baboon is likely to be the preferred model for future drug studies. The technique of inducing endometriosis allows the possibility of both prevention and treatment studies. In the former type the drug is given at the time of induction, and differences in endometriosis development between drug and control group can be assessed at follow-up laparoscopy. In treatment studies the drug is given to animals with already induced endometriosis, thereby making it possible to see the effects on established disease.

New promising compounds for the treatment of endometriosis include MMP inhibitors, antiangionetics, and anti-inflammatory drugs. So far, the only drug-effect study in the baboon model is a preliminary one on recombinant human tumor necrosis factor (TNF)-α-binding protein-1 (r-hTBP-1).[104] Fourteen baboons with induced endometriosis were randomized to TBP, a GnRH antagonist, or placebo. In both treatment groups the progression of endometriosis was partially inhibited, with a complete absence of endometriosis-associated adhesions. Furthermore, treatment with TBP did not result in inhibition of the follicular phase, ovulation, and/or menstruation. The result suggests a transition in medical treatment from hormonal suppression of endometriotic lesions to selective anti-inflammatory inhibition with maintenance of fertility potential.

FERTILITY

Endometriosis has clinically been associated with impaired fertility, and recent studies in humans show that endometriosis occurs in 30–40% of infertile women.[105] However, a causal relationship between endometriosis and infertility has been difficult to establish. Apart from a more obvious mechanism of endometriosis-associated adhesions in severe disease, minimal endometriosis is believed to affect fertility by ovulatory dysfunction,[106] or maybe through the luteinized unruptured follicle syndrome (LUF).[107] However, in baboons, minimal endometriosis appears not to be associated with infertility and could be a physiological phenomenon caused by cyclic retrograde menstruation.[108] In contrast, mild to severe disease is clearly associated with infertility, even in the absence of ovarian endometriotic cysts.[109]

Although the clinical definition of LUF is controversial,[1,62,110] studies in baboons suggest that repetitive LUF syndrome may be a cause of endometriosis-associated subfertility in baboons with mild endometriosis.[111]

The baboon model offers several advantages in fertility studies. First, trials can be standardized for the degree of disease (after the induction of endometriosis). Second, the presence of ovulation can be detected based on the perineal cycle. Third, timed intercourse with a male baboon of proven fertility is possible by behavioral observation and postcoital testing.[99,109]

CONCLUSION

Even though most of the studies in primates have been carried out on induced endometriosis, which differs somewhat from spontaneous disease, primate research offers an exclusive model for the study of endometriosis. The method of inducing endometriosis simplifies prospective placebo-controlled drug studies, which is, considering today's drug arsenal, a necessity in the development of successful treatments for endometriosis. With respect to the extrapolation of results from animal studies to humans, primates are definitely superior to rodents. Among primates, the baboon seems to be best suited for experimental studies.

OTHER ANIMAL MODELS

Few other animals have been used in endometriosis research; however, a chicken embryo chorioallantoic membrane (CAM) model has recently been used. It was demonstrated that human endometrial cells, after 3 days of incubation, could form endometriotic lesions in the mesenchymal layer of the CAM.[112] The importance of tissue integrity in the implantation of human endometrium in ectopic locations was demonstrated in the CAM model.[113] Tissue from stage III and IV ovarian endometriomas implanted in CAM expressed upregulated MMP-2 and MMP-9 mRNA compared to normal endometrium.[114] Implants from stage IV endometriomas also induced a more intense vasoproliferative response than those from stage III, whereas no vasoproliferative response was induced by the normal endometrium. The authors concluded that angiogenesis and the degradation of extracellular matrix occur together in endometriosis, and are more pronounced in severe endometriosis.[114]

FUTURE OF RESEARCH IN ENDOMETRIOSIS

Future research in endometriosis should continue to focus on pathogenesis, early interactions between endometrial and peritoneal cells in the pelvic cavity at the time of menstruation, and the development of new drugs for the treatment of endometriosis with associated infertility. For reasons discussed in this chapter, research should be conducted in non-human primate models, with special focus on the baboon model. More integration is needed between the areas of epidemiology and genetics, and important questions remain regarding the relationship between endometriosis and environmental factors. Pelvic inflammation in women with endometriosis could be the target for new diagnostic and therapeutic approaches. Systemic and extrapelvic manifestations of endometriosis must be analyzed carefully, and better tools are needed to measure quality of life in women with chronic pain caused by endometriosis.[115]

ETHICS OF PRIMATE RESEARCH IN THE AREA OF ENDOMETRIOSIS AND REPRODUCTION

Obviously, many important data would not be available if research was possible only in rodents or humans. Although the risks with modern laparoscopy are limited, repeated surgery for research purposes cannot be considered ethical in humans. In view of the ongoing debate on animal research, the importance of good animal care and high quality of study design must not be overlooked. The availability of well educated animal technicians, proper housing, and good anesthesia is vital for further development in animal models. Researchers should become more aware of the validation of animal models and participate more actively in the ethical discussion regarding the use of non-human primates in medical research. Most approaches for reproductive research in non-human primates in primate studies do not differ significantly from those in humans, but unfortunately this is not publicly known. It is of great importance to communicate correct information about modern primate research to the general public and to the media, and this should be the responsibility of those involved in non-human primate research. Only this way can patients and the public be assured about the scientific value and the high ethical standards used for reproductive research in non-human primates.

REFERENCES

1. D'Hooghe TM. Clinical relevance of the baboon as a model for the study of endometriosis. Fertil Steril 1997;68:613–25.
2. Schenken RS, Asch RH. Surgical induction of endometriosis in the rabbit: effects on fertility and concentrations of peritoneal fluid prostaglandins. Fertil Steril 1980;34:581–7.
3. Vernon MW, Wilson EA. Studies on the surgical induction of endometriosis in the rat. Fertil Steril 1985;44:684–94.
4. Steinleitner A, Lambert H, Suarez M et al. Periovulatory calcium channel blockade enhances reproductive performance in an animal model for endometriosis-associated subfertility. Fertil Steril 1991;55:26–31.
5. Nisolle M, Casanas-Roux F, Donnez J. Early-stage endometriosis: adhesion and growth of human menstrual endometrium in nude mice. Fertil Steril 2000;74:306–12.
6. Zamah NM, Dodson MG, Stephens LC et al. Transplantation of normal and ectopic human endometrial tissue into athymic nude mice. Am J Obstet Gynecol 1984;149:591–7.
7. Somigliana E, Vigano P, Rossi G et al. Endometrial ability to implant in ectopic sites can be prevented by interleukin-12 in a murine model of endometriosis. Hum Reprod 1999;14:2944–50.
8. Beliard A, Noël A, Goffin F et al. Role of endocrine status and cell type in adhesion of human endometrial cells to the peritoneum in nude mice. Fertil Steril 2002;78:973–8.

9. Hahn DW, Carraher RP, Foldesy RG et al. Development of an animal model for evaluating effects of drugs on endometriosis. Fertil Steril 1985;44:410–15.

10. Dunselman GAJ, Willebrand D, Land JA et al. A rabbit model for endometriosis. Gynecol Obstet Invest 1989;27:29–33.

11. Uchiide I, Ihara. T, Sugamata M. Pathological evaluation of the rat endometriosis model. Fertil Steril 2002;78:782–6.

12. Rossi G, Somigliana E, Moschetta M et al. Dynamic aspects of endometriosis in a mouse model through analysis of implantation and progression. Arch Gynecol Obstet 2000;263:102–7.

13. Bruner KL, Matrisian LM, Rodgers WH et al. Suppression of matrix metalloproteinases inhibits establishment of ectopic lesions by human endometrium in nude mice. J Clin Invest 1997;99: 2851–7.

14. Bruner-Tran KL, Eisenberg E, Yeaman GR et al. Steroid and cytokine regulation of matrix metalloproteinase expression in endometriosis and the establishment of experimental endometriosis in nude mice. J Clin Endocrinol Metab 2002;8710:4782–91.

15. Beliard A, Noel A, Goffin F et al. Adhesion of endometrial cells labled with 111Indium-tropoloante to peritoneum: a novel in vitro model to study endometriosis. Fertil Steril 2003;79:724–9.

16. Fang Z, Yang S, Gurates B. Genetic or enzymatic disruption of aromatase inhibits the growth of ectopic uterine tissue. J Clin Endocrinol Metab 2002;87:3460–6.

17. Rock JA, Markham SM. Pathogenesis of endometriosis. Lancet 1992;340:1264–7.

18. Iwabe T, Harada T, Tsudo T et al. Tumor necrosis factor-alpha promotes proliferation of endometriotic stromal cells by inducing interleukin-8 gene and protein expression. J Clin Endocrinol Metab 2000;85:824–9.

19. Witz CA, Monotoya-Rodriguez IA, Schenken RS. Whole explants of peritoneum and endometrium: a novel model of the early endometriosis lesion. Fertil Steril 1999;71:56–60.

20. Wieser F, Fabjani G, Tempfer C et al. Tumor necrosis factor-alpha promoter polymorphisms and endometriosis. J Soc Gynecol Invest 2002;9:313–18.

21. Harada T, Iwabe T, Tarakawa N. Role of cytokines in endometriosis. Fertil Steril 2001;76:1–10.

22. Bullimore DW. Endometriosis is sustained by tumour necrosis factor-alpha. Med Hypotheses 2003;60:84–8.

23. Altman GB, Gown AM, Luchtel DL et al. RANTES production by cultured primate endometrial epithelial cells. Am J Reprod Immunol 1999;42:168–74.

24. Hornung D, Fujii E, Lim KH et al. Histocompatibility leukocyte antigen-G is not expressed by endometriosis or endometrial tissue. Fertil Steril 2001;75:814–17.

25. Sillem M, Prifti S, Koch A et al. Regulation of matrix metalloproteinases and their inhibitors in uterine endometrial cells of patients with and without endometriosis. Eur J Obstet Gynecol Reprod Biol 2001;95:167–74.

26. Trinchieri G. Interleukin-12 and the regulation of innate resistance and adaptive immunity. Nat Rev Immunol 2003;3:133–46.

27. Koller BH, Marrack P, Kappler JW. Normal development of mice deficient in beta 2M, MHC class I proteins, and CD8+ T cells. Science 1990;248:1227–30.

28. Somigliana E, Vigano P, Filardo P et al. Use of knockout transgenic mice in the study of endometriosis: insights from mice lacking beta2-microglobulin and interleukin-12p40. Fertil Steril 2001;751:203–6.

29. Keenan JA, Williams-Boyce PK, Massey PJ. Regression of endometrial explants in a rat model of endometriosis treated with the immune modulators loxoribine and levamisole. Fertil Steril 1999;72:135–41.

30. Steinleitner A, Lambert H, Roy S. Immunomodulation with pentoxifylline abrogates macrophage-mediated infertility in an vivo model: a paradigm for a novel approach to the treatment of endometriosis-associated infertility. Fertil Steril 1991;55:26–31.

31. Schandene L et al. Differential effects of pentoxifylline on the production of tumor necrosis factor-alpha (TNF-alpha) and interleukin-6 (IL6) by monocytes and T cells. Immunology 1992;76:30–4.

32. Ota H, Rong H, Igarashi S. Suppression of natural killer cell activity by splenocyte transplantation in a rat model of endometriosis. Hum Reprod 2002;17:1453–8.

33. Bogdan C. The function of type I interferons in antimicrobial immunity. Curr Opin Immunol 2000;4:19–24.

34. Ingelmo J, Quereda F, Acien P. Intraperitoneal and subcutaneous treatment of experimental endometriosis with recombinant human interferon a-2b in a murine model. Fertil Steril 1999;71:907–11.

35. Hahn DW, Carraher RP, Foldesy RG et al. Development of an animal model for evaluating effects of drugs on endometriosis. Fertil Steril 1985;44:410–15.

36. Sharpe KL, Bertero MC, Muse KN et al. Spontaneous and steroid-induced recurrence of endometriosis after suppression by a gonadotropin-releasing hormone antagonist in the rat. Am J Obstet Gynecol 1991;164:187–94.

37. Jones RC. The effect of luteinizing hormone agonist (Wy-40,972), levonorgestrel, danazol and ovariectomy on experimental endometriosis in the rat. Acta Endocrinol 1984;106:282–8.

38. Golan A, Dargenio R, Winston RML. The effect of treatment on experimentally produced endometrial peritoneal implants. Fertil Steril 1986;46:954–8.

39. Stöckemann K, Hegele-Hartung C, Chwalisz K. Effects of the progesterone antagonists onapristone (ZK98) and ZK136 799 on surgically induced endometriosis in intact rats. Hum Reprod 1995;10:3265–71.

40. D'Antonio M, Martelli F, Peano S et al. Ability of recombinant human TNF binding protein-1 (r-hTBP-1) to inhibit the development of experimentally induced endometriosis in rats. J Reprod Immunol 2000;48:81–98.

41. Hornung D, Chao VA, Vigne JL. Thiazolidinedione inhibition of peritoneal inflammation. Gynecol Obstet Invest 2003;55:20–4.

42. Hull ML, Charnock-Jones DS, Chan CL et al. Antiangiogenic agents are effective inhibitors of endometriosis. J Clin Endocrinol Metab 2003;88:2889–99.

43. Mori T, Nakahashi K, Kyokuwa M et al. A matrix metalloproteinase inhibitor, ONO-4817, retards the development of mammary tumor and the progression of uterine adenomyosis in mice. Anticancer Res 2002;22:3985–8.

44. Hahn DW, Carraher RP, Foldesy RG et al. Experimental evidence for failure to implant as a mechanism of infertility associated with endometriosis. Am J Obstet Gynecol 1986;155:1109–13.

45. Donnez J, Wayembergh M, Casanas-Roux F et al. Effect on ovulation of surgically induced endometriosis in rabbits. Gynecol Obstet Invest 1987;24:131–7.

46. Kaplan CR, Carlton AE, Olive DL et al. Effect of ovarian endometriosis on ovulation in rabbits. Am J Obstet Gynecol 1989;160:40–4.

47. Dunselman GAJ, Land JA, Bouckaert PXJM et al. Effect of endometriosis on ovulation, ovum pick-up, fertilization and tubal transport in the rabbit. J Reprod Fertil 1988;82:193–7.

48. Dunselman GA, Land JA, Dumoulin JC et al. Effect of endometriosis on early embryonic development in the rabbit. Hum Reprod 1988;3:459–61.

49. Dunselman GA, Dumoulin JCM, Land JA et al. Lack of effect of peritoneal endometriosis on fertility in the rabbit model. Fertil Steril 1991;56:340–2.

50. Rajkumar K, Schott PW, Simpson CW. The rat as an animal model for endometriosis to examine recurrence of ectopic endometrial tissue after regression. Fertil Steril 1990;53:921–5.

51. Barragan JC, Brotons J, Ruiz JA et al. Experimentally induced endometriosis in rats: effect on fertility and the effects of pregnancy and lactation on the ectopic endometrial tissue. Fertil Steril 1992;58:1215–19.

52. Finaz C, Cochet C, de Grouchy J. Identité des caryotypes de *Papio papio* et *Macaca mulatta* en bandes R, G, C et Ag-NOR. Ann Genet 1978;21:149–51.

53. Dutrillaux B, Biemont M C, Viegas-Pequignot E et al. Comparison of the karyotypes of four Cercopithecoidae: *Papio papio, P. anubis, Macaca mulatta* and *M. fascicularis*. Cytogenet Cell Genet 1979;23:77–83.

54. Balner H. The major histocompatibility system of subhuman primate species. In: Götze D, ed. The Major Histocompatibility System in Man and Animals. Berlin: Springer-Verlag, 1977; 79–127.

55. Stone WH, Treichel RS, VandeBerg JL. Genetic significance of some common primate models in biomedical research. Prog Clin Biol Res 1987;229:73–93.

56. VandBerg JL, Williams-Blangero S. Strategies for using nonhuman primates in genetic research on multifactorial diseases. Lab Anim Sci 1996;46:146–51.

57. Zondervan K, Cardon L, Desrosiers R et al. The genetic epidemiology of spontaneous endometriosis in the rhesus monkey. Ann NY Acad Sci 2002;955:233–8.

58. Hadfield RM, Yudkin PL, Coe CL et al. Risk factors for endometriosis in the rhesus monkey (*Macaca mulatta*): a case–control study. Hum Reprod Update 1997;3:109–15.

59. Jacobson VC. The intraperitoneal transplantation of endometrial tissue in the rabbit. Arch Pathol Lab Med 1926;1:169–74.

60. Te Linde RW, Scott RB. Experimental endometriosis. Am J Obstet Gynecol 1950;60:1147–73.

61. Schenken RS, Williams RF, Hodgen G. Effect of pregnancy on surgically induced endometriosis in cynomolgus monkeys. Am J Obstet Gynecol 1987;157:1392–6.

62. Dmowski WP, Steele RN, Baker GF. Deficient cellular immunity in endometriosis. Am J Obstet Gynecol 1981;141:377–83.

63. Schenken RS, Asch RH, Williams RF et al. Etiology of infertility in monkeys with endometriois: luteinized unruptured follicles, luteal phase defects, pelvic adhesions, and spontaneous abortions. Fertil Steril 1984;41:122–30.

64. Rier SE, Martin DC, Bowman RE et al. Endometriosis in rhesus monkeys (*Macaca mulatta*) following chronic exposure to 2,3,7,8-tetrachlorodibenzo-*p*-dioxin. Fundam Appl Toxicol 1993;21:433–41.

65. Arnold DL, Nera EA, Stapley R et al. Prevalence of endometriosis in rhesus (*Macaca mulatta*) monkeys ingesting PCB (Aroclor 1254): review and evaluation. Fundam Appl Toxicol 1996;31:42–55.

66. Rier SE, Turner WE, Martin DC et al. Serum levels of TCDD and dioxin-like chemicals in rhesus monkeys chronically exposed to dioxin: correlation of increased serum PCB levels with endometriosis. Toxicol Sci 2001;59:147–59.

67. Yang JZ, Agarwal SK, Foster WG. Subchronic exposure to 2,3,7,8-tetrachlorodibenzo-*p*-dioxin modulates the pathophysiology of

68. Guo S. The link between exposure to dioxin and endometriosis: a comprehensive reappraisal of primate data. Gynecologic and Obstetric Investigation 2004; 57: 157–73.

69. Werlin LB, Hodgen GD. Gonadotropin-releasing hormone agonist suppresses ovulation, menses and endometriosis in monkeys: an individualized, intermittent regimen. J Clin Endocrinol Metab 1983;56:844–8.

70. Mann DR, Collins DC, Smith MM et al. Treatment of endometriosis in Rhesus monkeys: effectiveness of a gonadotropin-releasing hormone agonist compared to treatment with a progestational steroid. J Clin Endocrin Metab 1986;63: 1277–83.

71. Grow DR, Williams RF, Hsiu JG et al. Antiprogestin and/or gonadotropin releasing hormone agonist for endometriosis treatment and bone maintenance: a 1-year primate study. J Clin Endocrinol Metab 1996;81:1933–9.

72. Bambra C. Veterinary management and research techniques for reproductive studies in the baboon: a practical approach. Nairobi: Institute of Primate Research, 1993.

73. Isahakia MA, Bambra CS. Primate models for research in reproduction. In: Alexander NJ, Griffin D, Spieler JM, Waites G (eds) Gamete Interaction: Prospects for Immunocontraception. New York: John Wiley & Sons, 1990; 487–500.

74. D'Hoogh TM, Bambra CS, Cornillie FJ. Prevalence and laparoscopic appearance of spontaneous endometriosis in the baboon (*Papio anubis, Papio cynocephalus*). Biol Reprod 1991;45:411–16.

75. D'Hooghe TM, Bambra CS, De Jonge I et al. The prevalence of spontaneous endometriosis in the baboon increases with the time spent in captivity. Acta Obstet Gynecol Scand 1996;75:98–101.

76. D'Hooghe TM, Bambra CS, Raeymaekers BM et al. Intrapelvic injection of menstrual endometrium causes endometriosis in baboons (*Papio cynocephalus, Papio anubis*). Am J Obstet Gynecol 1995;173:125–34.

77. Folse DS, Stout LC. Endometriosis in a baboon. Lab Anim Sci 1978;28:217–19.

78. D'Hooghe TM, Bambra CS, Raeymaekers BM et al. Immunosuppression can increase progression of spontaneous endometriosis in baboons. Fertil Steril 1995;64:172–8.

79. Dick EJ, Hubbard GB, Martin LJ, Leland MM. Record review of baboons with histologically confirmed endometriosis in a large established colony. J Med Primatol 2003;32:39–47.

80. American Fertility Society. Revised American Fertility Society Classification of Endometriosis. Fertil Steril 1985;43:351–2.

81. D'Hooghe TM, Bambra CS, Raeymaekers BM et al. Serial laparoscopies over 30 months show that endometriosis is a progressive in captive baboons (*Papio anubis, Papio cynocephalus*). Fertil Steril 1996;65:645–9.

82. Sampson JA. Peritoneal endometriosis due to menstrual dissemination of endometrial tissue into the pelvic cavity. Am J Obstet Gynecol 1927;14:422–69.

83. D'Hooghe TM, Bambra CS, Raeymaekers BM et al. Increased incidence and recurrence of retrograde menstruation in baboons with spontaneous endometriosis. Hum Reprod 1996;11:2022–5.

84. Blumenkrantz MJ, Gallagher N, Bashore RA et al. Retrograde menstruation in women undergoing chronic peritoneal dialysis. Obstet Gynecol 1981;57:667–70.

85. Halme J, Becker S, Hammond MG et al. Retrograde menstruation in healthy women and in patients with endometriosis. Obstet Gynecol 1984;64:151–4.

86. D'Hooghe TM, Bambra CS, Suleman MA et al. Development of a model of retrograde menstruation in baboons (*Papio anubis*). Fertil Steril 1994;62:635–8.

87. McArthur JW, Ulfelder H. The effect of pregnancy upon endometriosis. Obstet Gynecol Surv 1965;20:709–33.

88. D'Hooghe TM, Bambra CS, De Jonge I et al. Pregnancy does not affect endometriosis in baboons (*Papio anubis, Papio cynocephalus*). Arch Gynecol Obstet 1997;261:15–19.

89. D'Hooghe TM, Bambra CS, Ling Xiao et al. The effect of menstruation and intrapelvic injection of endometrium on peritoneal fluid parameters in the baboon. Am J Obstet Gynecol 2001;184: 917–25.

90. Debrock S, Drijkoningen M, Goossens W et al. Quantity and quality of retrograde menstruation: red blood cells, inflammation and peritoneal cells. Annual Meeting of the American Society for Reproductive Medicine, San Diego, USA, 24 October 2000.

91. Osteen KG, Keller NR, Feltus FA et al. Paracrine regulation of matrix metalloproteinase expression in the normal human endometrium. Gynecol Obstet Invest 1999;48:2–13.

92. Spuijbroek MD, Dunselman GA, Menheere PP et al. Early endometriosis invades the extracellular matrix. Fertil Steril 1992;58:929–33.

93. Fazleabas AT, Brudney A, Gurates B et al. A modified baboon model for endometriosis. Ann NY Acad Sci 2002;955:308–17.

94. Haney AF, Muscato JJ, Weinberg JB. Peritoneal fluid cell populations in infertility patients. Fertil Steril 1981;35:696–8.

95. Halme J, Becker S, Hammond MG et al. Pelvic macrophages in normal and infertile women: the role of patent tubes. Am J Obstet Gynecol 1982;142:890–5.

96. Muscato JJ, Haney AF, Weinberg JB. Sperm phagocytosis by human peritoneal macrophages: a possible role of infertility in endometriosis. Am J Obstet Gynecol 1982;144:503–10.

97. Badawy SZA, Cuenca V, Stitzel A et al. Immune rosettes of T and B lymphocytes in infertile women with endometriosis. J Reprod Med 1987;32:194–7.

98. Hill JA, Faris HMP, Schiff I et al. Characterization of leucocyte subpopulations in the peritoneal fluid of women with endometriosis. Fertil Steril 1988;50:216–22.

99. D'Hooghe TM, Debrock S, Hill JA et al. Animal models for research in endometriosis. In: Tulandi T, Redwine D eds. Endometriosis: advances and controversies. Marcel Dekker: New York: 2004;p81–99.

100. D'Hooghe TM, Bambra CS, Hill JA et al. Effect on endometriosis and the menstrual cycle on white blood cell subpopulations in the peripheral blood and peritoneal of baboons. Hum Reprod 1996;11:1736–40.

101. Healy DL, Rogers PA, Hii L, Winfield M. Angiogenesis: a new theory for endometriosis. Hum Reprod Update 1998;4:736 –40.

102. D'Hooghe TM, Scheerlinck JP, Koninckx PR et al. Anti-endometrial lymphocytotoxicity and natural killer cell activity in baboons (*Papio anubis* and *Papio cynocephalus*). Hum Reprod 1995;10:558–62.

103. Oosterlynck D, Cornillie FJ, Waer M et al. Women with endometriosis show a defect in natural killer cell activity resulting in a decreased cytotoxicity to autologous endometrium. Fertil Steril 1991;56:45–51.

104. D'Hooghe TM, Nugent N, Cuneo S et al. Recombinant human TNF binding protein (r-hTBP-1) inhibits the development of endometriosis in baboons: a prospective, randomized, placebo- and drug-controlled study. General Program Prize Winning Paper and oral presentation at the Annual Meeting of the American Society for Reproductive Medicine, Orlando, USA, 22–24 October 2001. Fertil Steril 2001;76:O-2, S-1.

105. Taylor RN, Lundeeni SG, Giudice LC. Emerging role of genomics in endometriosis research. Fertil Steril 2002;78:694–8.

106. Tummon IS, Maclin VM, Radwanksa E et al. Occult ovulatory dysfunction in women with minimal endometriosis or unexplained infertility. Fertil Steril 1988;50:716–20.

107. Koninckx PR, Ide P, Vandenbroucke W et al. New aspects of the pathophysiology of endometriosis and associated fertility. J Reprod Med 1980;24:257–60.

108. D'Hooghe TM, Bambra CS, Koninckx PR. Cycle fecundity in baboons of proven fertility with minimal endometriosis. Gynecol Obstet Invest 1994;37:63–5.

109. D'Hooghe TM, Bambra CS, Raeymaekers BM et al. A prospective controlled study over 2 years shows a normal monthly fertility rate (MFR) in baboons with stage I endometriosis and a decreased MFR in primates with stage II and stage III–IV disease. Fertil Steril 1996;66:809–13.

110. Scheenjes E, te Velde ER, Kremer J. Inspection of the ovaries and steroids in serum and peritoneal fluid at various time intervals after ovulation in fertile women: implications for the luteinized unruptured follicle syndrome. Fertil Steril 1990;54:38–41.

111. D'Hooghe TM, Bambra CS, Raeymaekers BM et al. Increased incidence and recurrence of recent corpus luteum without ovulation stigma (luteinized unruptured follicle-syndrome?) in baboons (*Papio anubis, Papio cynocephalus*) with endometriosis. J Soc Gynecol Invest 1996;3:140–4.

112. Maas JW, Groothuis PG, Dunselman GA et al. Development of endometriosis-like lesions after transplantation of human endometrial fragments onto the chick embryo chorioallantoic membrane. Hum Reprod 2001;16:627–31.

113. Nap AW, Groothuis PG, Demir AY et al. Tissue integrity is essential for ectopic implantation of human endometrium in the chicken chorioallantoic membrane. Hum Reprod 2003;181:30–4.

114. Ria R, Loverro G, Vacca A et al. Angiogenesis extent and expression of matrix metalloproteinase-2 and -9 agree with progression of ovarian endometriomas. Eur J Clin Invest 2002;32:199–206.

115. D'Hooghe TM, Debrock S. Future directions in endometriosis research. Obstet Gynecol Clin North Am 2003;30:221–44.

11. Symptoms

Steven R. Lindheim

Endometriosis often presents with an array of clinical symptoms, including non-cyclic pain, dysmenorrhea, dyspareunia, abnormal uterine bleeding, and infertility (Table 11.1). Nearly 15% of American women between the ages of 18 and 50 suffer from symptoms related to endometriosis.[1] Although some of these symptoms are strongly suggestive of endometriosis, none is pathognomonic of the disorder and, conversely, can be present in 45–50% of asymptomatic women.[2] Moreover, these symptoms are not exclusive and can be associated with other conditions, such as intra-abdominal adhesions, chronic pelvic inflammatory disease, ovarian cysts, adenomyosis, irritable bowel syndrome, or interstitial cystitis (Table 11.2). This chapter will focus on the symptoms, their pathophysiology, and their correlation to disease.

CLINICAL PRESENTATION: PREVALENCE AND PATHOPHYSIOLOGY

PAIN

Symptomatic endometriosis most commonly involves the pelvis and the most consistent symptom is chronic pelvic pain. This is defined as the presence of non-menstrual pain below the navel for more than 3 months, or menstrual pain of at least 6 months in duration causing functional disability.[3] Pain has a reported prevalence of 30–70% in adults[1,4] and 45–58% in adolescents.[5,6] It may be either unilateral or bilateral, chiefly in the lower abdomen, but often diffuse, and tends to be aggravated premenstrually, leaving residual postmenstrual soreness.

The mechanism of pain, and specifically how endometriosis causes pain, is incompletely understood, but is thought to be principally due to an altered pain-processing system.[7–12] Noxious stimuli, including pressure, stretching, ischemia, or chemical irritation induce pain receptors that are transmitted by afferent myelinated and non-myelinated nerve fibers. These nerve fibers can be activated in somatic structures (including parietal perineum) or visceral structures (uterus, fallopian tubes, and ovaries) and reach their cell bodies in the posterior root ganglion of the corresponding spinal nerve. There they either form afferent components of a local reflex arc or pass to higher centers of the autonomic nervous center, where the perception of pain is further affected by descending neural pathways. Higher centers can modulate the pain response by increasing or decreasing nociceptive transmission, including

---

Table 11.1 Common presenting signs and symptoms of endometriosis

- Pelvic pain complaints
- Dysmenorrhea
- Dyspareunia
- Dysfunctional uterine bleeding
- Gastrointestinal
- Lower back pain
- Infertility

Table 11.2 Causes of chronic pain

Gastrointestinal	Psychiatric
• Functional bowel disease	• Depression
• Inflammatory bowel disease	• Somatization
• Cancer	• Hypochondriasis
	• Somatic delusions
Urinary	**Rheumatologic**
• Interstitial cystitis	• Fibromyalgia
• Urethral syndrome	• Regional pain disorders
• Chronic calculi	
Musculoskeletal	**Gynecologic**
• Abdominal hernia	• Endometriosis/adenomyosis
• Neuroma	• Uterine fibroids
• Lumbar disk disease	• Adhesions
• Orthopedic disorders	• Chronic infection

opioids or endorphins within the brain to activate descending neurons. Normally, activation of these descending analgesic pathways varies from person to person. When a reduction in the activity of pain-suppressing systems occurs it may reduce pain tolerance, accounting for individual differences to similar pain stimuli and the inability to tolerate pain.

In abnormal conditions, repeated stimulation of sensory pain fibers appears to cause changes in the nerve fiber chemical milieu, which results in lower thresholds for activation and altered excitability, referred to as peripheral sensitization. This can further lead to central sensitization, where connecting nerves in the dorsal horn of the spinal cord develop exaggerated responses to excitation, recruit higher central neurons, begin to self-sustain activation, and disable normal pain-inhibition pathways from dorsal horn nerves and higher central nerve centers. As a result, central sensitization ceases to rely on continued peripheral stimulation and allows for self-perpetuated pain. Moreover, this can explain why patients present with pain that seems inappropriate for the degree of pathology (hyperalgesia) or have pain that arises from non-noxious stimuli (allodynia).

Pain can also radiate to areas not involved in the initial pain. As pelvic pain sensations enter through afferent nerve fibers into the spinal cord they intermingle with neuronal inputs (afferent nerve fibers) innervating skin dermatomes. Often, this results in either muscular contractions or cutaneous discomfort in the region supplied by the affected dermatome. This phenomenon is called referred pain. The dermatomes to which pelvic pain can be referred are as follows:

- Ovarian afferents, which enter the spinal cord at T10, may result in periumbilical pain.
- Uterine afferents at T12 may result in lower abdominal pain.
- Bladder afferents at L1 can be referred to skin over the pubis.
- Vaginal afferents at L1 can be referred to skin over the groin.
- Vulvar afferents can be referred to skin over the lower back.

It has for many years been believed that endometriosis causes pain simply through the stretching of tissue that directly surrounds endometriotic implants. However, extravasated blood and desquamation of cells from the endometrium, as well as from active endometriotic implants during menstruation, may indirectly stimulate an inflammatory condition within the peritoneal cavity. On the other hand, the endometriotic implants themselves may secrete inflammatory substances, such as eicosanoids, cytokines, and growth factors, that initiate the chain of events that results in pain symptoms.[13–18]

In pain related to ovarian endometriomas, they are inclined to rupture or leak some of their entrapped blood into the peritoneal cavity. This may occur suddenly or intermittently. In either case the blood may produce a chemical peritonitis, with severe pain, rebound tenderness, and other signs of peritoneal irritation.

Confusion also lies in the fact that there is little correlation between extent of disease and clinical symptoms. Typically women with complaints of pelvic pain have deep or infiltrative lesions, and the depth of infiltration correlates directly with pain severity. Histologic assessment of endometriotic implants removed en bloc demonstrates that deep implants (>5 mm) are more likely to be found in women with complaints of pelvic pain, and implants >10 mm in depth are found almost exclusively in women with severe pain.[19] However, as depicted in Table 11.3, which shows the results of a study using one of the

Table 11.3 Percentage of patients with each symptom by endometriosis stage

	Stage				
	I	II	III	IV	P value
Pelvic pain	38	46	36	41	0.21
Dysmenorrhea	73	86	72	85	0.68
Dyspareunia	30	25	36	29	0.91

Data from Fedele et al. (1990)[88]

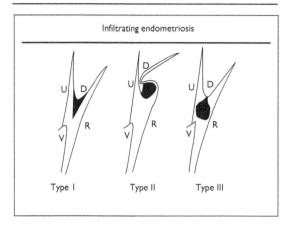

Figure 11.1 Tissue retraction secondary to endometriotic implants.

earlier American Fertility Society staging systems, no relationship was found between the presence of pain and other symptoms and the extent of endometriosis.[20]

Perhaps this can be explained by an altered pain-processing system as described above. However, the explanation may lie in the underestimation of the volume of disease seen at laparoscopy, as the depth of infiltration correlates poorly with visible surface area involvement. Tissue can retract around and over lesions, or lesions can occur as adenomyosis-like tissue 'müllerian rests' within tissue, resulting in pain despite little or no apparent disease (Figure 11.1). Another possible explanation is that minimal disease may appear as atypical lesions (red or clear) that may produce more prostaglandins than the typical black lesions,[21] but which may also be more easily overlooked by the surgeon.

DYSMENORRHEA

Dysmenorrhea is associated with endometriosis in more than 50% of adults[22] and up to 75% of adolescents.[5] The pain occurs with menstruation, is usually cramping and spasmodic, and is centered in the lower abdomen.

Classically, primary dysmenorrhea is a condition associated with the ovulatory cycle.[23] The pain is caused by myometrial contractions induced by prostaglandins (PGE_2 and $F_{2\alpha}$), which can be explained by a threefold increase of prostaglandins and metabolites into the systemic circulation from the follicular phase to the luteal phase, and further increasing during menstruation.[24] By comparison, secondary dysmenorrhea is associated with a variety of pathologic conditions, including structural anomalies, pelvic inflammatory disease, intrauterine devices, and endometriosis.[25]

The etiology of dysmenorrhea in women with endometriosis has remained speculative. Retrograde menstruation, once thought to be the cause of pain, does not appear to cause dysmenorrhea in controlled trials.[26–29] In human and experimental animals, endometriotic tissue contains and produces prostaglandins. Moreover, clinical trials[30] demonstrate that prostaglandin synthetase inhibitors substantially reduce dysmenorrhea symptoms in the treatment of endometriosis-associated pain. This suggests that endometriotic lesions do in fact cause pain.

DYSPAREUNIA

Dyspareunia is defined as recurrent or persistent genital pain upon penile penetration. This can cause anxiety and avoidance, thereby interfering with sexual intercourse. Dyspareunia may be related to the stimulation of pain fibers by traction on or stretching of scarred inelastic tissues, and/or by pressure on nodules of endometriosis embedded in fibrotic tissues.[31] The reported prevalence is highly variable, ranging from 4% to 55%.[32,33] Other etiologies of dyspareunia include hymeneal scarring, pelvic inflammatory disease, and various vulvar conditions, including vulvar vestibulitis.

The criteria for the diagnosis of dyspareunia specify that the disturbance be not caused by vaginismus (recurrent or persistent involuntary spasm of the musculature of the outer third of the vagina) or lack of lubrication. Vaginismus more often results from psychological disorders or traumatic events, including rape and physical abuse, or in women who have experienced vaginal pain secondary to infections, previous surgery, or chemical agents.

ANOVULATION AND ABNORMAL UTERINE BLEEDING

Anovulation is often linked to endometriosis with a prevalence of 9–27%, often resulting in abnormal uterine bleeding or infertility.[34–36] In the rabbit model, endometriosis is thought to impair ovulation primarily through periovarian adhesions.[37] In human studies, women with minimal and mild endometriosis have been shown to have occult ovulatory dysfunction with lower preovulatory and peak estradiol levels, and altered granulosa cell steroidogenic capacity in vitro has been reported.[38,39] Others have shown a delayed or decreased luteal progesterone secretion, abnormal serum and follicular LH secretory patterns, hyperprolactinemia, and inadequate luteolysis, with continued progesterone production from an active corpus luteum into the follicular phase of the following menstrual cycle.[40–44] Conversely, other studies have failed to demonstrate abnormal folliculogenesis and ovulation in women with minimal to mild disease.[45,46] Unfortunately, many of these studies lacked control groups and utilized inconsistent criteria for the diagnosis of anovulation, and addressed infertility as their endpoint. Furthermore, they have often not corrected for associated pelvic pathologies that might have been the source of the bleeding.[47,48] At present, a cause-and-effect relationship has not been clearly defined in the presence of endometriosis and abnormal uterine bleeding.

INFERTILITY

Infertility is a common symptom of endometriosis, though the true incidence is difficult to assess adequately. The rate of endometriosis in the infertile patient undergoing surgical evaluation has ranged from 20% to 68%.[4,49–54] Despite the apparent association, however, the mechanism by which endometriosis may cause infertility remains unclear.

When endometriosis produces anatomic distortion of the pelvic viscera or fallopian tube obstruction, the result is often infertility. This has been supported by animal models where surgically induced endometriosis-related adhesions reduce ovum recovery by the uterine horns.[55,56] In

---

Table 11.4 Possible causes for infertility in those with endometriosis

- Anatomic distortion
- Anovulation, luteal-phase defects, and hormonal abnormalities
- Galactorrhea/hyperprolactinemia
- Luteinized unruptured syndrome
- Autoimmune dysfunction
- Peritoneal inflammatory response
- Peritoneal fluid prostaglandins
- Spontaneous abortion and uterine receptivity abnormalities

---

women with more advanced stages of endometriosis, conservative surgery with pelvic restoration significantly improves pregnancy outcomes,[57,58] although results from such studies are retrospective, non-randomized, and should be viewed with caution. In a meta-analysis of conservative laparoscopic surgery for severe endometriosis, Candiani et al[59] reported a significant improvement in overall cumulative pregnancy rates of 48%. However, monthly fecundity rates only range from 2% to 3.3%.

A more common presentation for endometriosis is minimal to mild peritoneal and ovarian implants. A number of mechanisms (Table 11.4) that have been suggested regarding how endometriosis in the absence of pelvic distortion causes infertility, including ovulatory and endocrine defects[38–46] and alterations to the peritoneal immune environment.[60–63] However, the validity of these explanations remains unproven. In experimental animal models, transplanted endometrium has not been shown to decrease fertility in the absence of pelvic adhesions.[37,55] Many clinical studies have addressed this issue, but sample size and study design severely affect their interpretation.[64–69] Current surgical treatment data for early-stage disease suggest that lesions do impair fertility, and that surgical resection may achieve modest improvements over no therapy or medical suppression (see Chapter 15).

ATYPICAL SYMPTOMS

Atypical symptoms may be site specific when endometriosis is found in unusual locations outside the pelvis. Sciatica, cyclic leg pain, pain over the buttock, and paresthesia of the thighs and/or knees, exacerbated during menses, can be associated with the retroperitoneal presence of fibrotic endometriotic nodules. Sciatica pain may also represent referred pain originating from pelvic peritoneum rather than direct irritation of the lumbosacral plexus of the sciatic nerve.[70]

Disease in the iliac fossa may present as flank pain that may be secondary to endometriosis of the ureter. Involvement of the bladder or ureter may cause dysuria, hematuria, or ureteral obstruction, with the potential for kidney failure. Donnez et al reported ureteral stenosis in 11% of patients with rectovaginal nodules ≥3 cm and recommends preoperative intravenous pyelography (IVP) to prevent non-reversible loss of renal function.[71]

Intestinal endometriosis may present as irritable bowel-like symptoms, obstructive symptoms, or even acute symptoms such as appendicitis. Rectal bleeding has been noted to occur in about 20% of endometriosis patients with significant bowel involvement.[72] Right lower quadrant pain frequently correlates with endometriosis of the appendix, particularly with a positive preoperative Gastrografin enema.[73] Inguinal or umbilical endometriosis may mimic the signs of an incarcerated hernia.[74] Obstructive jaundice or ascites can result from hepatic endometriosis.[75]

Unusual symptoms can result from atypical disease locations. Pleuritic chest pain, pleural effusions, pneumothorax, or cyclic catamenial hemoptysis may be due to pulmonary involvement.[76,77] A traumatic intervention on the uterus is often found in the patient's history and the most commonly proposed mechanism involves hematogenic migration during a uterine procedure. Cyclic headaches or seizures may be secondary to brain lesions.[78]

Cutaneous involvement has also been noted on the perineum, vagina, or less commonly in the inguinal region, the umbilicus, or at the site of surgical scars.[79,80] These lesions are associated with cyclic pain, tenderness, swelling, and bleeding.

CORRELATION OF SYMPTOMS TO DISEASE

Although clinical symptoms can be suggestive of endometriosis, none are pathognomonic of disease. Epidemiologic studies suggest that symptoms of pain, dysmenorrhea, and dyspareunia, and the risk of endometriosis, are increased by the following:[81]

- Nulliparity;
- Menses which lasts more than 6 days;
- Menstrual cycle length less than 27 days;
- Sedentary lifestyle;
- Müllerian anomalies, including outflow tract narrowing or obstruction;
- Use of oral contraceptives with high doses of estrogen.

Because pelvic surgery is the current gold standard for diagnosis, validation studies are difficult to perform.[82] A few studies have attempted to assess the predictive value of clinical symptoms for endometriosis seen at surgery. Severe dysmenorrhea is the only symptom that is predictive of endometriosis in subfertile women.[83] Naish et al[84] reported that severe dysmenorrhea was better than dyspareunia and pelvic pain in predicting endometriosis (63% positive predictive value (PPV) and 95% negative predictive value (NPV)). In contrast, Fedele et al reported that the frequency of dysmenorrhea was similar in both those with endometriosis and infertile controls; however, deep dyspareunia was more prevalent regardless of disease stage,[85] although others have reported an inverse relationship with respect to dyspareunia or no relationship at all.[83,86]

In most studies pelvic pain is more common in those with endometriosis,[86] although Williams and Pratt[87] reported that in 1000 women undergoing celiotomy non-cyclic pelvic pain was less common in those with endometriosis. Frequency of pelvic pain has been correlated to extent of disease by Fedele et al,[88] but others report no association between extent of disease and severity of symptoms.[85]

Unfortunately, either retrospective analysis or the inclusion of infertile patients limits the reliability of these studies. A recent study by Eskenazi et al[89] provides a more rigorous scientific assessment. These authors prospectively evaluated the predictive value of preoperative non-invasive tools, including a detailed medical history and grading of endometriosis-related symptoms (pelvic pain, dysmenorrhea, dyspareunia, and infertility), to determine whether surgical diagnosis of endometriosis could be predicted in those undergoing laparoscopy for pelvic pain, infertility, tubal ligation, or masses in the adnexae or uterus. Moderate success was seen in predicting a surgical diagnosis of endometriosis with a sensitivity of 66% for women who present with any symptoms (pelvic pain, dysmenorrhea, dyspareunia, or infertility) prior to surgery, with a 56% positive predictive value and a 78% negative predictive value. Patients with dysmenorrhea were more correctly diagnosed with endometriosis (68%) than those with pelvic pain (63%), dyspareunia (54%), and infertility (52%). However, these clinical signs only seemed to be reliable predictors for ovarian endometriosis (66% correctly classified) rather than non-ovarian endometriosis (38% correctly classified).

CONCLUSION

Many women suffer from an array of symptoms related to endometriosis. Although each is suggestive of endometriosis, they are not exclusive to the disease and can be associated with other conditions. A comprehensive history can certainly raise a clinician's suspicion for endometriosis.

REFERENCES

1. Mathias SD, Kuppermann M, Lieberman RF et al. Chronic pelvic pain: prevalence, health-related quality of life, and economic correlates. Obstet Gynecol 1996;87:321–7.
2. Balacsch J, Creus M, Fabreques F et al. Visible and non-visible endometriosis at laparoscopy in fertile and infertile women and in patients with chronic pelvic pain: a prospective study. Hum Reprod 1996;11:387–91.
3. American College of Obstetricians and Gynecologists. Medical management of endometriosis. ACOG Practice Bulletin #11 Washington DC: American College of Obstetricians and Gynecologists, 1999.
4. Koninckx PR, Meuleman C, Demeyere S et al. Suggestive evidence that pelvic endometriosis is a progressive disease, whereas deeply infiltrating endometriosis is associated with pelvic pain. Fertil Steril 1991;55:759–65.
5. Chatman DL, Ward AB. Endometriosis in adolescents. J Reprod Med 1982;27:22–7.
6. Goldstein DP. Acute and chronic pelvic pain. Pediatr Clin North Am 1989;36:573–80.
7. Woolf CJ, Decosterd I. Implications of recent advances in the understanding of pain pathophysiology for the assessment of pain in patients. Pain 1999;Aug (Suppl 6): S141–7.
8. Nurmikko TJ, Nash TP, Wiles JR. Recent advances: control of chronic pain. Br Med J 1998;317:123–33.
9. Russo CM, Brose WG. Chronic pain. Annu Rev Med 1998;49:123–33.
10. Smith BL, Hopton JL, Chambers WA. Chronic pain in primary care. Fam Pract 1999;16:475–82.
11. Bennet RM. Emerging concepts in the neurobiology of chronic pain: evidence of abnormal sensory processing in fibromyalgia. Mayo Clin Proc 1999;74:385–99.
12. Elbadawi A. Neuromorphologic basis of vesicourethral function: I. Histochemistry, ultrastructure, and function of intrinsic nerves of the bladder, and urethra. Neurourol Urodyn 1982;1:3–50.
13. Taketani Y, Kuo TM, Mizuno M. Comparison of cytokine levels and embryo toxicity in peritoneal fluid from infertile women with untreated and treated endometriosis. Am J Obstet Gynecol 1992;167:265–70.
14. Hill JA, Anderson DJ. Lymphocyte activity in the presence of peritoneal fluid from fertile women and infertile women with and without endometriosis. Am J Obstet Gynecol 1989;161:861–4.
15. Koyama N, Matsuura K, Okamura H. Cytokines in the peritoneal fluid of patients with endometriosis. Int J Gynecol Obstet 1993;43:45–50.
16. Halme J. Role of peritoneal inflammation in endometriosis infertility. Ann NY Acad Sci 1991;622:266–74.
17. Giudice LC, Tazuke SI, Swiersz L. Status of current research on endometriosis. J Reprod Med 1998;43:252–62.
18. Oral E, Arici A. Peritoneal growth factors and endometriosis. Semin Reprod Endocrinol 1996;14:257–67.
19. Vernon MW, Beard JS, Graves K, Wilson EA. Classification of endometriotic implants by morphologic appearance and the capacity to synthesize prostaglandin. Fertil Steril 1986;46:801–6.
20. Fedele L, Parazzini F, Bianchi S et al. Stage and localization of pelvic endometriosis and pain. Fertil Steril 1990;53:155–8.
21. Stripling MC, Martin DC, Chatman DL et al. Subtle appearance of endometriosis. Fertil Steril 1988;49:427–31.
22. Pittaway DE. Diagnosis of endometriosis. Infertil Reprod Med Clin North Am 1992;3:619–31.
23. Wilson L, Kurzrok R. Studies on the motility of the human uterus in vivo. Endocrinology 1938;23:79–86.
24. Pickles VR, Hall W, Best FA et al. Prostaglandins in endometrium and menstrual fluid from normal and dysmenorrheic subjects. Br J Obstet Gynecol 1965;72:185–92.
25. Liu DT, Hitchcock A. Endometriosis: its association with retrograde menstruation, dysmeorrhea, and tubal pathology. Br J Obstet Gynaecol 1986;93:859–62.
26. Moon YS, Leung PCS, Yeun BH et al. Prostaglandin F in human endometriotic tissue. Am J Ostet Gynecol 1981;141:344–5.
27. Schenken RS, Asch RH, Williams RF et al. Etiology of infertility in monkeys with endometriosis. Measurement of peritoneal fluid prostaglandins. Am J Obstet Gynecol 1984;150:349–53.
28. Vernon MS, Beard JS, Graves K et al. Classification of endometriotic implants by morphologic appearance and capacity to synthesize protaglandin F. Fertil Steril 1986;46:801–6.
29. Kauppila A, Pualakka J, Ylikorkala O. Prostaglandin biosynthesis inhibitors and endometriosis. Prostaglandins 1979;18:655–61.
30. Leiblum S. Sexual pain disorders. In: Gebbard G, ed. Treatment of Psychiatric Disorders. Washington, DC: American Psychiatric Press, 1996;1941–58.
31. Vercellini P, Bocciolone L, Vendola N et al. Peritoneal endometriosis: morphologic appearance in women with chronic pelvic pain. J Reprod Med 1991;36:533–6.

32. Meana M, Binik Y. Painful coitus: a review of female dyspareunia. J Nerv Ment Dis 1994;18:264–72.

33. Steege J, Ling F. Dyspareunia: a special type of chronic pelvic pain. Obstet Gynecol Clin North Am 1993;20:779–93.

34. Soules MR, Malinak LR, Bury R et al. Endometriosis and anovulation: a coexisting problem in the infertile female. Am J Obstet Gynecol 1976;125:412–17.

35. Badawy SZ, Nusbaum M, Taymour E et al. Ovulatory dysfunction in patients with endometriosis. Diag Gynecol Obstet 1981;3:305–7.

36. Dmowski WP, Radwanska E, Binor Z et al. Mild endometriosis and ovulatory dysfunction: effect of danazol treatment on success of ovulation induction. Fertil Steril 1986;46:784–9.

37. Kaplan CR, Eddy CA, Olive DL et al. Effect of ovarian endometriosis on ovulation in rabbits. Am J Obstet Gynecol 1989;160:40–4.

38. Tummon IS, Maclin VM, Radwanska E et al. Occult ovulatory dysfunction in women with minimal endometriosis or unexplained infertility. Fertil Steril 1988;50:716–20.

39. Cahill DJ, Hull MG. Pituitary–ovarian dysfunction and endometriosis. Hum Reprod Update 2000;6:56–66.

40. Williams CA, Oak MK, Eelstein M. Cyclical gonadotropin and progesterone secretion in women with minimal endometriosis. Clin Reprod Fertil 1986;4:259–68.

41. Ji H. Luteal function in patients with endometriosis. Zhongguo Yi Xue Ke Xue Yuan Xue Bao 1989;11:344–8.

42. Cahill DJ, Wardie PG, Maile LA et al. Ovarian dysfunction in endometriosis-associated and unexplained infertility. J Assist Reprod Genet 1997;14:554–7.

43. Cunha-Filho JS, Gross JL, Lemos NA et al. Prolactin and growth hormone secretion after thyrotrophin-releasing hormone infusion and dopaminergic (DA2) blockade in infertile patients with minimal/mild endometriosis. Hum Reprod 2002;17:960–5.

44. Ayers JW, Birenbaum, Menon KM. Luteal phase dysfunction in endometriosis: elevated progesterone levels in peripheral and ovarian veins during the follicular phase. Fertil Steril 1987;47:925–9.

45. Mahmood TA, Templeton A. Folliculogenesis and ovulation in infertile women with mild endometriosis. Hum Reprod 1991;6:227–31.

46. Mahmood TA, Messinis IE, Templeton A. Follicular development in spontaneous and stimulated cycles in women with minimal–mild endometriosis. Br J Obstet Gynaecol 1991;98:783–8.

47. Djursing H, Peterson K, Weberg E. Symptomatic postmenopausal endometriosis. Acta Obstet Gynecol Scand 1981;60:529–30.

48. Ranney B. Endometriosis. III. Complete operations. Reasons, sequelae, treatment. Am J Obstet Gynecol 1971;109:1137–44.

49. Matorras R, Rodriquez F, Pijoan JI et al. Epidemiology of endometriosis in infertile women. Fertil Steril 1995;63:34–8.

50. Gruppo Italiano per lo Studio dell' Endometriosis. Prevalence and anatomical distribution of endometriosis in women with selected gynecological conditions: results from a multicentric Italian study. Hum Reprod 1994;9:1158–62.

51. Mahumood TA, Templeton A. Prevalence and genesis of endometriosis. Hum Reprod 1991;6:544–9.

52. Pauerstein CJ. Clinical presentation and diagnosis. In: Schenken RS, ed. Endometriosis: contemporary concepts in clinical management. Philadelphia: JB Lippincott, 1989; 127–44.

53. Burns WN, Schenken RS. Pathophysiology. In: Schenken RS, ed. Endometriosis: contemporary concepts in clinical management. Philadelphia: JB Lippincott, 1989; 83–126.

54. Strathy JH, Molgaard CA, Coulam CB et al. Endometriosis and infertility: a laparoscopic study of endometriosis among fertile and infertile women. Fertil Steril 1982;38:667–72.

55. Schenken RS, Asch RH, Williams RF et al. Etiology of infertility in monkeys with endometriosis. Fertil Steril 1984;41:122–30.

56. Werlin LB, DiZerga GS, Hodgen GD. Endometriosis: effect of ovulation, ovum pickup, and transport in monkeys: an interim report. Fertil Steril 1981;35:263 [abstract].

57. Luciano AA, Lowney J, Jacobs SL. Endoscopic treatment of endometriosis-associated infertility. Therapeutic, economic, and social benefits. J Reprod Med 1992;37:573–6.

58. Olive DL, Lee KL. Analysis of sequential treatment protocols for endometriosis-associated infertility. Am J Obstet Gynecol 1986;154:613–19.

59. Candiani GB, Vercellini P, Fedele L et al. Conservative surgical treatment for severe endometriosis in infertile women: are we making progress? Obstet Gynecol Surv 1991;46:490–8.

60. Surrey ES, Halme J. Effect of peritoneal fluid from endometriosis patients on endometrial stromal cell proliferation in vitro. Obstet Gynecol 1990;76:792–7.

61. Morcos RN, Gibbons WE, Findley WE. Effect of peritoneal fluid on in vitro cleavage of 2-cell mouse embryos: possible role of infertility associated endometriosis. Fertil Steril 1985;44:678–83.

62. Miller KS, Pittaway DE, Deaton JL. The effect of serum from infertile women with endometriosis on fertilization and early embryonic development in a murine in vitro fertilization model. Fertil Steril 1995;64:623–6.

63. Damewood MD, Hesla JS, Schlaff WD et al. Effect of serum from patients with minimal to mild endometriosis on mouse embryo development in vitro. Fertil Steril 1990;54:917–20.

64. Bayer SR, Seibel MM, Saffan DS et al. The efficacy of danazol treatment for minimal endometriosis in an infertile population: a prospective, randomized study. J Reprod Med 1988;33:179–83.

65. Telimaa S. Danazol and medroxyprogesterone acetate inefficacious in the treatment of endometriosis associated infertility. Fertil Steril 1988;50:872–5.

66. Adamson GD, Pasta DJ. Surgical treatment of endometriosis-associated infertility: meta-analysis compared with survival analysis. Am J Obstet Gynecol 1994;171:1488–504.

67. Hughes EG, Fedorkow DM, Collins JA. A quantitative overview of controlled trial in endometriosis-associated infertility. Fertil Steril 1993;59:963–70.

68. Marcoux S, Maheux R, Berube S. Laparoscopic surgery in infertile women with minimal or mild endometriosis. N Engl J Med 1997;337:217–22.

69. Gruppo Italiano per lo Studio dell Endometriosis. Ablation of lesions or no treatment in minimal–mild endometriosis in infertile women: a randomized trial. Hum Reprod 1999;14:1332–4.

70. Vilos GA, Vilos AW, Haebe JJ. Laparoscopic finding, management, histopathology, and outcome of 25 women with cyclic leg pain. J Am Assoc Gynecol Laparosc 2002;9:145–51.

71. Donnez J, Nisolle M, Squifflet J. Ureteral endometriosis: a complication of rectovaginal endometriotic (adenomyotic) nodules. Fertil Steril 2002;77:32–7.

72. Schenken RS. Treatment of human infertility: the special case of endometriosis. In: Adashi EY, Rock JA, Rosenwaks Z, eds. Reproductive Endocrinology. Surgery, and Technology. Philadelphia: Lippincott-Raven, 1995; 2121–39.

73. Harris RS, Foster WG, Surrey MW et al. Appendiceal disease in women with endometriosis and right lower quadrant pain. J Am Gynecol Laparosc 2001;8:536–41.

74. Yeun JS, Chow PK, Koong HN et al. Unusual sites (thorax and umbilical hernial sac) of endometriosis. J Roy Coll Surg Edin 2001;46:313–15.

75. Jeanes AC, Murray D, Davidson B et al. Case report: hepatic and retroperitoneal endometriosis presenting as obstructive jaundice with ascites: a case report and review of the literature. Clin Radiol 2002;57:226–9.

76. Yu Z, Fleishman JK, Rahman HM et al. Catamenial hemoptysis and pulmonary endometriosis: a case report. Mt Sinai J Med 2002;69:261–3.

77. L'huillier JP, Slat-Baroux J. A patient with pulmonary endometriosis. Rev Pneumol Clin 2002;58:233–6.

78. Gomi IM, Hiranouchi N, Fujimoto K et al. A case of cerebral endometriosis causing catamenial epilepsy. Neurology 1993;43:2708–9.

79. Sataloff DM, LaVorgna KA, McFarland MM. Extrapelvic endometriosis presenting as a hernia, clinical reports and review of the literature. Surgery 1989;105:109–12.

80. Michowitz M, Baratz M, Stavorovsky M. Endometriosis of the umbilicus. Dermatologica 1983;167:326–30.

81. Cramer DW. Epidemiology of endometriosis. In Wilson EA, ed. Endometriosis. New York: Alan R. Liss,1987; 5–22.

82. Eskanazi B, Warner M. Epidemiology of endometriosis. Obstet Gynecol Clin North Am 1997;24:235–58.

83. Forman RG, Robinson JN, Mehta Z et al. Patient history as a simple predictor of pelvic pathology in subfertile women. Hum Reprod 1993;8:53–5.

84. Naish CE, Kennedy BH, Barlow DH. Correlation between pain symptoms and laparoscopic findings. In: Brosens IA, Donnez J, eds. Program and abstracts of the Third World Congress on Endometriosis, 1–3 June 1993, Brussels.

85. Fedele L, Bianchi S, Bocciolone L et al. Pain symptoms associated with endometriosis. Obstet Gynecol 1992;79:767–9.

86. Vercellini P, Tresidi I, Giorgi OD et al. Endometriosis and pelvic pain: relation to disease stage and localization. Fertil Steril 1996;65:299–304.

87. Williams TJ, Pratt JH. Endometriosis in 1,000 consecutive celiotomies: incidence and management. Am J Obstet Gynecol 1977;129:245–50.

88. Fedele L, Parazzini F, Bianchi S et al. Stage and localization of pelvic endometriosis and pain. Fertil Steril 1990;53:155–8.

89. Eskanazi B, Warner M, Bonsignore L et al. Validation study nonsurgical diagnosis of endometriosis. Fertil Steril 2001;76:929–35.

12. Diagnosis

Steven R. Lindheim

Endometriosis is a disease that has always been thought to almost exclusively affect women of reproductive age. It often presents with an array of clinical symptoms, including pain, dysmenorrhea, dyspareunia, cyclic pain, abnormal uterine bleeding, and infertility. The reported prevalence is over 70% in those who complain of pelvic pain and more than 80% of women evaluated for a combination of pelvic pain and infertility,[1] though this can vary depending on the age, race, and socioeconomic status of the defined population.[2] With the increased use of laparoscopy, the prevalence of endometriosis is even more common among adolescents than previously thought, which has been reported to be 45–58% of adolescents who present with abdominal pain and dysmenorrhea.[2,3] The youngest reported histologically confirmed case of endometriosis is 10.5 years old.[4]

Of all the above symptoms, pain is the most commonly associated with endometriosis, affecting nearly 15% of American women between the ages of 18 and 50.[5] Chronic pelvic pain (CPP), defined as non-menstrual pain of at least 3 months' duration, or menstrual pain of at least 6 months' duration, is typically confined to the lower abdomen and below the umbilicus, interfering with normal daily function.[6] Altered daily function can have variable extremes, including work-related concentration abilities, or habits related to intercourse and recreational activities. At the other extreme, women with CPP can be confined to bed, to the point where it has been described that one in four spend at least one half day in bed each month, primarily because of the pain associated with endometriosis.[5] Attempts have been made to differentiate cyclical pain from pain that is independent of the menstrual cycle, but from a treatment standpoint the most important feature is the degree of disability it causes.

There are many disorders associated in women with CPP (Table 12.1). This chapter will focus on the differential diagnosis of CPP and the diagnostic approach, including history, physical examination, laboratory testing, and imaging studies.

Table 12.1 Differential diagnosis of chronic pelvic pain

Gynecologic
- Endometriosis
- Adenomyosis
- Chronic pelvic infection
- Hydrosalpinx
- Degenerating leiomyomata uteri

Gastrointestinal
- Irritable bowel syndrome
- Diverticulitis
- Inflammatory bowel disease

Urinary
- Interstitial cystitis
- Urethral syndrome
- Detrusor dyssynergia
- Chronic calculi

Musculoskeletal/rheumatologic
- Fibromyalgia
- Hernia
- Disc disease
- Arthritis
- Scoliosis

Psychiatric
- Depression
- Physical or sexual abuse
- Hypochondriasis
- Somatization
- Drug dependency
- Factitious

Adapted from Scialli AR.

ETIOLOGIES ASSOCIATED WITH CPP

GASTROINTESTINAL TRACT

Disorders of the intestinal tract are often accompanied by symptoms of nausea, vomiting, constipation, or diarrhea, but pain may be the only or the most prominent symptom. Various etiologies of the intestinal tract that can cause chronic pelvic pain include irritable bowel syndrome, inflammatory bowel disease (including Crohn's disease or ulcerative colitis), chronic infection (*Giardia lamblia*), malabsorptive conditions, chronic appendicitis, diverticular disease, or colorectal cancer.

IRRITABLE BOWEL SYNDROME

Irritable bowel syndrome (IBS) is a functional bowel disorder characterized by abnormal motility and sensation. It affects 15–20% of American adults and is a diagnosis of exclusion. Two sets of criteria are used to diagnose IBS. The Manning criteria consist of abdominal pain associated with looser, frequent stools at the onset of pain that is relieved by defecation associated with mucous discharge and a feeling of incomplete evacuation.[7] The Rome criteria are more objective and include recurrent or continuous abdominal pain of 3 months' duration that is relieved by defecation and associated with a change in the frequency and consistency of stools, including diarrhea alone, constipation alone, or a combination of both.[8,9] The pain, including abdominal bloating, is typically worse after eating and can be associated with either constipation (25%) or diarrhea (15%), together with a sense of incomplete rectal emptying. More recently, new criteria (Rome II) have been established which allow for the identification of subgroups of IBS.[10]

To further confuse the picture, symptoms may vary with the menstrual cycle, causing affected women to present to a gynecologist.[11,12] The association between IBS and dysmenorrhea has been well documented by Crowell et al,[13] who reported that women who had dysmenorrhea were more likely to have functional bowel disorders (61%)

than those who did not (20%). The menses-related exacerbations of IBS symptoms are thought to be due to excessive prostaglandins, though this has not been validated.[14] The patient's clinical response to prostaglandin inhibitors may help to distinguish IBS from dysmenorrhea.[15]

Treatment has focused on the use of fiber and peppermint oil, but clinical trials are flawed and do not support the use of these agents.[16,17] In those in whom constipation is the predominant symptom treatment has focused on osmotic laxatives (cisapride), which have had variable success.[18] New therapies, including antimuscarinic agents (M3 selective antagonists), serotonin antagonists (fedotozine), CCK antagonists, and GnRH antagonists, are all being evaluated as therapies for IBS.[19–21]

INFLAMMATORY BOWEL DISEASE/COLORECTAL CANCER

Whereas irritable bowel syndrome represents a functional bowel disorder, inflammatory bowel disease represents abnormalities of the bowel mucosa or the entire bowel wall. Inflammatory bowel disease encompasses a wide spectrum of clinical and pathologic entities. Symptoms may be limited to the gastrointestinal tract and include diarrhea, abdominal pain, tenesmus, and bloody stools. When severe, diarrhea and inflammation can give rise to systemic symptoms of anorexia, weight loss, malnutrition, and general debilitation.

Although the etiology of inflammatory bowel disease remains unknown, the most popular theory is that the body's immune system reacts to a virus or a bacterium by causing ongoing inflammation in the intestine. Two types often distinguished are ulcerative colitis and Crohn's disease (also known as regional enteritis).[22,23] Ulcerative colitis is an inflammatory disease of the colon that causes a diffuse mucosal inflammation virtually always involving the rectum. Patients usually present with diarrhea, the passage of blood and mucus in the stool, and abdominal pain, though the clinical presentation is extremely variable and is characterized by acute attacks followed by periods of remission. Crohn's disease is a full-thickness inflammation of the intestinal wall and typically affects young adults. As a result, the formation of adhesions between adjacent loops of bowel and other abdominal organs is common, with fistulae from bowel segment to bowel segment, bladder, abdominal wall, and skin, including the abdominal wall, flank, or in the perineum. The presence of anal fissures is characteristic of Crohn's disease. Clinically, Crohn's disease presents with vague abdominal pain, mild diarrhea, gastrointestinal bleeding, anorexia, fatigue, and lethargy. Although it is similar to ulcerative colitis, symptoms can be vague.

A number of extraintestinal manifestation are seen with inflammatory bowel disease, and these include arthritic complaints in up to 25% of patients; erythema nodosum in 20% of patients; pyoderma gangrenosum (poorly healing indolent ulcers) generally confined to the extremities; stomatis; conjunctivitis; and uveitis.[24]

Colorectal cancer can also manifest itself as crampy abdominal pain and altered bowel habits, although symptoms of anemia (fatigue, lethargy) are more common owing to occult gastrointestinal bleeding. It is rare to see colorectal cancer in patients under the age of 50, although patients with ulcerative colitis have an abnormally high incidence.[25]

Radiographic findings can be suggestive of bowel disease. In patients under 50 years of age a sigmoidoscopy and CBC with erythrocyte sedimentation rate are recommended. Colonoscopy or barium enema are recommended in patients with a history suggestive of a more proximal colonic pathology or in those over 50 years of age having nocturnal diarrhea, or with blood in the stool.

In patients with inflammatory bowel disease the goals of therapy are to reduce the abdominal discomfort, control diarrhea, and decrease the inflammation. Sulfasalazine and glucocorticoids are the mainstays of drug therapy for both ulcerative colitis and Crohn's disease, although newer antibody therapy should be considered in patients who fail standard therapies. Roughage should be eliminated and antidiarrheal agents should be prescribed with caution.[26]

URINARY TRACT CAUSES OF PELVIC PAIN

Urinary symptoms, including frequent urination and dysuria, are the typical presentation of disorders of the urinary system. However, chronic midline suprapubic pain may be the only or the most prominent symptom of urinary tract disease. Various etiologies include interstitial cystitis, urethral syndrome, or chronic ureteral calculi.

INTERSTITIAL CYSTITIS

Interstitial cystitis (IC) is difficult to diagnose and treat and is estimated to affect from 10 to 500 per 100 000.[27–30] Typically, IC is diagnosed in the later reproductive years. However, many suffer from symptoms similar to those of a chronic urinary tract infection (UTI), including nocturia and urgency (average number of voids per day is 16, compared to six in normal subjects), for many years prior to their diagnosis. The pain is experienced suprapubically and is exacerbated by a full bladder and relieved to some extent by voiding. On examination, more than 95% will have a tender bladder base on bimanual pelvic examination. Some patients with advanced disease have tenderness and spasm of the levator ani and pubococcygeus muscles. Historically, the diagnosis has required cystoscopy to identify bladder mucosal changes, including pinpoint petechial hemorrhages, and to assess for bladder capacity using hydrodistension, which is typically reduced.[31] A simple office-based test, the potassium sensitivity challenge, uncovers uroepithelial dysfunction in up to 90% of cases.[32]

The etiology of IC remains controversial; potential causes include autoimmune abnormalities, allergic reaction, and infection. Normally, a film of mucin consisting largely of glycosaminoglycans (GAG), is secreted by bladder epithelial cells and serves as a protective coat covering the luminal surface of the bladder. In IC, this layer is believed to be functionally defective. It is further thought that noxious substances (primarily potassium ions) in urine permeate the bladder wall, resulting in tissue irritation leading to symptoms of IC.

Treatment has focused on bladder retraining and modification. Pharmacologic treatment involves the use of pentoan polysulfate sodium (Elmiron) 100 mg/tid. This FDA-approved oral agent is analogous to naturally occurring GAG, which block uroepithelial permeability.

URETHRAL SYNDROME

Urethral syndrome is caused by chronic inflammation of tissue around the urethra. This condition may produce pain with intercourse and can occur with or without a full bladder. It is often misdiagnosed as recurrent UTI, as the classic symptoms mimic those of an infection (pressure, urgency, and frequency), although nocturia and negative urine cultures are often present. Clinical suspicion should arise when a thickening around the urethra (rope-like) in the midline is appreciated. The etiology is often infection, including *Chlamydia, Mycoplasma*, or herpes. Confirmation is typically made with evidence of inflammation on urinalysis, though cultures are usually negative. Treatment entails long-term antibiotics (up to 3 months) or urethral dilation, which generally produce good results.

URETERAL STONES

Ureteral stones can cause severe flank pain, with radiation to the groin. However, with stones in the distal ureter, anterior pain can be a presenting complaint. Typically stones are acute in nature and are passed within a few days of clinical presentation, but a chronic picture is possible. Hematuria is seen, and the disorder is typically confirmed with an intravenous pyelogram.

MUSCULOSKELETAL CAUSES OF PELVIC PAIN

Pain arising from the abdominal wall or back is often interpreted as originating from the peritoneal cavity. Pathology includes abdominal wall hernia, neuroma, disk herniation, and orthopedic conditions.

ABDOMINAL WALL HERNIA

Defects in the abdominal wall (e.g. hernias) can cause peritoneum or intestine to become trapped, producing visceral pain. Abdominal hernias occur in women as well as men. Detection is easiest with the patient in the standing position, but if the woman is only examined in the supine position, or with her feet in stirrups, the presence of a hernia may be easily overlooked.

NEUROMA

A neuroma results in a hypersensitive nerve ending, which is often found in a surgical incision. Women with a history of surgery who subsequently develop pain at the site of the surgical scar may have an incisional hernia or neuroma. Careful palpation with the patient both standing and supine may help distinguish the two conditions. Neuromas may also respond well to local anesthetic injection.

DISK HERNIATION

Herniation of a lumbar disk may compress a nerve root, producing shooting pain along the distribution of the root. Classic sciatica is characterized by back pain radiating around the flank and into the groin or leg, but abdominal pain can also occur. Weakness or decreased muscle spindle reflexes in the distribution of the compressed root can aid in the diagnosis. Pain on percussion over the affected vertebral region is also common.

ORTHOPEDIC CONDITIONS

Other orthopedic problems may produce pain in the abdomen. Abnormal posture has been proposed as a cause of pain by stretching of the abdominal muscles, thoracolumbar fascia and muscles of the lower back and thighs.[33] Asymmetric leg length may also produce abdominal muscle stretching, leading to pain.[34] Posture and whether the pelvis is tilted can be assessed by observing the patient standing or walking. Leg lengths can be measured directly.

RHEUMATOLOGIC CAUSES OF PELVIC PAIN

FIBROMYALGIA

Fibromyalgia is a generalized state of hyperalgesia involving multiple parts of the body, and affects 3–6% of women of reproductive age. Although it is categorized as a rheumatologic disorder, fibromyalgia is actually due to an abnormality in pain processing[35] and not an abnormality in the body wall. As a result of abnormal pain processing, pain signals may not be suppressed or may be inappropriately augmented. This condition results in widespread pain and diffuse tenderness on examination, though the pain tends to be most severe in one or two regions of the body.

Diagnostic criteria established by the American College of Rheumatology[36] include pain in all four quadrants of the body. Areas overlying the axial skeleton and tenderness must be present in at least 11 of 18 defined tender points. Patients often experience associated sleep and mood disturbances, including depression, although they typically do not meet full DSM-IV criteria for depression. Further confusing the diagnosis is the overlap of visceral pain associated with disorders including irritable bowel syndrome and interstitial cystitis.[37]

The most effective medical treatment has included the use of tricyclic compounds (e.g. nortriptyline, cyclobenzaprine), analgesics, and low-impact aerobic exercise. Selective serotonin reuptake inhibitors (SSRI) have been shown to be marginally effective. Cognitive–behavioral therapy, which addresses maladaptive behavior(s), has been shown to be efficacious.[38]

REGIONAL PAIN SYNDROMES

Regional pain syndromes are closely related to fibromyalgia, but the abnormal pain processing typically involves isolated regions of the body. It is thought that the abnormal pain processing is due to episodes of intense stimulation of pain fibers. A history of sexual or physical abuse leading to CPP may be due to a triggering of abnormal neurologic pain processing. As with fibromyalgia, treatment addresses primarily cognitive processes and maladaptive behaviors, not psychiatric issues.[39]

PSYCHIATRIC CAUSES OF PELVIC PAIN

CPP has been associated with psychiatric etiologies, and mood disturbances are an important element to address when patients present with CPP.

DEPRESSION

Depression is a common disease and a common cause of CPP.[40,41] Criteria for the diagnosis of depression are listed in Table 12.2, which is from the DSM-IV Primary Care Edition. For non-psychiatric primary care practitioners to make the diagnosis is supported by the American Psychiatric Association, the American Academy of Family Physicians, the American Academy of

---

Table 12.2 Criteria for depression

1. At least 5 of the following symptoms have been present nearly every day during the same 2-week period and represent a change from previous functioning. At least one of the symptoms must be either depressed mood or loss of interest or pleasure.
   - Depressed mood (or irritable mood in children or adolescents)
   - Markedly diminished interest or pleasure in all, or almost all, activities
   - Significant weight loss or weight gain when not dieting
   - Insomnia or hypersomnia
   - Psychomotor agitation or retardation
   - Fatigue or loss of energy
   - Feelings of worthlessness or excessive or inappropriate guilt
   - Diminished ability to think or concentrate
   - Recurrent thoughts of death, recurrent suicidal ideation without a specific plan, or a suicide attempt or specific plan for committing suicide
2. Symptoms are not better accounted for by a mood disorder due to general medical condition, a substance-induced mood disorder or bereavement (normal reaction to the death of a loved one)
3. Symptoms are not better accounted for by a psychiatric disorder (e.g. schizoaffective disorder)

Data from American Psychiatric Association

Pediatrics, the American Board of Family Practice, the American College of Obstetricians and Gynecologists, the American College of Physicians, the American Medical Association, the Association of Departments of Family Medicine, the Society of General Internal Medicine, and the Society of Teachers of Family Medicine.[41] Treatment with antidepressants has been shown to improve symptoms of CPP, suggesting that pain may be due to psychiatric disease.[42,43]

SOMATIZATION

Somatization refers to physical manifestations of psychologic distress. This disorder is diagnosed in patients with multiple physical complaints, but somatization cannot be attributed to any other known general medical condition.[41] DSM-IV criteria include:

- At least four different sites of pain
- At least two gastrointestinal symptoms (e.g. nausea and diarrhea)
- At least one neurologic symptom (e.g. impaired coordination)
- At least one sexual or reproductive organ symptom (e.g. irregular menses or altered libido).

HYPOCHONDRIASIS

Hypochodriasis is a preoccupation with fears of having a serious disease despite appropriate medical examinations and reassurance by a healthcare provider.[44] These patients spend an excessive amount of time on their complaints, often presenting with detailed diaries covering months or years; however, many patients also fear they will receive upsetting information if evaluated, and thus avoid consultations and remain preoccupied with physiologic events, believing they are physically ill. It may reflect a means of socializing by the patient. Cognitive–behavioral therapy has been shown to be an effective form of treatment.

SOMATIC DELUSIONS

Somatic delusions are erroneous beliefs.[41] For example, a somatic delusion can be a belief that a creature is living inside a patient's abdomen and eating away at internal organs. This disorder is unusual as a complaint of CPP and is often associated with other evidence of disordered thoughts.

CONTROLLED SUBSTANCE ABUSE

The complaint of factitious chronic pain is associated with a substance abuse problem and is a way for the patient to obtain medications for abusive purposes. The healthcare provider should always be alert to this problem, and DMS-IV symptoms listed in Table 12.3 may be present in those with problematic substance abuse.[41] Although patients with true CPP may use analgesics for pain relief, they typically obtain relief without increasing the dose of analgesia and/or do not experience any of the psychosocial dysfunction that is often characteristic of problematic substance abuse.

SEXUAL DYSFUNCTION

Sexual pain disorders typically result in pain associated with sexual intercourse, referred to as dyspareunia. Estimates place the incidence around 10–15% of women. The etiology can result from a number of physical conditions or psychogenic causes.

PHYSICAL CAUSES

There are a host of physical conditions that can cause dyspareunia, including hymeneal scarring,

---

Table 12.3 Symptoms associated with problematic substance abuse

- Impaired control of substance use
- Guilt or regret about use, efforts to cut down, complaints or concerns from others
- Recent substance use with resultant neurologic symptoms, cardiovascular symptoms, confusion, anxiety, sleep disturbance, depressed mood, or sexual dysfunction
- Psychosocial dysfunction (e.g. family conflict) related to substance use
- Tolerance (the need for increasing amounts to achieve effect)

Data from American Psychiatric Association

---

pelvic inflammatory disease, vulvar conditions including vulvar vestibulitis, and chronic lack of lubrication.[45] Associated with dyspareunia is the condition known as vaginismus, which refers to the recurrence of persistent involuntary spasm of the outer third of the vagina, interfering with sexual intercourse and causing marked interpersonal difficulty or distress. Rates have been reported to range from 12% to 17% of females reporting to sexual therapy clinics.[46] This has been known to occur in women with a history of infections, surgeries, or use of chemical agents.

PSYCHOGENIC CAUSES

Most female sexual disorders are caused or maintained by psychological rather than physical factors, and have their origin with respect to the following:[47]

- Developmental factors, including those that associate sex with guilt and shame, religious taboos, misinformation about sex
- Traumatic factors, including rape or other sexual or gynecological trauma, childhood sexual or physical abuse
- Relational factors, including resentment and antagonistic feelings toward one's sexual partner, inadequate foreplay and time for arousal, personal upsets, and anxieties that prevent concentration on sensual exchange and fantasies, with a focusing on negative or unattractive aspects of one's partner.

For organic causes of sexual dysfunction both surgical and pyschopharmacologic interventions have been found to be helpful.[48,49] For psychogenic causes, some combination of systemic desensitization couples' therapy, pubococcygeal muscle exercises, and vaginal self-dilation in well-motivated patients with supportive partners has a good prognosis.[47,49]

GYNECOLOGIC DISORDERS OF
PELVIC PAIN

A number of gynecologic conditions, as listed in Table 12.4, may result in pelvic pain. However,

Table 12.4 Gynecologic conditions resulting in pelvic pain

- Endometriosis
- Adenomyosis
- Chronic pelvic inflammatory disease (PID)
- Ovarian cyst
- Leiomyomata
- Pelvic varicosities
- Ovarian remnant syndrome

most conditions typically result in acute pelvic symptoms, and only endometriosis and adenomyosis are clearly associated with CPP.

ADENOMYOSIS

Adenomyosis is the presence of endometrial glands and stroma in the muscle wall of the uterus, and can result in symptoms suggestive of endometriosis. However, these two conditions are very different and are only found concomitantly 20% of the time.[50] The pathogenesis of adenomyosis remains unclear, but the barrier between the endometrium and the myometrium is broken, resulting in a direct extension of endometrial components at least 4 mm beneath the endomyometrial junction.[51] Adenomyosis is usually observed in older and multiparous women, and although the majority of women are asymptomatic, symptoms include secondary dysmenorrhea and menorrhagia. The uterus tends to enlarge symmetrically and become tender, especially just prior to the onset of menses.

Diagnosis has classically been confirmed by histological examination. In cases of extensive adenomyosis, hysterosalpingography can reveal glandular filling within myometrial tissue, but this is only present in 25% of cases as myometrial glandular components do not generally communicate with the endometrial cavity.[52] Transabdominal or transvaginal ultrasound can reveal diffuse uterine enlargement without focal abnormalities, or diffuse areas of heterogeneity or poorly defined hypoechoic areas (smooth muscle hypertrophy) and tiny myometrial cysts (owing to dilated ectopic glands).[53,54] MRI is superior to ultrasound, with higher sensitivity and specificity for diagnosing adenomyosis, particularly in premenopausal women because of the improved definition of the junctional zone.[52,55] Adenomyomas can often be distinguished from fibroids because they are typically oval and poorly defined, whereas fibroids are round and well marginated.[56]

No satisfactory treatment exists and the condition is thought to be due to the relative deficiency of progesterone and estrogen receptors in the adenomyomatous cells compared to endometrial cells. Although some investigators have suggested the use of GnRH agonists, the deficiency in receptors may explain the diminished response to ovarian hormone suppression.[57] Occasionally women may respond to prostaglandin synthetase inhibitors; these tend to be most efficacious if therapy is commenced 1–2 days before the onset of menses. Hysterectomy is the most successful form of definitive therapy for patients with adenomyosis. However, making an accurate diagnosis prior to hysterectomy depends largely on the index of suspicion.

ADHESIONS/PELVIC INFECTION

Some believe that adhesions themselves can be a cause of CPP, as they cause anatomic distortion and nerve compression; however, support in the literature is lacking. Chronic pelvic infection is also thought to result in CPP, but this too lacks support in the literature. Anecdotal reports of improvement with antibiotics may be related to the anti-inflammatory effect of these drugs.

LEIOMYOMAS

Uterine leiomyomas (fibroids) occur in one of 4–5 women during their reproductive life and are the most common solid tumor of the female pelvis. They are believed to originate directly from the myometrium. It is estimated that between 20% and 50% of women will experience symptoms, the severity of which appears to be related to the size and location of the fibroids; symptoms include menorrhagia, pelvic pain, pressure, and urinary symptoms. The exact relationship between uterine leiomyomas and pelvic pain is unclear. Large uterine fibroids can cause pressure symptoms, and with cystic degeneration can cause acute symptoms, but their role in CPP is questionable. Diagnosis is typically made with ultrasound and MRI.[58]

Assessment of the uterine cavity is also recommended, as endometrial pathology, including leiomyomas, polyps, scarring, and cervical stenosis, has been found in up to 30% of patients with a primary diagnosis of CPP.[59,60] Evaluation using sonohysterography, hysterosalpingography, or hysteroscopy may improve the diagnosis and treatment of CPP.

MAKING A DIAGNOSIS OF ENDOMETRIOSIS

Given the wide array of medical conditions associated with CPP, a systematic approach, including a focus on the principles of physical diagnosis (history and physical examination), is a key component of making a correct diagnosis. There are a number of clinical and physical clues that are suggestive of endometriosis. However, the key to diagnosis is for the physician to evaluate the patient completely, whether he or she is a gynecologist, internist, surgeon, or urologist. A comprehensive approach to the evaluation of a woman with pelvic pain, paying attention to somatic, psychologic, dietary, environmental, and other factors, results in outcomes superior to those of a standard approach directed primarily at the pelvic organs.[61]

THE EVALUATION: HISTORY AND PHYSICAL EXAMINATION

The most important part in evaluating the patient with CPP is the history and physical examination, and in most instances the former gives the most valuable information. Each question must be directed at all organ systems, as many diseases/disorders can present as pelvic pain. Unfortunately, given the practical time constraints in daily medical practice, a few salient points should be considered when evaluating patients with CPP:

- Schedule the patient for as many subsequent visits as necessary. Patients appreciate this and feel you are being thorough in your evaluation.
- Use a questionnaire to elicit a focused and complete history prior to the patient's initial visit. This offers the advantages of soliciting specific information from the patient and permitting her sufficient time and privacy to reflect on her answers.
- Listen to the patient. Open-ended questioning is of great value in eliciting a description of the patient's chief complaints.
- Using a pain map (see Figure 12.6) can also be helpful and may help identify non-pelvic sites of pain.[62]

In addition to the description of the pain, its quality, where it radiates, its severity, and its timing (PQRST),[63] open-ended questions are of great value in eliciting a description of the chief complaint. A complete history should include a review of all organ systems (see Table 12.1). A menstrual history is important because pelvic and abdominal pain is usually cyclical, and its relationship to menstrual function should be assessed.

The psychological history should include questions about psychiatric illnesses, familial dysfunction, and sexual and physical abuse, the latter of which has been found to occur in up to 75% of patients with CPP.[64] Addressing issues included in Table 12.2 will help to assess for clinical depression. Numerous psychological tests are also available, including the Beck Depression Inventory (BDI), a standardized and validated, 21-question written test that measures specific symptoms of depression. Other tests include the Minnesota Multiphasic Personality Inventory (MMPI), which screens patients for a wide range of psychopathologies. The McGill Pain Questionnaire and the West Haven–Yale Multidimensional Pain Inventory (WHY MPI) are useful tests to assess how the pain affects the patient on a day-to-day basis. The former assesses the complexity of the pain experience, how it

changes over time, and its intensity.[65] The latter assesses the patient's perception of the impact of pain on her everyday life, how it affects others in her life, and her general activity level.[65] It is recommended that, if required, a mental health professional should administer this component of the overall assessment.

PHYSICAL EXAMINATION

The elements of the physical examination are familiar to most physicians. Attention to areas outside the scope of expertise is key, as one may overlook other organ systems. Table 12.5 presents features of the physical examination that may be helpful in evaluating patients with CPP to rule out abnormalities outside the pelvis. An examination should include the head, eyes, ears, nose, throat, and neck, with specific attention to the thyroid gland, as the side effects of hypo- or hyperthyroidism may contribute to the symptoms of lethargy or anxiety often experienced by patients with CPP.

GENERAL

The physical evaluation, which typically takes place with the patient in a supine position, should be performed in the erect position to help identify any abnormalities of the musculoskeletal system. A careful breast examination should be performed and any areas of tenderness noted.

Auscultation of the heart and lungs should follow, as endometriosis can occur in almost every organ of the body.[66] It is believed that this may be due to vascular or lymphatic transport of endometrial fragments. Pulmonary endometriosis can be manifested as asymptomatic nodules or as pneumothorax, hemothorax, or hemoptysis during menses.[67] Assessment for any costovertebral angle tenderness is important to exclude an indolent pyelonephritis.

Endometriosis should be included in the differential diagnosis of CPP that involves abdominal scar lesions.[68,69] Previous abdominal surgical incisions involving a hysterotomy from a cesarean section or myomectomy that involve

Table 12.5 Features of the physical examination that are useful in the evaluation of the woman with CPP

- General
  Appearance
  Affect
- Back
  Point tenderness (spine, trigger points)
  Range of motion
- Chest wall
  Point tenderness (trigger points)
  Asymmetry
- Abdomen
  Appearance
  Defects of the abdominal wall (standing and supine)
  Consistency
  Tenderness
  Organ enlargement
  Masses
  Bowel sounds
  Bruits
- Pelvic examination
  External genitalia: appearance
  Vagina: appearance, discharge
  Urethral/periurethral: tenderness, discharge, mass
  Cervix: appearance, discharge, tenderness to motion
  Uterus: size, shape, consistency, tenderness, mobility
  Adenexa: mass, ovarian size, tenderness
  Rectal: mass, uterosacral ligament nodularity/tenderness, stool (color, mucus, occult blood)
- Extremities
  Leg length
  Tenderness with straight leg raising against resistance
  Tenderness with abduction at the hip
  Strength and sensation
  Gait

cyclical pain emanating from a mass in the vicinity of an abdominal surgical scar or umbilicus should not be overlooked. Although this is a rare occurrence, it is not well recognized and often mistaken for a suture granuloma, lipoma, abscess, cyst, or incisional hernia.

There are a number of non-gynecologic findings that occur more often in women with endometriosis and which should be considered in the general assessment, including scoliosis,[70] dysplastic nevi,[71] and red hair.[72,73] Dysplastic nevi and scoliosis have been reported to be respectively five and 10 times more likely in women with endometriosis than in controls. In women with a family history of melanoma, those with CPP had a three times greater likelihood of having endometriosis.

ABDOMEN

Abdominal assessment with rectus tensing is an important part of the examination to help differentiate between abdominal wall pain and intraperitoneal pain. However, evaluating areas in abdominal quadrants away from the area of tenderness helps the patient to relax and gain confidence that the examination will be gentle. Having the patient voluntarily contract and relax her abdominal muscles prior to the examination, particularly in those who exhibit considerable guarding, is a useful technique.[74]

Rectus tensing involves the patient lying in the supine position with the hips flexed or the legs straight. The legs are then lifted about six inches from the horizontal plane while the chin is touched to the chest, ensuring that the rectus muscle is contracted. If the pain is in the abdominal wall and the pain site palpated, pain will be experienced. If the pain is intraperitoneal, pushing on the abdominal wall will not produce pain, allowing the differentiation of superficial pain from intraperitoneal cavity pain.[75]

PELVIC/RECTAL

A pelvic examination may reveal the presence of masses or fixed organs, suggesting the presence of organic disease within the abdomen or pelvis. The rectal examination provides superior access to any small masses of the posterior cul de sac or uterosacral or broad ligaments, indicating the presence of endometriosis. Rectal tenderness or heme-positive stools may suggest the presence of bowel disease.

Assessment of the cervix is often overlooked. Lateral displacement of the cervix, first described 30 years ago,[75] is defined as the presence of the entire cervix lateral to the vaginal midline. Lateral displacement of the cervix is often associated with pelvic pathology, specifically endometriosis. It is felt that this displacement occurs because of shortening of one of the uterosacral ligaments by lesions causing asymmetric fibrosis. Batt et al[75] reported cervical displacement in 17% of cases of Stage 3 disease, and 14% of Stage 4 disease, and

Barbieri et al[76] reported that 28% of women with endometriosis had lateral displacement of the cervix. This is confirmed on digital or speculum examination, though the latter can artificially displace the cervix laterally and should be placed carefully when examining the patient.[77]

The diameter of the external cervical os can also be suggestive of pelvic pathology. Normally menstrual blood flow exits the uterus either by traversing the cervical canal or by retrograde menstruation through the tubal ostia. It has been estimated that when the diameter of the cervical os is less than 4.5 mm there is significantly more retrograde menstruation than when the diameter is more than 4.5 mm,[78] and as a reference most nulliparous women have a cervical diameter greater than 5 mm. A recent study revealed that 19% of women with endometriosis had cervical stenosis, with a diameter less than 4.75 mm.[78]

Using a cotton-tipped applicator can help make the diagnosis of cervical stenosis. An applicator has a maximal tip diameter of approximately 4.75 mm. If this will not pass through the external os, a presumptive diagnosis of cervical stenosis can be made.[78]

PAIN MEASUREMENT

Pain mapping as depicted in Figure 12.1 has been described to determine the exact location and severity of suspected locations.[74] Pain ratings can be based on a scale of 0–10, where 0 represents no pain and 10 represents the worst pain ever experienced.

The area map to assess abdominal tenderness is shown in Figure 12.2. The abdomen is divided into nine locations, and following palpation the lowest to highest score is recorded. The patient is then asked to close her eyes and point to the one place where it hurts the most; 50% of patients will point to one single area.

To localize a specific area of pain/discomfort on pelvic examination a paracervical map is used, as shown in Figure 12.3. The paracervical map is divided into eight areas as on a clock face: 12:00, 1:30; 3:00, 4:30, 6:00, 7:30, 9:00, and 10:30 o'clock. A long

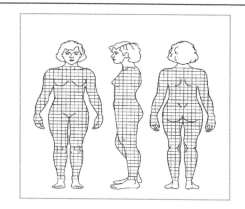

Figure 12.1 Pain Map. Patients are instructed to mark squares representing the location of their pain. (Reprinted from Carter.[58])

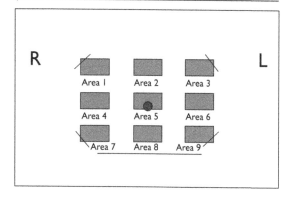

Figure 12.2 Area map to assess tenderness. (Reproduced from Pelvic Pain Clinic, Yale University School of Medicine.)

Q-tip is meticulously pressed against the tissue in each of these areas, again recording the intensity of pain on a scale of 0–10. These areas are further evaluated on bimanual examination, allowing further assessment of the type of pain and the presence of any abnormalities in the suspected areas.

Focal tenderness on pelvic examination has been correlated with pelvic pathology. In a prospective study by Ripps et al[79] pathology was seen in 97% (68 of 70) of patients who had focal tenderness on pelvic examination. Endometriosis was found in 68% (45 of 68) at the site of tenderness, and 96% of lesions were fibrotic. Conversely, tenderness was found at the site of endometriosis

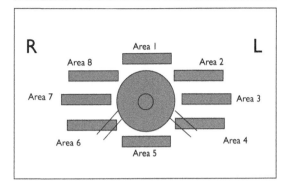

Figure 12.3 Pericervical map to localize discomfort during pelvic exam. (Reproduced from Pelvic Pain Clinic, Yale University School of Medicine.)

Table 12.6 Laboratory tests in patients with chronic pelvic pain
Strongly recommended tests
• Complete blood count, including differential
• Urinalysis
• Testing for gonorrhea and *Chlamydia*
Tests that may be indicated based on findings of the history and physical examination
• Vaginal wet smear
• Sedimentation rate
• Antinuclear antibody, rheumatoid factor, and other tests for autoantibodies
• Stool testing for infectious agents

From Scialli AR.[61]

in 76% (45 of 59) in patients with endometriosis. Two patients had endometriosis at other sites, and 12 others had endometriosis but no tenderness. In those with focal tenderness, the average depth of infiltration was greater (5.4 mm) than in non-tender lesions (3.4 mm), but not significantly different. If focal tenderness was associated with negative *Chlamydia* titers, endometriosis was seen in 83% of patients.

LABORATORY TESTING

Although the history and physical examination are the most important components of the evaluation in patients with CPP, selected laboratory studies may be helpful. Certain tests are strongly recommended (see Table 12.6) whereas others are based on findings from the history and physical examination (see Table 12.5).[61] This is based on a clinical trial in which this battery of screening tests was employed.[80]

Blood markers, including CA-125, CA 19-9, and serum protein PP14 (glycodelin), have been used to screen for endometriosis but overall lack sensitivity and specificity. Specifically, CA-125 is an antigen that is expressed by cell lines derived from coelomic epithelium, which develops into müllerian derivatives. An elevated concentration has been found in some women with endometriosis and seems to correlate with extent of disease,[81] but extensive evaluation has found that CA-125 levels

lack the sensitivity or specificity to be useful as a screening test.[82–86] This is because elevated serum CA-125 can also be found in other gynecologic conditions, including pelvic inflammatory disease, uterine fibroids, ovarian cysts, and ovarian cancer. Peritoneal fluid CA-125 from women in all stages of endometriosis has been shown to be consistently elevated even in the presence of normal serum levels, and may prove to be a useful marker. However, despite being useful to screen early-stage endometriosis that may be missed at laparoscopy,[87] it still requires a surgical procedure, minimizing its utility as a screening test.

Serum PP14, which varies during the menstrual cycle and originates almost exclusively in human secretory endometrium, has been shown to be greatest with advanced endometriosis, but its utility as a diagnostic test warrants further investigation.[88] Most recently, serum CA 19-9 levels have been shown to correlate in patients at all stages of endometriosis and are significantly higher than in those without endometriosis; they may thus prove a useful marker for determining the severity of disease.[89]

IMAGING STUDIES

Imaging techniques have been used in an attempt to diagnose pelvic pathology, particularly endometriosis. The most commonly performed is ultrasonography, although according to the ACOG

Table 12.7 Differential diagnosis of pelvic mass with similar echogenic appearance on ultrasound

- Hemorrhagic corpus luteum
- Tuberculous ovarian abscess
- Mature benign cystic teratoma (dermoid)
- Mucinous cystadenoma
- Granulosa-cell carcinoma

Technical Bulletin guidelines it is not essential in all women with CPP, as its value in evaluation is limited.[6] However, findings on physical examination that are suggestive of pathology should lead the physician to order an ultrasonographic evaluation of the pelvis. Such findings include obesity, where adequate assessment is difficult, or in the uncooperative patient.

The most easily recognized sonographic feature associated with endometriosis is an endometrioma. The presence of homogeneous low-level echoes in a cystic pelvic mass is strongly suggestive of disease. Using this finding alone, transvaginal ultrasound (TVS) has a sensitivity of 79–86% and a specificity of 89–98%.[90,91] Less frequently, septations (29%) and fluid levels (5%) can also be identified in endometriomas.[92] The differential diagnosis of pelvic masses with similar echogenic appearances is depicted in Table 12.7.

On the other hand, extraovarian focal implants, which account for over 45% of endometriotic disease, are very difficult and challenging to detect by ultrasound.[93] The use of power Doppler has been reported to aid in the diagnosis.[94] However, this technique relies on the presence of implants with vascular activity, but as the majority of implants are scarified and have no significant vascular activity, power Doppler appears to have limited value in most patients, particularly with respect to broad ligament endometriosis. In those with involvement of the uterosacral ligament, thickness seems to be associated with the degree of involvement. Obha et al reported that the average uterosacral ligament thickness was 11.2 ± 2.1 mm in non-affected patients, 12.8 ± 4.7 mm with superficial disease, and 14.5 ± 3.5 mm with deep infiltrative disease, though the authors reported this using

transrectal ultrasound.[95] It is also recognized that pelvic fluid is associated with endometriosis, although a discriminatory volume of pelvic fluid has not been determined.[96,97] Involvement of the rectum and cervix has also been described as homogeneous masses with and without cystic areas; and if the cervix is involved, as complex multicystic masses. Correct prediction of these lesions has been reported to be >80%.[98,99] None the less, the diagnosis of extraovarian endometriosis is particularly challenging and should not reliably be used to identify focal implant disease unless in experienced hands.

Magnetic resonance imaging (MRI) has been suggested as a diagnostic tool because of the differences in signal intensity of endometrium compared to other pelvic tissues, though this technique has proved to be of limited value.[100] A newer technique of fat-saturated MRI has been shown to be useful in detecting small endometrial implants and has excellent sensitivity, specificity, and predictive value compared to conventional MRI.[101,102]

Endometrial cavitary defects, including polyps and myomas, have been noted in up to 30% of patients with CPP. Evaluation using hysterosalpingography, sonohysterography, or hysteroscopy may provide useful information and may improve the diagnosis and treatment of CPP.[103,104]

Contrast studies, including intravenous pyelography, computed tomography (CT), and/or a barium enema of the urinary or intestinal tracts may occasionally be indicated depending on history and physical examination findings.

LAPAROSCOPY

Laparoscopy and visual detection have been the 'gold standard' for diagnosing endometriosis. This is based on the presumption that laparoscopy allows the visualization of the pelvis, and if pathology is encountered the procedure affords the opportunity to treat any disease surgically. However, given the wide array of appearances, laparoscopy can often miss disease because the implant characteristics can be microscopic, deep in penetration, and not visible from the peritoneal surface owing to its subtle appearance.[105,106]

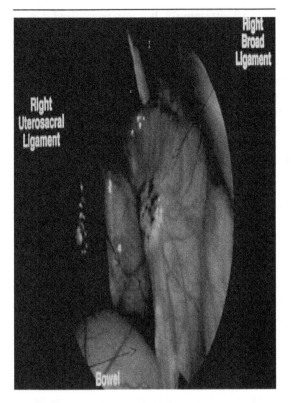

Figure 12.4 Classic 'powder burn' implants. (Reproduced with permission from TAP Phramaceutical.)

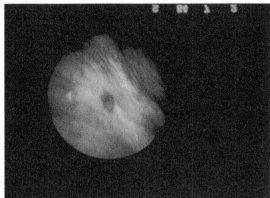

Figure 12.5 Atypical appearance: white opacifications. (Reproduced with permission from TAP Phramaceutical.)

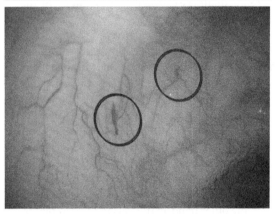

Figure 12.6 Atypical appearance: red flame-like peritoneal lesions. (Reproduced with permission from TAP Phramaceutical.)

The typical implant appears as a stellate, reddish-blue puckered 'powder-burn' lesion (Figure 12.4). However, atypical appearances have been appreciated, including white opacifications (Figure 12.5), red flame-like peritoneal lesions (Figure 12.6), translucent glandular excrescences (Figure 12.7), peritoneal petechiae, and yellow-brown patches. Peritoneal defects (Figure 12.8) are sometimes associated with endometriosis beneath the surface of the peritoneum. Tissue resection will often reveal endometriosis.

On the other hand, not all lesions represent endometriosis. The clear vesicles in Figure 12.9 are actually remnants of the wolffian duct system. The powder-like lesions in the anterior cul de sac in Figure 12.10 represent psamma bodies (previous *Chlamydia* infection). Not all red lesions are endometriosis implants, as seen in Figure 12.11, where the reddish areas in the cul de sac are actu-

ally vascular abnormalities. Such areas should be studied closely by pressing on them with a probe to see if they blanch, indicating vascularity. Given that a colorless manifestation is not uncommon, a technique that has been described as useful is the painting of peritoneal surfaces with bloody peritoneal fluid, whereupon colorless endometriotic lesions can be highlighted. It is these suspected areas that should be excised and histologically examined.[107]

Theoretically, laparoscopy should have high sensitivity and specificity for diagnosing endo-

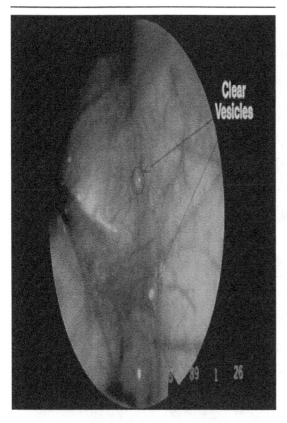

Figure 12.7 Atypical appearances: translucent glandular excrescences. (Reproduced with permission from TAP Phramaceutical.)

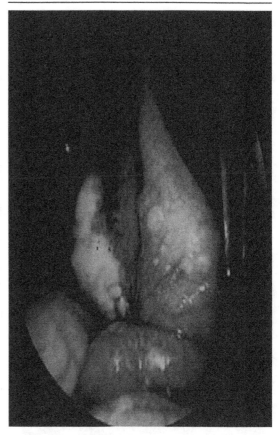

Figure 12.9 Remnants of the Wolffian duct system suggestive of atypical endometriosis. (Reproduced with permission from TAP Phramaceutical.)

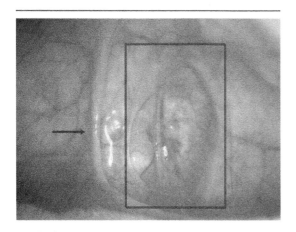

Figure 12.8 Atypical appearances: Peritoneal defects. (Reproduced with permission from TAP Phramaceutical.)

metriosis. However, using pathological confirmation of disease as the 'gold standard', the specificity of laparoscopy for diagnosing endometriosis ranges at best from 40% to 80% among various surgeons.[108,109] This is most likely due to the many visual manifestations, making it difficult to identify all endometriotic lesions reliably.

PHARMACOLOGIC DIAGNOSIS OF ENDOMETRIOSIS

A newly evolving approach to the diagnosis of endometriosis is based on clinical suspicion and the use of empiric 'pharmacotherapy'. This has recently been evaluated in a placebo-controlled

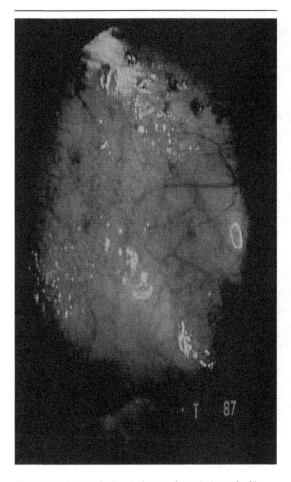

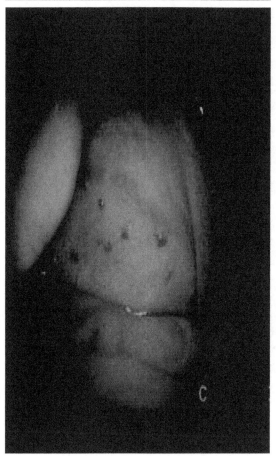

Figure 12.10 Psamma bodies similar to endometriotic powder-like lesions. (Reproduced with permission from TAP Phramaceutical.)

Figure 12.11 Vascular abnormalities similar to atypical endometriosis. (Reproduced with permission from TAP Phramaceutical.)

randomized study where Ling et al[77] identified 100 women with CPP using strict inclusion and exclusion criteria. The women were randomized to receive either monthly injections of depot leuprolide acetate or placebo for a total of 3 months. Pain was measured with the 4-point Biberoglu–Behrman scale.[77] At the end of 3 months all women underwent laparoscopy to assess for pelvic pathology. At laparoscopy, it was determined that 87% of the women in the placebo group and 78% in the leuprolide group had endometriosis. The reduced incidence in the latter is probably attributed to the presence of smaller lesions as a result of the leuprolide treatment that were harder to identify. More than 80%

of women experienced an improvement in pain or tenderness on GnRH-agonist therapy, compared to 40% of women on placebo. Moreover, 8 of 11 women using GnRH agonists had pain improvement without visible disease.

Based on these findings, it has been advocated that after non-gynecologic causes of CPP are excluded, empiric pharmacologic hormone therapy is a reasonable and cost-effective approach to the clinical diagnosis of endometriosis. With this algorithm, laparoscopy might best be reserved for women with CPP who fail to respond to antiendometriosis therapy.[6]

CONCLUSION

CPP in women can be due to a number of disorders of different organ systems, though endometriosis is the most likely cause of pain. History, physical examination, and selected laboratory and imaging studies can effectively diagnose many of these disorders. Although laparoscopy remains the 'gold standard' for diagnosis, endometriosis has many subtle visual appearances, making direct visualization difficult and challenging. Empiric therapy is a new and reliable approach for diagnosing the cause of CPP and should be considered in the evaluation and management of women with this condition.

REFERENCES

1. Balasch J, Creus M, Fabreugues F, et al. Visible and non-visible endometriosis at laparoscopy in fertile and infertile women and in patients with chronic pelvic pain: aprospective study. Hum Reprod 1996;11:387–91.

2. Houston DE. Evidence for the risk of pelvic endometriosis by age, race, and socioeconomic status. Epidemiol Rev 1984;6:167–91.

3. Kraus F. Female genitalia. In: Kissane J, ed, Anderson's Pathology. St Louis: CV Mosby, 1990, 1620–1725.

4. Goldstein DP, DeCholnoky C, Emans SJ. Adolescent endometriosis. J Adol Health Care 1980;1:37–41.

5. Mathias SD, Kuppermann M, Lieberman RF, et al. Chronic pelvic pain: prevalence, health-related quality of life, and economic correlates. Obstet Gynecol 1996;87:321–27.

6. American College of Obstetricians and Gynecologists. Medical management of endometriosis. ACOG Practice Bulletin #11 Washington DC: American College of Obstetricians and Gynecologists, 1999.

7. Levitan Z, Eibschitz I, Devries K. The value of laparoscopy in women with chronic pelvic pain and a "normal pelvis". Int J Gynecol Obstet 1985;23:71–4.

8. Lee NC, Dicker RC, Rubin GL, et al. Confirmation of the preoperative diagnosis for hysterectomy. Am J Obstet Gynecol 1984;150:283–7.

9. Manning AP, Thompson WG, Heaton KW, et al. Towards positive diagnosis of the irritable bowel. Br Med J 1978;2:653–4.

10. Drossman DA, Thompson WG, Talley NJ, et al. Identification of sub-groups of functional gastrointestinal disorders. Gastroenterol Int 1990;3:159–72.

11. Drossman DA, Whitehead WE, Camilleir M. Irritable bowel syndrome: a technical review for practical guideline development. Gastroenterology 1997;112:2120–37.

12. Thompson WG, Longstreth GF, Drossman, et al. Functional bowel disorders and functional abdominal pain. Gut 1999;45 (suppl 2):II43–7.

13. Hogston P. Irritable bowel syndrome as a cause of chronic pain in women attending a gynecology clinic. Br Med J 1987;294:934–5.

14. Whitehead WE. Gastrointestinal disorders. In: Steege JF, Metzger DA, Levy BS, eds. Chronic Pelvic Pain: An Integrated Approach. Philadelphia: WB Saunders:, 1998, 205–13.

15. Crowell MD, Dubin NH, Robinson JC, et al. Am J Gastrenterol 1994;89:1973–7.

16. Advincula AP. Irritable Bowel Syndrome. Female Patient 2000;25:18–29.

17. Longstreth GF, Fox DD, Youkeles L, et al. Psyllium therapy in the irritable bowel syndrome: a double-blind trial. Ann Intern Med 1981;95:53–6.

18. King TS, Elia M, Hunter JO. Abnormal colonic ferrmentation in irritable bowel syndrome. Lancet 1998;352:1187–9.

19. Pittler MH, Ernst E. Peppermint oil for irritable bowel syndrome: a critical review and meta-analysis. Am J Gastroenterol 1998;93:1131–5.

20. Farching MJ. New drugs in the management of the irritable bowel syndrome. Drugs 1998;56:11–21.

21. Houghton LA, Rogers J, Whorwell PJ, et al. Zamifenacin (UH-76,654) a potent gut M3 selective muscarinic antagonist reduces colonic motor activity in patients with irritable bowel syndrome. Ailment Pharmacol Ther 1997;11:561–8.

22. Read NW, Abitol JL, Bardhan KD, et al. Efficacy and safety of the peripheral kappa agonist fedotozine versus placebo in the treatment of functional dyspepsia. Gut 1997;41:664–8.

23. Mathias JR, Clench MH, Abell TL, et al. Effect of leuprolide acetate in treatment of abdominal pain and nausea in premenopausal women with functional bowel disease; a double-blind placebo controlled, randomized, study. Dig Dis Sci 1998;43:1347–55.

24. Dobbins WO 3rd. Current status of the precancer lesion in ulcerative colitis. Gastroenterology 1977;73:1431–3.

25. Mekhjian HS, Switz DM, Melnyk CS, et al. Clinical features and natural history of of Crohn's disease. Gastroenterology 1979;77:898–906.

26. Greenstein AJ, Janowitz HD, Sachar DB. The extraintestinal complications of Crohn's disease and ulcerative colitis: a study of 700 patients. Medicine 1976;55:401–12.

27. Fawaz KA, Glotzer DJ, Goldman H, et al. Ulcerative colitis and Crohn's disease of the colon – a comparison of the long term postoperative courses. Gastroenterology 1976;71:372–8.

28. Lennard-Jones JE, Powell-Tuck J. Drug treatment of inflammatory bowel disease. Clin Gastroenterol 1979;8:187–217.

29. Oravisto KJ. Epidemiology of interstitial cystitis. Ann Chir Gynaecol Fenn 1975;64:75–7.

30. Held PJ, Hanno PM, Wein AJ, et al. Epidemiology of interstitial cystitis: 2. In: Hanno PM, Staskin DR, Kranne RJ, Wein AJ, eds. Interstitial Cystitis. New York: Springer-Verlag, 1990, 29–48.

31. Joones CA, Nyberg L. Epidemiology of interstitial cystitis. Urology 1997;49(suppl 5A):2–9.

32. Curhan GC, Speizer FE, Hunter DJ, et al. Epidemiology of interstitial cystitis: a population based study. J Urol 1999;161:549–52.

33. Kaufman DM. The Genitourinary Perspective: Chronic Pelvic Pain and Lower Urinary Tract Disorders. Changing Perspectives, a new outlook on gynecologic disorders. Series Proceeding 2001, Sponsored by Medical Education Collaborative, pp 25–9.

34. King PM, Myers CA, Ling FW, et al. Musculoskeletal factors in chronic pelvic pain. J Psychosom Obstet Gynecol 1991;12:87–98.

35. Sicuranza BJ, Richards J, Tisdale LH. The short leg syndrome in obstetrics and gynecology. Am J Obstet Gynecol 1970;10:217–18.

36. Clauw DJ, Chrousos GP. Chronic pain and fatigue syndromes: overlapping clinical and neuroendocrine features and potential pathogenic mechanisms. Neuroimmunomodulation 1997;4:134–53.

37. Wolfe F, Smythe HA, Yunus MB, et al. The American College of Rheumatology 1990 Criteria for the Classification of Fibromyalgia. Report of Multicenter Criteria Committee. Arthritis Rheum 1990;33:160–72.

38. Wallace DJ. Genitourinary manifestations of fibrositis: an increased association with the female urethral syndrome. J Rheumatol 1990;17:238–9.

39. Yunus MB. Towards a model of pathophysiology of fibromyalgia: aberrant central pain mechanisms with peripheral modulation. J Rheumatol 1992;19:846–50.

40. Blumer D, Heilbronn M. Chronic pain as a variant of depressive disease: the pain-prone disorder. J Nerv Ment Dis 1982;170:381–406.

41. Walker EA, Katon WJ, Harrop-Griffiths J, et al. Relationship of chronic pelvic pain to psychiatric diagnosis and childhood sexual abuse. Am J Psychiatry 1988;145:75–80.

42. American Psychiatric Association. Diagnostic and Statistical Manual of Mental Disorders. Fourth Edition. Primary Care Version. Washington, DC: The American Psychiatric Association; 1995.

43. Abramovitz JS, Schwartz SA, Whiteside SP. A contemporary conceptual model of hypochondriasis. Mayo Clin Proc 2002;77:1323–30.

44. Steege J, Ling F. Dyspareunia: a special type of chronic pelvic pain. Obstet Gynecol Clin North Am 1993;20:779–93.

45. Spector I, Carey M. Incidence and prevalence of the sexual dysfunctions: a critical review of the empirical literature. Arch Sex Behav 1990;19:389–408.

46. Lazarus A. Dyspareunia: a multimodal psychotherapeutic perspective. In: Leiblum S, Rosen R, eds. Principles and Practice of Sex Therapy: An Update for the 1990s. New York: Guilford Press, 1989, 92–111.

47. Marinoff SC, Turner ML. Vulvar vestibulitis syndrome: an overview. Am J Obstet Gynecol 1991;165:1228–33.

48. Leiblum SR, Pervin LA, Campbell EH. The treatment of vaginismus: success and failure. In: Leiblum SR, Rosen RC, eds. Principles and Practice of Sex Therapy: An Update for the 1990s. New York: Guilford Press, 1989, 113–18.

49. Emge LA. The elusive adenomyosis of the uterus. Am J Obstet Gynecol 1962;83:1541–63.

50. Reinhold C, McCarthy S, Bret PM, et al. Diffuse adenomyosis: comparison of endovaginal ultrasound and MR imaging with histopathologic correlation. Radiology 1996;199:151–8.

51. Yoder IC. Diagnosis of uterine anomalies: relative accuracy of MR imaging, endovaginal sonography, and hysterosalpingography. Radiology 1992;185:343, discussion 344.

52. Siedler D, Laing FC, Jeffrey RB, et al. Uterine adenomyosis: a difficult sonographic diagnosis. J Ultrasound Med 1987;6:345–9.

53. Reinhold C, Atri M, Mehio A, et al. Diffuse uterine adenomyosis: morphologic criteria and diagnostic accuracy of endovaginal sonography. Radiology 1995;197:609–14.

54. Ascher SM, Arnold LL, Patt RH, et al. Adenomyosis: a prospective comparison of MR imaging and transvaginal sonography. Radiology 1994;190:803–6.

55. Schnall MD. Magnetic resonance evaluation of acquired benign uterine disorders. Semin Ultrasound CT MR 1994;15:18–26.

56. Yen SS. Clinical applications of gonadotropin-releasing hormone and gonadotropin-releasing hormone analogs. Fertil Steril 1983;39:257–66.

57. Winkel CA. Diagnosis and treatment of uterine pathology. In: Carr BR and Blackwell RE eds, Textbook of Reproductive Medicine. Norwalk: Appleton & Lange, 1993, 481–505.

58. Carter J. Combined hysteroscopic and laparoscopic findings in patients with chronic pelvic pain. J Am Assoc Gynecol Laparosc 1994;2:43–7.

59. Nezhat F, Nezhat C, Nezhat CH, et al. Use of hysteroscopy in addition to laparsocopy for evaluating chronic pelvic pain. J Reprod Med 1995;40:431–4.

60. Peters AAW, van Dorst E, Jellis B, et al. A randomized clinical trial to compare two different approaches in women with chronic pelvic pain. Obstet Gynecol 1991;77:740–4.

61. Scialli AR for the Pelvic Pain Expert Working Group. Evaluating Chronic Pelvic Pain (A Consensus Recommendation). J Reprod Med 1999;44:945–52.

62. Bates B, Hoekelman RA. Interviewing and the health history. In: Bates BJB, eds. A Guide to Physical Examination. Philadelphia: Lippincott Company, 1979, 1–24.

63. Toomey TC, Hernandez JT, Gittleman DF, et al. Relationship of sexual and physical abuse to pain and psychological assessment variables in chronic pelvic pain patients. Pain 1993;53:105–9.

64. Melzack R. The McGill pain questionnaire: major properties and scoring methods. Pain 1975;1:277–99.

65. Rock JA, Markham SM. Extra pelvic endometriosis. In: Wilson EA, ed. Endometriosis. New York, Alan R. Liss, Inc., 1987,185–206.

66. Foster DC, Stern JL, Buscema J, et al. Pleural and parenchymal pulmonary endometriosis. Obstet Gynecol 1981;58:552–6.

67. Purvis RS, Tyring SK. Cutaneous and subcutaneous endometriosis. Surgical and hormonal therapy. J Dermatol Surg Oncol 1994;20:693–5.

68. Nirula R, Greaney GC. Incisional endometriosis: an under appreciated diagnosis in general surgery. J Am Coll Surg 2000;190:404–7.

69. Cramer DW, Hornstein MD, Ng WG, et al. Endometriosis associated with the N314D mutation of galactose-1-phosphate uridyl transferase. Mol Human Reprod 1996;2:149–52.

70. Hornstein MD, Thomas PP, Sober AJ, et al. Association between endometriosis, dysplastic nevi, and history of melanoma in women of reproductive age. Human Reprod 1997;12:143–5.

71. Woodworth SH, Singh M, Yussman MA, et al. A prospective study on the association between red hair color and endometriosis in infertile patients. Fertil Steril 1995;64: 651–2.

72. Frisch RE, Wyshak G, Albert LS, et al. Dysplastic nevi, cutaneous melanoma, and gynecologic disorders. Int J Dermatol 1992;31:331–5.

73. Steege J. The evaluation and treatment of women with pelvic pain. In: Sciarra J, ed. Gynecology and Obstetrics. Philadelphia: Harper & Row, 1984,1–11.

74. Olive DL. Initial Evaluation of the Patient. In: An Integrated Approach to the Management of Chronic Pelvic Pain. Killingworth: Pharmedica Press, 1997, 15–20.

75. Batt RE, Naples JD. Observations with hyserosalpingography and culdoscopy in management of infertility. Med Digest 1969;15:34–7.

76. Barbieri RL, Propst AM. Physical examination findings in women with endometriosis: uterosacaral ligament abnormalities, lateral cervical displacement and cervical stenosis. J Gynecol Techniques 1999;4:1–3.

77. Barbieri RL, Callery M, Perez SE. Directionality of menstrual flow: cervical os diameter as a determinant of retrograde menstruation. Fertil Steril 1992;57:727–30.

78. Barbieri RL. Stenosis of the external cervical os: an association with endometriosis in women with chronic pelvic pain. Fertil Steril 1998;70:571–3.

79. Ripps BA, Martin DC. Focal Pelvic Tenderness, Pelvic Pain, and Dysmenorrhea in Endometriosis. J Reprod Med 1991;36:470–72.

80. Ling FW. Randomized controlled trial of depot leuprolide in patients with pelvic pain and clinically suspected endometriosis. Obstet Gynecol 1999;93:51–8.

81. Cheng YM, Wang ST, Chou CY. Serum CA-125 in preoperative patients at high risk for endometriosis. Obstet Gynecol 2002;99:375–80.
82. Pittaway DE, Fayez JA. The use of CA-125 in the diagnosis and management of endometriosis. Fertil Steril 1986;46:790–5.
83. Malkasian GD Jr, Podratz KC, Stanhope CR et al. Ca-125 in gynecologic practice. Am J Obstet Gynecol 1986;155:515–18.
84. Patton EP, Field CS, Harms RW, et al. CA-125 levels in endometriosis. Fertil Steril 1986;45:770–3.
85. Gurgan T, Kisnisci H, Yatali H, et al. Serum and peritoneal fluid CA-125 levels in early stage enometriosis. Gynecol Obstet Invest 1990;30:105–8.
86. Kauppila A, Telimaa S, Ronnberg L, et al. Placebo-controlled study on serum concentrations of CA-125 before after treatment of endometriosis with danazol or high-dose medroxyprogesterone acetate alone or after surgery. Fertil Steril 1988;49:37–41.
87. Krasnicki D. Serum and peritoneal fluid CA-125 levels in patients with endometriosis. Ginekol Pol 2001;72:1365–9.
88. Telimaa S, Kauppila A, Ronnberg L, et al. Elevated serum levels of endometrial secretory protein PP14 in patients with advanced endometriosis. Suppression by treatment with danazol and high-dose medroxyprogesterone acetate. Am J Obstet Gynecol 1989;161:866–71.
89. Harada T, Kubota T, Aso T. Usefulness of CA19-9 versus CA125 for the diagnosis of endometriosis. Fertil Steril 2002;78:733–9.
90. Volpi E, DeGrandis T, Zuccaro G, et al. Role of transvaginal sonography in the detection of endometriomata. J Clin Ultrasound 1995;23:163–7.
91. Mais V, Guerriero S, Ajossa S, et al. The efficiency of transvaginal ultrasonography in the diagnosis of endometrioma. Fertil Steril 1993;60:776–80.
92. Kupfer MC, Schwimer SR, Lebovic J. Transvaginal sonographic appearance of endometriomata: spectrum of findings. J Ultrasound Med 1992;11:129–33.
93. Jenkins S, Olive DL, Haney AF. Endometriosis: pathogenic implication of the anatomic distribution. Obstet Gynecol 1986;37:335–8.
94. Papadimitriou A, Kalogirou D, Antoniou G, et al. Power Doppler ultrasound: a potentially useful alternative in diagnosing pelvic pathology conditions. Clin Exp Obstet Gynecol 1996;23:229–32.
95. Ohba T, Mizatani H, Maeda T, et al. Evaluation of endometiosis in uterosacral ligaments by transrectal ultrasonography. Human Reprod 1996;11:2014–17.
96. Rock JA, Dubin NH, Ghodgaonkar RB, et al. Cul-de-sac fluid in women with endometriosis; fluid volume, protein, and prostanoid concentration during the proliferative phase – days 8 to 12. Fertil Steril 1982;37:747–50.
97. Rezai N, Ghodgaokar RB, Zacur HA, et al. Cul-de-sac fluid in women with endometriosis; fluid volume, protein, and prostanoid concentration during the peri-ovulatory period – days 13 to 18. Fertil Steril 1987;48:29–32.
98. Hauge C, Nielsen MB, Rasmussen OO, et al. Clinical findings and endosonographic appearance of endometriosis in the anal sphincter. J Clin Ultrasound 1993;21:48–51.
99. Veiga-Ferreira MM, Leiman G, Dunber F, et al. Cervical endometriosis: Facilitated diagnosis by fine needle aspiration cytologic testing. Am J Obstet Gynecol 1987;157: 849–56.
100. Bryan PJ, Butler HE, LiPuma JP. Magnetic resonance imaging of the pelvis. Radiol Clin North Am 1984;22:897–915.
101. Takahashi K, Okada M, Okada S, et al. Studies on the detection of small endometrial implants by magnetic resonance imaging using a fat saturation technique. Gynecol Obstet Invest 1996;41:203–6.
102. Takahashi K, Okada M, Ozaki T, et al. Diagnosis of pelvic endometriosis by magnetic resonance imaging using "fat saturation" technique. Fertil Steril 1994; 62:973–7.
103. Nezhat F, Nezhat C, Nezhat CH, et al. Use of hysteroscopy in addition to laparoscopy for evaluating chronic pelvic pain. J Reprod Med 1995;40:431–4.
104. Carter JE. Combined hysteroscopic and laparoscopic findings in patients with chronic pelvic pain. J Am Assoc Gynecol Laparosc 1994;2:43–7.
105. Jansen RP, Russell P. Nonpigmented endometriosis: Clinical, laparoscopic, and pathologic definition. Am J Obstet Gynecol 1986;155:1154–9.
106. Stripling MC, Martin DC, Chatman DL, et al. Subtle apearance of pelvic endometriosis. Fertil Steril 1988;49:427–31.
107. Redwine DB. Peritoneal blood painting: An aid in the diagnosis of endometriosis. Am J Obstet Gynecol 1989;161:865–6.
108. Moen MH, Halvosen TB. Histologic confirmation of endometriosis in different peritoneal lesions. Acta Obstet Gynecol Scanda 1992;1:337–42.
109. Murphy AA, Green WR, Bobbie D, et al. Unsuspected endometriosis documented by scaanning electron microscopy in visually normal peritoneum. Fertil Steril 1986;46:522–4.

13. Assessing Health Status in Endometriosis

Lisa Story, Nik Taylor, Enda McVeigh, Crispin Jenkinson and Stephen Kennedy

INTRODUCTION

Endometriosis is one of the most common gynecologic conditions and is associated with distressing symptoms such as dysmenorrhea, chronic pelvic pain (CPP), and dyspareunia. Consequently, researchers often measure pain levels in endometriosis patients, particularly to assess treatment efficacy in clinical studies and randomized controlled trials (RCTs). However, the overall effects on health-related quality of life (HRQoL) have largely been neglected, and there have been few attempts to measure HRQoL using reliable instruments.

It has certainly been suggested that mental health is more severely affected than physical functioning in endometriosis,[1] and various factors unrelated to disease severity, such as hormonal status, may influence the emotional distress and impact on the woman's life caused by pain symptoms.[2] Walker et al,[3] Hawkridge,[4] and Wigfall-Williams[5] all suggest that a patient's emotional reaction to the diagnosis is similar to that of bereavement: initial shock, disbelief, and anxiety, followed by either denial and inaction, or information gathering and steps towards treatment. Weinstein[6] also argues that endometriosis leads to pain, anxiety, and distress which form a vicious circle, ultimately producing an acute sense of helplessness, hopelessness, and despair, and Hawkridge[4] maintains that the pain, disability, anxiety, fear, isolation, and confusion that many sufferers experience lead to an inability to cope with the necessary changes in lifestyle and goals brought about by having the disease.

The life changes include effects upon a woman's career, as time off work may be needed because of ill health or hospital visits, and upon relationships, as dyspareunia affects intimacy and the disease is associated with infertility. Dyspareunia can be a particularly distressing symptom because it often results in marital difficulties precisely at the time a woman needs support from her partner the most.[7] Furthermore, the anticipation of pain during intercourse can be as debilitating as the pain itself, and the cycle of pain, fear, and more pain can lead to an avoidance of intercourse altogether and a withering of intimate relationships as a consequence.

Added to these problems is the requirement to cope with the side effects and complications of medical intervention: persistent interruptions to daily life because of hospital visits and surgery, and the emotional strain of not knowing whether a particular treatment will be successful. Weinstein[6] refers to the 'treatment carousel' which eclipses the daily life of the endometriosis sufferer as she constantly repeats phases of decision-making, treatment, contention with side effects and consequences, and the movement between relief, recurrence, and frustration. In fact, Damario and Rock[8] argue that the quality of life of women with endometriosis can only improve with greater focus on achieving long-term pain relief, thereby preventing the cycle of adverse effects on physical activity, work productivity, sexual fulfillment, and mood. Clearly, therefore, being able to measure pain effectively is an essential prerequisite in assessing a woman's health status and the efficacy of any medical intervention.

GENERAL PAIN MEASURES

Pain is a very subjective phenomenon, influenced by context, cultural beliefs, and other psychological variables. It is a multidimensional entity, far more complex than simply being the consequence of the activation of nociceptive pathways. Pain cannot therefore be observed directly by the clinician, and assessment is reliant upon the patient's own reports. These can be harnessed in the form of self-report scales that provide an important outcome measure, especially in clinical trials.

The three most commonly used instruments to assess pain intensity are verbal rating, numerical rating and visual analog scales. A verbal rating scale (VRS) consists of a list of adjectives, in order of intensity, describing a component of pain. The patient must select the word she feels describes her pain most appropriately; the words are usually assigned a numerical value, which allows a score to be derived. VRS are easy to administer and score, and they are acceptable to patients; there is also good evidence for construct validity. Disadvantages include forcing the patient to choose only one word or phrase, which may not adequately reflect her pain experience, and making the assumption that the intervals between adjectives, or grades of intensity, are equal (i.e. the patient's perception of the magnitude of difference between minimal to mild and mild to moderate may not be equal, although in a scoring system of 0–3 they would appear to be so). This can present a problem, particularly when the VRS is used as a quantitative outcome measure in clinical trials.

A numerical rating scale (NRS) is similar to a VRS but the patient is required to rank components of her pain with a numerical value. This may be between 0 and 10 (11-point scale), 0 and 20 (21-point scale), or 0 and 100 (101-point scale), with endpoints representing the extremes of pain. NRS are easy to administer and score; they can also have many response categories. There is good evidence for construct validity, but scores do not necessarily have ratio qualities.

A visual analog scale (VAS) consists of a line, usually 10 cm long, the ends of which are labeled with the extremes of a pain variable. Gradations may be marked with adjectives (verbal graphic rating scale) or numbers (numerical graphic rating scale). The patient must mark the place on the line that she feels corresponds best with her level of pain. Such a scale does present many response categories and the scores do have ratio qualities. There is also good evidence for construct validity. They can, however, be quite time-consuming to interpret.

However, all of these scales are unidimensional, which means they can only address one component of pain at a time. Multidimensional scales have therefore been devised to explore the components of pain in more depth, taking into account psychological effects such as emotional arousal. One of the most frequently used is the McGill Pain Questionnaire,[9] which gives lists of adjectives in three categories: sensory, affective, and evaluative assessments, together with an overall pain rating index. Each word in these categories is given a numerical rating, depending upon its position within the word set. The patient must select words she feels are appropriate to her experience. From this choice, the total pain rating index (PRI) can be derived based on the rank values of words selected, as well as separate PRI for each of the descriptive categories. The McGill Pain Questionnaire has been shown to be reliable, valid, and consistent, although it is quite complicated and time-consuming to use.

The way that pain affects a patient's life can also be assessed in a more global way, both quantitatively in terms, for example, of rescue analgesia needed in a clinical trial, and qualitatively by assessing the effect of pain of daily activities.

PAIN MEASURES USED IN ENDOMETRIOSIS STUDIES

Three specific pain symptoms – dysmenorrhea, dyspareunia, and non-cyclical pelvic pain – tend to be assessed either alone or in combination in clinical studies and RCTs using linear scales such as VRS, NRS, and VAS. Multidimensional verbal rating scales have also been devised specifically for use in endometriosis to provide a more global picture of the pain. The most widely used has been a clinician-devised four-point scale known as the Biberoglu–Behrman Scale (Table 13.1), for three symptoms (dysmenorrhea, dyspareunia and pelvic pain), and two signs (pelvic tenderness and induration) associated with endometriosis.[10]

Dysmenorrhea is classified on the basis of loss of work efficiency and need for bed rest (absence of pain, 0; some loss of work efficiency, mild, 1; in

Table 13.1 Endometriosis severity profile scoring system, based on the Biberoglu–Behrman Scale[10]

Dysmenorrhea	Absent	(0) No discomfort
	Mild	(1) Some loss of work efficiency
	Moderate	(2) In bed part of one day, occasional loss of work
	Severe	(3) In bed one or more days, incapacitation
	Not applicable	(4) Amenorrhea
Dyspareunia	Absent	(0) No difficulty or pain
	Mild	(1) Tolerated discomfort
	Moderate	(2) Intercourse painful to point of interruption of intercourse
	Severe	(3) Avoids intercourse because of pain
	Not applicable	(4) Not sexually active, or prefers not to answer
Pelvic pain	Absent	(0) No discomfort
	Mild	(1) Occasional pelvic discomfort
	Moderate	(2) Noticeable discomfort for most of cycle
	Severe	(3) Requires strong analgesics, persistent during cycle other than during menstruation
Pelvic tenderness	Absent	(0) No tenderness
	Mild	(1) Minimal tenderness on palpation
	Moderate	(2) Entensive tenderness on palpation
	Severe	(3) Unable to palpate because of tenderness
Induration	Absent	(0) No induration
	Mild	(1) Uterus freely mobile, induration in the cul-de-sac
	Moderate	(2) Thickened and indurated adnexa and cul-de-sac, restricted mobility
	Severe	(3) Nodular adnexa and cul-de-sac, uterus frequently frozen

bed for part of 1 day, occasional loss of work, moderate, 2; in bed for 1 or more days, incapacitation, severe, 3); non-menstrual pain in relation to discomfort and analgesic usage (absence of pain, 0; occasional pelvic discomfort, mild, 1; noticeable discomfort for most of the cycle, moderate, 2; pain continuing throughout the cycle or requiring strong analgesics, severe, 3); and dyspareunia according to limitations of sexual activity (no impact, 0; tolerated discomfort, mild, 1; intercourse painful to the point of interruption, moderate, 2; intercourse avoided because of pain, severe, 3). Findings on examination are pelvic tenderness (no tenderness, 0; minimal tenderness on palpation, mild, 1; extensive tenderness on palpation, moderate, 2; severe tenderness on palpation, severe, 3) and induration (no abnormality, 0; uterus freely mobile, induration in the cul de sac, mild, 1; thickened and indurated adnexa and cul de sac, restricted uterine mobility, moderate, 2; nodular adnexa and cul de sac, uterus frequently frozen, severe, 3). A score

is calculated for all three symptoms combined or for all five components together to produce a single outcome measure; in one study, the scale was used to assess dyspareunia alone.[11]

Andersch and Milson[12] devised a more multidimensional questionnaire specifically for young women with dysmenorrhea, which defines pain using a number of different parameters: systemic symptoms, analgesia use, and impact on daily activities. This was modified and used as an outcome measure in one RCT[11] in which pain was defined by limitations imposed on the ability to work (unaffected, 0; rarely affected, 1; moderately affected, 2; clearly inhibited, 3), the presence of systemic symptoms (absent, 0; present, 1), and the need for analgesia (none, 0; rarely, 1; regularly, 2; ineffective, 3). Scores were then summed, giving a total out of 7 (mild, 1–3; moderate, 4–5; severe, 6–7).

The methods used to assess pain as an outcome measure in endometriosis are summarized in Table 13.2. Only studies included in Cochrane

Table 13.2 Summary of the pain scales, where available, that were used in RCTs included in Cochrane Reviews[13–18]

Study	Summed NRS 0–30 for dysmenorrhea, dyspareunia and pelvic pain	10 cm VAS	VRS/NRS 0–3, absent, mild, moderate, severe for symptoms – dysmenorrhea, dyspareunia and pelvic pain		Pelvic signs, 0–3, absent, mild, moderate, severe for pelvic tenderness and induration totalled with symptoms score (0–15 scale)	Biberlogu–Behrman		Modified Biberlogu–Behrman – dysmenorrhea, dyspareunia and pelvic pain only		Biberlogu–Behrman for dyspareunia only	Andersch and Milson	Patient questioned re symptoms – details not specified	Analgesic usage
			Individual breakdown of scores	Total score of pelvic symptoms		Individual breakdown of scores	Sum total of scores	Individual breakdown of scores	Sum total of scores				
Bromham 1995			x										
Dlugi 1990						x							x
Dmowski 1989				x									
Fedele 1989						x						x	
GISG 1995		x				x							
Henzl 1988					x								
Hornstein 1990						x						x	
Hornstein 1995							x						
Howell 1995									x				
Kiilholma 1995				x	x								
Lemay 1995						x						x	
Makarainen 1996				x									
NEET 1992			x		x								
Overton 1994												x	
Rock 1991												x	

164

Table 13.2 Continued

Study	Summed NRS 0–30 for dysmenorrhea, dyspareunia and pelvic pain	10 cm VAS	VRS/NRS 0–3, absent, mild, moderate, severe for symptoms – dysmenorrhea, dyspareunia and pelvic pain		Pelvic signs, 0–3, absent, mild, moderate, severe for pelvic tenderness and induration totalled with symptoms score (0–15 scale)	Biberlogu–Behrman		Modified Biberlogu–Behrman – dysmenorrhea, dyspareunia and pelvic pain only		Biberlogu–Behrman for dyspareunia only	Andersch and Milson	Patient questioned re symptoms – details not specified	Analgesic usage
			Individual breakdown of scores	Total score of pelvic symptoms		Individual breakdown of scores	Sum total of scores	Individual breakdown of scores	Sum total of scores				
Shaw 1992			x		x								
Sutton 1994		x											
Tummon 1989	x												
Vercellini 1993		x				x					x		
Vercellini 1996		x						x					
Wheeler 1992							x					x	x

165

Reviews assessing treatment have been included.[13-18] In some RCTs a combination of scales[11,19-23] has been used, including one developed by Glick[24] to measure the need for analgesics.[22,23] As different tools have been used it is difficult to make comparisons between studies, especially as it is often unclear how the tools are administered, for example whether patients are typically asked to relate their pain experience to their worst, baseline, or current level of pain, and whether patients are consistently asked the questions in the same way at each assessment.

Another major problem concerns the way in which pain scores are summarized. For example, although multidimensional questionnaires usually ask patients about the three different components of pain in endometriosis, results are often expressed as a single total pain score. It is therefore possible that a large improvement in one symptom may mask deterioration in another, which applies particularly if dysmenorrhea is a major component of the pain, given that treatment often stops menstruation. Generating a score of 0 with treatment also presupposes a direct effect on the disease itself, which of course may not be the case.

In addition, some of the outcome measures used in the multidimensional tools are rather crude and somewhat limiting. The Biberoglu–Behrman Scale[10] considers severe dysmenorrhea to be associated with the need to remain in bed for 1 or more days. This is obviously subject to variation between individuals, and although a woman may wish to rest in bed because of excruciating pain the opportunity may not arise, owing to the demands of her life. However, another woman with a different lifestyle may be able to afford a lower threshold for bed rest. Where dyspareunia is concerned, the Biberoglu–Behrman questionnaire does not make allowances for the fact that abstinence from intercourse may occur for reasons other than the fact that it is painful.

Although questions can be raised about the validity of the tools used to assess pain in endometriosis, the scales are widely accepted and used in RCTs. Implementation of more refined testing is hampered by the reliance of regulatory authorities on these methods, and especially by their need to compare the effectiveness of novel compounds with existing treatments using the same outcome measures.

HEALTH AND QUALITY OF LIFE MEASUREMENT

No single definition of HRQoL exists. Rather it is considered a multidimensional concept incorporating general health, cognitive function, mental health, emotional state, subjective wellbeing, life satisfaction, and social support.[25] The measurement of HRQoL, once largely the remit of the social sciences, is gradually being adopted in clinical medicine because it is now being increasingly recognized that traditional outcome measures, such as pain levels, may not adequately assess the patient's experience or related aspects of health, which are important to patients. This change in approach – moving away from assessing outcomes largely from the clinician's perspective – has resulted in the generation of instruments (usually questionnaires) to measure subjective health status in a meaningful and reliable way.[25]

MEASURING HRQoL IN ENDOMETRIOSIS

HRQoL has not often been measured in endometriosis, which is surprising given the distressing nature of the disease. However, in a few studies, general instruments or parts of instruments designed to assess common, benign gynecologic conditions have been used.[26-28] As most are not specific to endometriosis or standardized instruments with established psychometric properties of reliability and validity, it is unlikely that they are measuring HRQoL systematically.[29]

A number of general instruments have also been utilized to study the psychological profiles of endometriosis patients. For example, Waller and Shaw[30] compared three groups: women with minimal/mild disease, women with pelvic pain and no obvious pathology, and women undergoing sterilization as controls, using the Beck Depression Inventory,[31] the Speilberger State-

Trait Anxiety Inventory,[32] and the Golombok–Rust Inventory of Sexual Satisfaction.[33] They reported that women with pelvic pain had similar scores on the Beck Depression Inventory, whether they had mild endometriosis or a normal pelvis. These scores were significantly higher than those of women with asymptomatic disease and normal controls. Women with symptomatic mild endometriosis also suffered with depressive symptoms and disorders of sexual functioning. Overall, they concluded that women with pelvic pain have substantial distress leading to abnormalities of psychological functioning.

To investigate whether women with endometriosis have a specific psychological profile, Low et al[34] studied 81 women with pelvic pain, of whom 40 had disease and the remainder had other gynecologic problems. The Eysenck Personality Questionnaire,[35] the Beck Depression Inventory,[31] the General Health Questionnaire,[36] the Speilberger State-Trait Anxiety Inventory,[32] the Golombok–Rust Inventory,[33] and the Short Form McGill Pain Questionnaire[9] were used to assess the patients. They reported that the women with endometriosis had higher psychoticism, introversion, and anxiety scores than the other women with pelvic pain, although the two groups had similar pain ratings. Both groups obtained neuroticism, anxiety, and psychiatric morbidity scores that were elevated relative to normative data.

Peveler et al[37] used the Brief Symptom Inventory,[38] the Eysenck Personality Questionnaire,[35] and the Social Adjustment Scale[39] to compare 51 women with medically unexplained pain and 40 women with endometriosis. They found that those with and without endometriosis could not be distinguished by mood symptoms or personality traits, and that based on the parenting role scores and overall adjustment scores there was significantly poorer social adjustment in endometriosis patients and greater social dysfunction.

Lewis et al[40] employed an interview schedule drawn from the Hamilton Rating Scale for Depression,[41] the Schedule for Affective Disorders and Schizophrenia,[42] the Beck Depression Inventory,[31] and criteria listed in DSM-III to investigate links between endometriosis and mood disorders in 16 women with confirmed disease. Twelve of the 16 women with laparoscopically confirmed disease met DSM-III criteria for a mood disorder; two women had equivocal diagnoses, and two showed no evidence of mood disorder.

MEASURING TREATMENT EFFECTS IN ENDOMETRIOSIS

The overall effectiveness of the clinical management of endometriosis was assessed in the 1997 Gynaecology Audit Project in Scotland.[43] The impact of treatment on HRQoL was studied using a condition-specific measure developed by seven clinical experts, and a general measure, the Short Form 36 (SF-36) health survey.[44] Postal questionnaires were sent to 273 women at diagnosis and 6 months later. There was a high correlation between the scores obtained using both instruments, which confirmed the validity of the condition-specific measure; the condition-specific scores also related well to the clinicians' assessment of disease severity and the need for further treatment. At 6 months' follow-up the changes conformed to expected hypotheses, demonstrating the responsiveness of both measures. However, the condition-specific measure was more responsive than the SF-36 to treatment-induced changes in pain symptoms.

In a recently published study, Abbott et al[45] analyzed outcomes in 176 women with endometriosis up to 5 years following laparoscopic surgery. VAS scores on an 11-point scale for dysmenorrhoea, non-menstrual pelvic pain, dyspareunia, and dyschezia were obtained and the following questionnaires were administered: the EQ-5D index and EQ-5D VAS, measures of physical functioning and patients' self-rated assessment;[46] the Short-Form 12 (SF-12), which measures both physical and mental health,[47] and a sexual activity questionnaire relating to pleasure, habit, and discomfort with intercourse.[48] Pain scores were all significantly reduced and HRQoL was improved as assessed by the EQ-5D index and the EQ-5Q VAS. Sexual pleasure and habit improved, and discomfort decreased.

Comparable results were obtained in a recent RCT comparing laparoscopic surgery for endometriosis with and without uterosacral ligament resection.[49] Both groups experienced similar and significant improvements in pain scores and HRQoL, assessed using the SF-36,[44] the Hospital Anxiety and Depression Scale,[50] and the revised Sabbatsberg Sexual Rating Scale,[51] which evaluates various aspects of sexual functioning separately, including libido, arousal, orgasm capacity, and satisfaction. Thus, the authors argued that the addition of uterosacral ligament resection to conservative laparoscopic surgery was of no benefit.

HRQoL instruments have only been used in a few studies assessing medical treatment. For example, in an RCT comparing nafarelin and medroxyprogesterone acetate, Bergqvist et al[52] used items from the General Health Questionnaire,[36] the Women's Health Questionnaire,[53] the 'Coping Wheel',[54] the Inventory of Social Support and Integration,[55] the demand–control questionnaire,[56] the Nottingham Health Profile Questionnaire,[57] and two psychosocial questionnaires assessing working conditions[58] and sleep.[59] Most psychosocial parameters, as well as emotional balance, improved in both groups during the study period. Interestingly, anxiety/depression and sleep disturbance were significantly more common in the 18 dropouts than in the 30 women who participated in the whole study. Lastly, in an RCT comparing cyproterone acetate and a continuous monophasic pill after conservative surgery, Vercellini et al[60] reported that both treatments produced a significant improvement in HRQoL, as assessed by the SF-36,[44] the Hospital Anxiety and Depression Scale,[50] and the revised Sabbatsberg Sexual Rating Scale.[51]

ENDOMETRIOSIS-SPECIFIC HRQoL INSTRUMENTS

In the small number of studies assessing the effect of treatment on HRQoL, mostly generic

measures have been used. However, a limitation of using generic measures is that they may not be sensitive enough to assess changes in specific illnesses, as they were designed to measure health status across a variety of diseases.

The condition-specific measure used in the Scottish Gynaecology Audit Project[43] was developed by seven clinicians with 'expertise in managing endometriosis'. The measure contains 16 questions which were constructed to reflect topics that might be covered in assessing women with the disease clinically: menstrual symptoms, impact of pelvic pain on functioning and wellbeing, and side effects of medical treatment. Colwell et al[61] have also developed a 95-item HRQoL questionnaire containing generic and endometriosis-specific scales and items based on a review of the published literature, and discussions with clinician and patient panels.[61] The final questionnaire included primarily validated scales, as well as items from the Medical Outcomes Study[47] relating to general health, comparative health, physical and emotional role functioning, bodily pain, anxiety, depression, behavioural and emotional control, general positive affect, emotional ties, and loneliness. The reliability, validity, and responsiveness of the instrument were tested in an open-label study comparing two doses of leuprolide: HRQoL was shown to vary in a manner consistent with clinician-rated measures of pelvic pain and dysmenorrhea, and with patient-reported levels of pain.

Therefore, although disease-specific instruments have been developed in endometriosis, most of the items contained in the questionnaires were not derived from patients with the disease. A patient-generated questionnaire would be preferable because, in general, the assessments patients make about their own health differ from the proxy reports healthcare professionals make about their patients' wellbeing.[62] In addition, disease-specific patient-generated questionnaires should be more responsive to changes in health status.[63]

The Endometriosis Health Profile-30 (EHP-30) is the first disease-specific instrument with established measurement properties that addresses the dimensions of HRQoL considered important to women with the disease.[64] The EHP-30 was developed in three stages: Stage 1 included open-ended exploratory interviews with 25 women to generate the items on the questionnaire; Stage 2 was an 87-item questionnaire administered in a postal survey to identify the most salient dimensions of HRQoL, and the reliability and validity of the questionnaire were then evaluated in Stage 3. The final instrument consists of a core questionnaire with 30 items and five scales: pain, control and powerlessness, emotional wellbeing, social support, and self-image. Six modular parts consisting of 23 questions were also developed and measure the areas of sexual intercourse, work, relationships with children, feelings about the medical profession, treatment, and infertility. All the scales achieved high internal reliability, and the intraclass correlation coefficients to evaluate the test–retest reliability were also high. Content validity was demonstrated as the questionnaire was developed from interviews with patients rather than the existing literature and/or clinical scales. Construct validity was demonstrated by showing high correlation between the EHP-30 and the relevant SF-36 scales. The EHP-30 is sensitive to change[65] and should prove useful in clinical trials as a means of assessing the impact of different medical and surgical interventions upon HRQoL. It has been translated into a number of different languages, and a short form, the EHP-5, has been developed which contains five items from the core and six items from the modular questionnaire.[66]

CONCLUSION

There are a large number of instruments that have been used in observational studies, clinical trials, and RCTs to assess pain, health status, and HRQoL in women with endometriosis. The adequacy of many of these instruments is questionable, as most were derived by clinicians, and it is now increasingly recognized that the most reliable instruments are those that have been generated by patients themselves. The routine use of valid and reliable tools in the future should facilitate the assessment of new treatments and surgical interventions.

REFERENCES

1. Low WY, Edelmann RJ. Psychosocial aspects of endometriosis: a review. J Psychosom Obstet Gynaecol 1990;12:3–12.
2. Mabbett L. Emotional aspects of endometriosis. National Endometriosis Society, 1998.
3. Walker E, Katon W, Jones LM, Russo J. Relationship between endometriosis and affective disorder. Am J Psychiatry 1989; 146:380–1.
4. Hawkridge C. Understanding endometriosis. London: MacDonald and Co., 1989.
5. Wigfall-Williams W. Hysterectomy: learning the facts, coping with the feelings, facing the future. New York: Michael Kesend, 1986.
6. Weinstein K. The emotional aspects of endometriosis: what the patient expects from her doctor. Clin Obstet Gynecol 1988;31:866–73.
7. Houston DE. Evidence for the risk of pelvic endometriosis by age, race and socioeconomic status. Epidemiol Rev 1984;6:167–91.
8. Damario MA, Rock JA. Pain recurrence: a quality of life issue in endometriosis. Int J Gynecol Obstet 1995;50 Suppl 1:S27–S42.
9. Melzack R. The short form of the McGill Pain Questionnaire. Pain 1987;27:191–7.
10. Biberoglu KO, Behrman SJ. Dosage aspects of danazol therapy in endometriosis: short-term and long-term effectiveness. Am J Obstet Gynecol 1981;139:645–54.
11. Vercellini P, Trespidi L, Colombo A et al. A gonadotropin-releasing hormone agonist versus a low-dose oral contraceptive for pelvic pain associated with endometriosis. Fertil Steril 1993;60:75–9.
12. Andersch B, Milson I. An epidemiologic study of young women with dysmenorrhea. Am J Obstet Gynecol 1982;144:655–60.
13. Moore J, Kennedy S, Prentice A. Modern combined oral contraceptives for pain associated with endometriosis. In: The Cochrane Library, Issue 3, 2003. Oxford: Update Software 2003.
14. Prentice A, Deary AJ, Goldbeck WS, Farquhar C, Smith SK. Gonadotrophin-releasing hormone analogues for pain associated with endometriosis. In: The Cochrane Library, Issue 3, 2003. Oxford: Update Software, 2003.
15. Prentice A, Deary AJ, Bland E. Progestogens and anti-progestogens for pain associated with endometriosis. In: The Cochrane Library, Issue 3, 2003. Oxford: Update Software, 2003.
16. Hughes E, Fedorkow D, Collins J, Vandekerckhove P. Ovulation suppression for endometriosis. In: The Cochrane Library, Issue 3, 2003. Oxford: Update Software, 2003.
17. Jacobson TZ, Barlow DH, Garry R, Koninckx P. Laparoscopic surgery for pelvic pain associated with endometriosis. In: The Cochrane Library, Issue 3, 2003. Oxford: Update Software, 2003.
18. Selak V, Farquhar C, Prentice A, Singla A. Danazol for pelvic pain associated with endometriosis. In: The Cochrane Library, Issue 3, 2003. Oxford: Update Software, 2003.
19. Vercellini P, De GO, Oldani S et al. Depot medroxyprogesterone acetate versus an oral contraceptive combined with very-low-dose danazol for long-term treatment of pelvic pain associated with endometriosis. Am J Obstet Gynecol 1996;175:396–401.
20. Sutton CJ, Ewen SP, Whitelaw N, Haines P. Prospective, randomized, double-blind, controlled trial of laser laparoscopy in the treatment of pelvic pain associated with minimal, mild, and moderate endometriosis. Fertil Steril 1994;62:696–700.

21. Gestrinone Italian Study Group. Gestrinone versus a gonadotropin-releasing hormone agonist for the treatment of pelvic pain associated with endometriosis: a multicenter, randomized, double-blind study. Fertil Steril 1996;66:911–19.

22. Wheeler JM, Knittle J, Miller JD. Depot leuprolide versus danazol in the treatment of women with symptomatic endometriosis: I. Efficacy results. Am J Obstet Gynecol 1992;167:1367–71.

23. Dlugi AM, Miller JD, Knittle J. Lupron depot (leuprolide acetate for depot suspension) in the treatment of endometriosis: a randomized, placebo-controlled, double-blind study. Lupron Study Group. Fertil Steril 1990;54:419–27.

24. Glick JH. Analgesic use scale. Cancer Treat Rep 1983;64:813–19.

25. Jenkinson C, McGee M. Health Status Measurement – a Brief but Critical Introduction. Oxford: Radcliffe Medical Press, 1998.

26. Doyle DF, Li TC, Richmond MN. The prevalence of continuing chronic pelvic pain following a negative laparoscopy. J Obstet Gynaecol 1998;18:252–5.

27. Kadir RA, Sabin CA, Pollard D, Lee CA, Economides DL. Quality of life during menstruation in patients with inherited bleeding disorders. Haemophilia 1998;4:836–41.

28. Zhao SZ, Kellerman LA, Francisco CA, Wong JM. Impact of nafarelin and leuprolide for endometriosis on quality of life and subjective clinical measures. J Reprod Med 1999;44:1000–6.

29. Jones GL, Kennedy SH, Jenkinson C. Health-related quality of life measurement in women with common benign gynecologic conditions: A systematic review. Am J Obstet Gynecol 2002;187:2–11.

30. Waller KG, Shaw RW. Endometriosis, pelvic pain, and psychological functioning. Fertil Steril 1995;63:796–800.

31. Beck AT, Steer RA. Beck Depression Inventory Manual. San Antonio, TX: The Psychological Corporation, Harcourt Brace Jovanovich, 1987.

32. Speilberger CD. Manual for the State-Trait Anxiety Inventory. Palo Alto, CA: Consulting Psychologists Press Inc, 1983.

33. Rust J, Golombok S. The Golombok–Rust inventory of sexual satisfaction. London: NFER-Nelson, 1986.

34. Low WY, Edelmann RJ, Sutton C. A psychological profile of endometriosis patients in comparison to patients with pelvic pain of other origins. J Psychosom Res 1993;37:111–16.

35. Eysenck HJ, Eysenck SBG. Eysenck Personality Questionnaire manual. San Diego, CA: Educational and Industrial Testing Service, 1975.

36. Goldberg D. Manual of the General Health Questionnaire. London: NFER-Nelson, 1979.

37. Peveler R, Edwards J, Daddow J, Thomas E. Psychosocial factors and chronic pelvic pain: a comparison of women with endometriosis and with unexplained pain. J Psychosom Res 1996;40:305–15.

38. Derogatis LR, Melisaratos N. The Brief Symptom Inventory: an introductory report. Psychol Med 1983;13:595–605.

39. Weissman MM, Bothwell S. Assessment of social adjustment by patient self report. Arch Gen Psychiatry 1976;33:1111–15.

40. Lewis DO, Comite F, Mallouh C et al. Bipolar mood disorder and endometriosis: preliminary findings. Am J Psychiatry 1987;144:1588–91.

41. Hamilton M. A rating scale for depression. Psychiatry 1960;23:56–62.

42. Endicott J, Spitzer RL. A diagnostic interview: the schedule for affective disorders and schizophrenia. Arch Gen Psychiatry 1978;35:837–44.

43. Bodner CH, Garratt AM, Ratcliffe J, Macdonald LM, Penney GC. Measuring health-related quality of life outcomes in women with endometriosis – results of the Gynaecology Audit Project in Scotland. Health Bull Edinb 1997;55:109–17.

44. Ware JE, Snow KK, Kosinski M, Gandek B. SF-36 Health Survey Manual and Interpretation Guide. Boston, MA: The Health Institute, New England medical Center, 1993.

45. Abbott JA, Hawe J, Clayton RD, Garry R. The effects and effectiveness of laparoscopic excision of endometriosis: a prospective study with 2–5 year follow-up. Hum Reprod 2003;18:1922–7.

46. Brooks R, EuroQOL Group. EuroQOL: the current state of play. Health Policy 1997;37:53–72.

47. Ware J, Kosinski M, Keller S. A 12-item short-form health survey. Construction of scales and preliminary tests of reliability and validity. Med Care 1995;34:220–33.

48. Thirlaway K, Fallowfield L, Cuzick J. The sexual activity questionnaire: a measure of women's sexual functioning. Qual Life Res 1996;5:81–90.

49. Vercellini P, Aimi G, Busacca M et al. Laparoscopic uterosacral ligament resection for dysmenorrhea associated with endometriosis: results of a randomized, controlled trial. Fertil Steril 2003;80:310–19.

50. Zigmond AS, Snaith RP. The Hospital Anxiety and Depression Scale. Acta Psychiatr Scand 1983;67:361–70.

51. Garratt AM, Torgerson DJ, Wyness J, Hall MH, Reid DM. Measuring sexual function in premenopausal women. Br J Obstet Gynaecol 1995;102:311–16.

52. Bergqvist A, Theorell T. Changes in quality of life after hormonal treatment of endometriosis. Acta Obstet Gynecol Scand 2001;80:7–37.

53. Wiklund I, Karlberg J, Lindgren R, Sandin K, Mattsson L-A. A Swedish version of the Women's Health Questionnaire. A measure of postmenopausal complaints. Acta Obstet Gynecol Scand 1993;72:648–55.

54. Haggmark C, Theorell T, Elk B. Coping and social activity patterns among relatives of cancer patients. Social Sci Med 1987;25:1021–5.

55. Henderson S, Duncan-Jones P, Byrne D. The interview schedule for social interaction. Psychol Med 1980;10:723–34.

56. Karasek RA. Job demands, job decision latitude and mental strain: implications for job redesign. Admin Sci Q 1978;24:285–307.

57. Hunt SM, McEven J. The development of a subjective health indicator. Sociol Health Illness 1980;12:231–45.

58. Unden A-L, Orth-Gomer K. Development of a social support instrument for use in population surveys. Social Sci Med 1989;29:1387–92.

59. Akerstedt T, Torsvall L. Experimental changes in shift schedules – their effects on well-being. Ergonomics 1978;21:849–56.

60. Vercellini P, De Giorgi O, Mosconi P et al. Cyproterone acetate versus a continuous monophasic oral contraceptive in the treatment of recurrent pelvic pain after conservative surgery for symptomatic endometriosis. Fertil Steril 2002;77:52–61.

61. Colwell HH, Mathias SD, Pasta DJ, Henning JM, Steege JF. A health-related quality-of-life instrument for symptomatic patients with endometriosis: a validation study. Am J Obstet Gynecol 1998;179:47–55.

62. Fitzpatrick R, Davey C, Buxton M, Jones DR. Patient-assessed outcome measures. In: Black N, Brazier J, Fitzpatrick R, eds. Health Services Research Methods. London: BMJ Publications, 1998;13–22.

63. Patrick DL, Deyo RA. Generic and disease-specific measures in assessing health status and quality of life. Med Care 2003;27:S217–232.

64. Jones G, Kennedy S, Barnard A, Wong J, Jenkinson C. Development of an endometriosis quality-of-life instrument: The Endometriosis Health Profile-30. Obstet Gynecol 2001;98:2–64.

65. Jones GL, Jenkinson C, Kennedy SH. Evaluating the sensitivity to change of the Endometriosis Health Profile Questionnaire: The EHP-30. Qual Life Res 2004;13:705–13.

66. Jones GL, Jenkinson C, Kennedy SH. Development of the Short Form Endometriosis Health Profile Questionnaire: The EHP-5. Qual Life Res 2004;13:695–704.

14. Medical Therapy of Endometriosis

David L. Olive

INTRODUCTION

Medical therapy is an integral part of the treatment armamentarium for endometriosis. The ability to attack this disease without surgical intervention is critical to the effective treatment strategy for many. However, drug treatment of endometriosis is far from perfect in terms of outcome measures. This chapter is designed to thoroughly discuss all available medical treatments of endometriosis, as well as the role of each in the treatment of this disease (Table 14.1). Experimental therapies will also be previewed, with an assessment of their current status. Finally, the role of medical therapy in conjunction with surgical treatment will be reviewed in an attempt to determine the advisability of this approach.

ESTABLISHED MEDICAL TREATMENTS OF ENDOMETRIOSIS

DANAZOL

The first drug to be approved for the treatment of endometriosis in the United States was danazol, an isoxazol derivative of 17α-ethinyl testosterone. It was originally thought to produce a pseudomenopause, but subsequent studies have shown the drug to act primarily by suppressing the midcycle luteinizing hormone (LH) surge,[1,2] creating a chronic anovulatory state. Additional actions include the inhibition of multiple enzymes in the steroidogenic pathology,[3] and an increase in free serum testosterone.[4] The recommended dosage of danazol for the treatment of endometriosis is 600–800 mg/day; however, these doses have substantial androgenic side effects, such as increased hair growth, mood changes, adverse serum lipid profiles, deepening of the voice (possibly irreversible), and rarely, liver damage (possibly irreversible and life-threatening) and arterial throm-

Table 14.1 Medical therapies for endometriosis

Established treatments
Danazol
Progestogens
Oral contraceptives
GnRH agonists
Gestrinone

Experimental treatments
Progesterone receptor modulators
GnRH antagonists
Aromatase inhibitors
TNF-α inhibitors
Angiogenesis inhibitors
Matrix metalloproteinase inhibitors
Immunomodulators
Estrogen receptor β agonists

bosis.[5,6] Studies of lower doses as primary treatment for endometriosis-associated pain have been uncontrolled or with small numbers, and thus contain information of limited value.[7] However, because of the many side effects of the drug, alternative routes of administration have been sought. Recently, the use of danazol vaginal suppositories[8] and a danazol-impregnated vaginal ring[9] has been described in small, uncontrolled trials. Preliminary results suggest that side effects may be less severe with the transvaginal approach.

PROGESTOGENS

Progestogens are a class of compound that produce progesterone-like effects on endometrial tissue. A large number of progestogens exist, ranging from those chemically derived from progesterone (progestins), such as medroxyprogesterone acetate (MPA), to 19-nortestosterone derivatives such as norethindrone and norgestrel. The proposed mechanism of action of these compounds is initial decidualization of endometrial tissue followed by eventual atrophy. This is believed to be due to a direct suppressive effect of progestogens on the estrogen receptors of the endometrium. Recent evidence suggests that another mechanism of action at the molecular level is the suppression of matrix metalloproteinases, enzymes important in the implantation and growth of ectopic endometrium.[10]

The most extensively studied progestational agent for the treatment of endometriosis is medroxyprogesterone. This drug was originally used orally for the treatment of endometriosis, with doses ranging from 20 to 100 mg daily; published randomized studies are limited to 100 mg daily. However, the depot formulation has also been used, in a dose of 150 mg every 3 months. The side effects of medroxyprogesterone are many and varied, yet even in high doses it seems to be better tolerated metabolically than danazol. A common side effect is transient breakthrough bleeding, which occurs in 38–47% of cases. This is generally well tolerated and, when necessary, can be adequately treated with supplemental estrogen or an increase in the progestogen dose. Other side effects include nausea (0–80%), breast tenderness (5%), fluid retention (50%), and depression (6%).[11] In published trials few patients have discontinued the medications because of side effects. In contrast to danazol, all of the abovementioned adverse effects resolve upon discontinuation of the drug.

Norethindrone acetate has also been used as a treatment for endometriosis. This 19-nortestosterone derivative has only been analyzed in a retrospective, uncontrolled trial of 52 women,[12] each of whom was treated initially with 5 mg daily, with increases of 2.5 mg increments up to a maximum dose of 20 mg daily, until amenorrhea was achieved. Side effects were similar to those seen with medroxyprogesterone.

Other progestational agents have also been used in the occasional study. Levonorgestrel, the active ingredient of Norplant, has also been used recently via an intrauterine device delivery system.[13] The drug has been shown to effectively decrease vascular endothelial growth factor (VEGF) and blood vessel proliferation, providing the rationale for its use in endometriosis.[14] It has recently been suggested as a desirable treatment for rectovaginal endometriosis, although the evidence thus far is uncontrolled.[13]

Progestogens may adversely affect serum lipoprotein levels.[15–17] Whether alterations in serum lipoprotein levels for 4–6 months have any clinical significance is unclear.

ORAL CONTRACEPTIVES (COMBINATION ESTROGEN–PROGESTOGEN)

The combination of estrogen and progestogen for the treatment of endometriosis – the so-called 'pseudopregnancy' regimen – is believed to produce initial decidualization and growth of endometrial tissue, followed in several months by atrophy. This has been observed in women[18] but is in direct conflict with data from the rhesus monkey.[19]

Pseudopregnancy regimens have been administered both orally and parenterally. Combination oral contraceptive pills such as norethynodrel and mestranol, norethindrone acetate and ethinyl estradiol, lynestrenol and mestranol, and norgestrel plus ethinyl estradiol have all been tried. Parenteral combinations have included 17-hydroxyprogesterone or depot medroxyprogesterone acetate paired with stilbestrol or conjugated estrogens.

The side effects of pseudopregnancy are often quite impressive, and include those encountered with progestogens alone, as well as estrogenic- and androgenic-related effects. Estrogens may cause nausea, hypertension, thrombophlebitis, and uterine enlargement. The 19-nortestosterone-derived progestogens may cause androgenic effects such as acne, alopecia, increased muscle mass, decreased breast size, and deepening of the voice. Noble and Letchworth, in a comparative trial of norethynodrel and mestranol versus danazol, found that 41% of the pseudopregnancy group failed to complete their course of therapy because of side effects of the medication.[20] However, dosages generally involved more estrogen and progestogen than are found in modern contraceptive preparations. The oral contraceptives commonly prescribed today for combination therapy are most likely to produce a progestogen-dominant picture similar to that of progestogen alone, with a low rate of adverse effects.

Today, oral contraceptives are the most commonly prescribed treatment for endometriosis symptoms. Despite this, there are few data regarding mechanism of action. One recent investigation suggests that oral contraceptives suppress proliferation and enhance programmed cell death (apoptosis) in endometrial tissue, perhaps providing a mechanistic clue to the action of these drugs.[21]

GnRH AGONISTS

Gonadotropin-releasing hormone agonists (GnRH agonists) are analogs of the hormone GnRH. This hypothalamic hormone is responsible for stimulating the pituitary gland to secrete follicle-stimulating hormone (FSH) and luteinizing hormone (LH), two hormones necessary for normal ovarian function. GnRH is secreted in a pulsatile manner; the correct pulse results in stimulation of FSH and LH release, whereas too high or too low a pulse rate results in a decrease in pituitary hormone secretion. GnRH agonists are modified forms of GnRH that bind to the pituitary receptors and remain for a lengthy period. Thus, they are identified by the pituitary as rapidly pulsatile GnRH and, after initial stimulation of FSH and LH secretion, result in a shutdown (downregulation) of the pituitary and no resulting stimulation of the ovary. The result is a hypoestrogenic state similar to that of menopause, producing endometrial atrophy and amenorrhea. It is also possible that the drug affects ectopic endometrium via additional mechanisms: animal studies have suggested alterations in plasminogen activators and matrix metalloproteinases, factors important in the development of endometriosis.[22]

The agonist can be given intranasally, subcutaneously, or intramuscularly, depending upon the specific product, with frequency of administration ranging from twice daily to every 3 months. The side effects are those of hypoestrogenism, such as transient vaginal bleeding, hot flashes, vaginal dryness, decreased libido, breast tenderness, insomnia, depression, irritability and fatigue, headache, osteoporosis, and decreased skin elasticity.[23]

A recent modification of GnRH-agonist treatment is to 'add back' small amounts of steroid hormone in a manner similar to that used in the treatment of postmenopausal women. The theory is that the requirement for estrogen is greater for endometriosis than is needed by the brain (to prevent hot flashes), the bone (to prevent osteoporosis), and other tissues deprived of this hormone.[24] Interestingly, this 'threshold hypothesis' appears to be true, with estrogen–progestogen or progestogen-only add-back therapy resulting in an equivalent rate of pain relief with far fewer side effects than with GnRH agonists alone. Estrogen as a solitary add-back, however, is less effective and thus not indicated.[25] Currently, only levonorgestrel add-back therapy has been approved by the US Food and Drug Administration, although regimens of conjugated estrogens and medroxyprogesterone have also been demonstrated to be effective.

GESTRINONE

Gestrinone (ethylnorgestrienone, R2323) is an antiprogestational steroid used extensively in Europe for the treatment of endometriosis, but not currently available in the United States. Its effects include androgenic, antiprogestogenic, and antiestrogenic actions, although the latter are not mediated by estrogen receptor binding.

This steroid is believed to act by inducting a progesterone withdrawal effect at the endometrial cellular level, thus enhancing lysosomal degradation of the cell structure. There is a rapid decrease in estrogen and progesterone receptors in normal endometrium following the administration of gestrinone, as well as a sharp increase in 17β-hydroxysteroid dehydrogenase. Interestingly, these cellular effects did not occur in samples of endometriotic tissue.[26]

Gestrinone may also inhibit ovarian steroido-genesis. A 50% decrease in serum estradiol level is noted after administration, perhaps related to the associated significant decline in sex hor-mone-binding globulin concentration (an andro-genic or antiprogestogenic effect).[27] No effect on adrenal function or prolactin secretion has been noted.

Gestrinone is administered orally in doses of 2.5–10 mg weekly, on a daily, twice-weekly, or three-times-weekly schedule. Side effects include androgenic and antiestrogenic sequelae. Although most side effects are mild and tran-sient, several, such as voice changes, hirsutism, and clitoral hypertrophy, are potentially irre-versible.

RESULTS OF MEDICAL TREATMENT

TYPES OF TREATMENT TRIAL

Although many studies have been published regarding the medical treatment of endometrio-sis, it is important to realize that not all are of equal importance. There is a hierarchy of clinical trial design that should be relied upon for assess-ing a study's validity and applicability.[28] These study designs, and their place in the hierarchy, are listed in Table 14.2.

Uncontrolled trials have limited value other than to suggest hypotheses to be tested by more rigorous designs. The same is true for historically controlled studies and concurrently controlled non-randomized trials, each of which introduces significant biases into the results. The gold stan-dard today is the randomized clinical trial (RCT), where subjects are randomly allocated to one of several treatment groups, often in a blinded man-ner such that the assignment is unknown to the patient or the physician until the conclusion of the trial. This design is the least biased of all approaches, and results in the most reliable conclusions.

Unfortunately, many RCT are too small to reach a negative conclusion with any degree of confidence. The results of RCT may also differ from one another, owing to slight differences in study design, different patient populations, or even as a result of chance events. For these rea-sons, when multiple randomized trials exist they can often be combined into a single evaluation called a meta-analysis.[29] The meta-analysis allows us to obtain a single, best answer to a question with a higher level of confidence than is usually possible with individual studies. However, it is important to bear in mind that a meta-analysis is only as good as the studies included in it: if poor-quality trials are placed into a meta-analysis, the resulting conclusions are as tenuous as those of the component studies.

ASSESSING EFFICACY

The value of a particular medical treatment varies according to the therapeutic goal of the intervention. With regard to endometriosis, three outcomes can be assessed to determine drug efficacy: the anatomic manifestations of the dis-ease, pain symptomatology, and infertility status.

The anatomic manifestations of endometrio-sis, implants, and adhesions, can be assessed before and after therapy to determine whether the intervention is of value. However, such a sim-ple comparison makes two assumptions. First, it is assumed that endometriosis is an invariably progressive disease, never to regress on its own; this is unfortunately incorrect, as the disease has in fact been noted to regress in both baboons and humans.[30,31] Second, the above comparison pre-supposes that once regression has occurred as a result of medical therapy, it is stable. This, too, is not the case, as implant and adhesion regrowth

---

Table 14.2 Hierarchy of evidence from clinical studies

I	Meta-analysis or large randomized clinical trial
II	Small randomized clinical trial
III	Non-randomized, concurrently controlled trial
IV	Historically controlled trial
V	Case–control study or cohort study
VI	Time–series study or anecdotal case reports
VII	Expert opinion

are both time-dependent phenomena. Thus, to adequately address the effect of a medical treatment upon endometriosis lesions, a proper control group for comparison is needed, with longitudinal follow-up.

A second outcome of interest is the effect upon pain. The first requirement of quality pain evaluation is a valid method of assessing pain.[32] A second necessity in pain research is longitudinal evaluation, as pain recurrence is a time-dependent phenomenon. Finally, to determine the efficacy of a drug in relieving pain, a large placebo effect must be accounted for. This phenomenon of relief by inactive drug may occur in as many as 55% of women with endometriosis-associated pain.[33] Thus, placebo-controlled trials are needed to determine absolute efficacy; comparative studies between drugs will allow the determination of relative efficacy.

The final outcome of interest is fertility enhancement. Unfortunately, it is rare that the woman with endometriosis-associated infertility has absolute infertility owing to the disease, as is the case with bilateral tubal blockage or azoospermia. Instead, most women suffering from endometriosis-associated infertility have a relative reduction in fecundity.[31] Thus they are able to conceive, albeit at a slower rate. To demonstrate improved fertility status after intervention, a comparison group of untreated women is clearly needed. Finally, as fertility is time dependent, longitudinal assessment is again critical.

From the above discussion, it is clear that optimal trials are properly controlled and randomized. In addition, it is important to have studies that have lengthy follow-up so that we can determine the long-term course post treatment. Studies such as these will be primarily relied upon in the subsequent discussion.

MEDICAL TREATMENT OF ENDOMETRIOSIS IMPLANTS

The effect of medications on implant volume, number, and extensiveness has been examined for a number of drugs in a number of ways. Many are poorly controlled or uncontrolled investigations, and often the observation searching for effect is carried out while the patient is taking the drug. Thus, what occurs after drug discontinuation is often unknown.

An effect of danazol on endometriotic implants has been consistently observed. Uncontrolled trials have demonstrated implant resolution in the vast majority of treated patients.[34,35] Studies have shown a mean decrease of 61–89% of implant volume[36,37] and a 43% decrease in classification score.[38] A single placebo-controlled RCT examined the effect upon implants 6 months after the completion of drug therapy and found resolution in 18% of the placebo group and 60% of the danazol treatment group.[39]

Although progestogens clearly affect ectopic endometrium, there is limited information on their histologic effect on endometriosis. In the rhesus monkey, levonorgestrel has been shown to decrease lesion size. In humans a single randomized prospective trial demonstrated that MPA 100 mg daily for 6 months produced complete resolution of implants in 50% of patients and a partial resolution in 13%, whereas corresponding figures for placebo were 12% and 6%, respectively.[39]

Several randomized trials have assessed the ability of gestrinone to reduce anatomic endometriosis. The drug has been shown to reduce the amount of disease comparably to danazol,[40] and doses as low as 1.25 mg twice weekly can accomplish this.[41,42]

GnRH agonists have been shown in numerous studies to decrease the classification score of endometriosis in patients on the drug; similar decreases were seen with the complete AFS classification, as well as a modified scoring system that excluded points for adhesions.[43,44] Thus, the effect is limited to causing a lessening of implant volume. In comparative trials the decreased AFS score is comparable to that seen with danazol treatment.[45] No study has evaluated the persistent effect of GnRH on implants after discontinuation of the drug, however. GnRH agonist plus add-back therapy has also been shown to decrease the AFS classification score, and to a degree similar to that seen with GnRH agonists alone.[46]

MEDICAL TREATMENT OF ENDOMETRIOSIS-ASSOCIATED PAIN

Pain relief has also been well demonstrated with danazol, with 84–92% of women responding.[47] A placebo-controlled RCT proved that danazol reduced pain significantly better than no treatment for up to 6 months following discontinuation of the drug.[39] No good data exist for longer follow-up periods. Recent evidence suggests that the median time to pain recurrence following discontinuation of the medication is 6.1 months.[48]

Few randomized trials exist to evaluate the effects of progestational agents on endometriosis-associated pain. Telimaa and colleagues[39] evaluated the effect of medroxyprogesterone acetate 100 mg/day for 6 months. The medication produced a significant and substantial improvement in pain scores while patients were receiving the drug, as well as up to 6 months following discontinuation. In fact, the relative attributable experimental effect (percentage decrease in pain severity attributable solely to treatment) was 50–74% at the conclusion of follow-up. Randomized comparative trials suggest medroxyprogesterone to be comparable in efficacy to danazol, although lynestrenol performed less well than a GnRH agonist for all aspects of endometriosis-associated pain.[49]

Numerous uncontrolled trials have evaluated pain relief with oral contraceptives, generally demonstrating an improvement in 75–89%.[11] A recent randomized clinical trial compared cyclic low-dose oral contraceptives to a GnRH agonist and found no substantial difference in the degree of relief afforded by the two drugs, except that the GnRH agonist provided greater relief of dysmenorrhea and possibly dyspareunia.[50] An uncontrolled trial of continuous OCP following failure of cyclic therapy suggested that this regimen may be superior, as 80% responded with pain relief.[51] However, no RCT have as yet assessed continuous administration.

The effectiveness of GnRH agonists in the treatment of endometriosis-associated pain has been demonstrated in both placebo-controlled and comparative randomized trials. The one placebo-controlled study demonstrated greater effectiveness of the drug at 3 months, at which time those in the placebo group still suffering from pain were allowed to opt out of the study.[52] In comparative trials, GnRH agonists and danazol were equally effective in relieving pain.[45,53–67] Oral contraceptives have also been compared with GnRH agonists: in a study of 57 women designed to have 80% power to detect a 35% difference in effect, cyclic oral contraceptive treatment was significantly less effective than GnRH agonist treatment for the relief of dysmenorrhea, nearly as effective for the relief of dyspareunia (statistically significantly different using one of two rating scales, but of questionable clinical importance), and equally efficacious in relieving nonspecific pelvic pain.[50]

Whereas the above studies randomized patients for initial therapy of endometriosis-associated pain, one study has examined the value of GnRH agonists in patients failing primary therapy. Ling and colleagues treated women having failed to obtain relief with OCP using either GnRH agonist or placebo.[68] Those treated with the active drug responded significantly better than those given placebo, with more than 80% experiencing pain relief in 3 months. Of interest is the fact that the therapy seemed to be beneficial whether or not endometriosis was seen at laparoscopy.

Several trials have addressed the efficacy of combined add-back therapy and GnRH agonist treatment during 6-month treatment periods.[69–74] In general, pain was relieved as effectively with the combination as with GnRH agonists alone, and it significantly reduced the side effects of the GnRH agonist (Figure 14.1). The results were similar in three longer trials of approximately 1 year's duration.[46,75,76] It seems clear that add-back therapy can be added to GnRH agonist treatment without loss of efficacy but with a substantial amelioration of hypoestrogenic symptoms. This seems to be the case even when the add-back therapy is begun during the first month of treatment, suggesting that an 'add-back free'

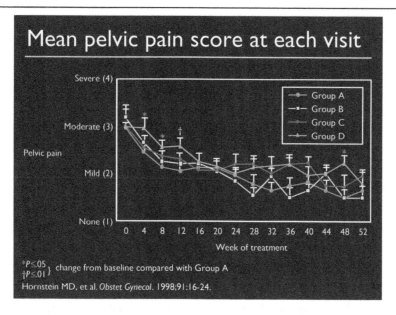

Figure 14.1 Pain relief with GnRH agonist with and without add-back therapy. Group 1 = GnRH agonist alone, Group 2 = GnRH agonist plus norethindrone, Group 3 = GnRH agonist plus low-dose conjugated estrogen/norethindrone, Group 4 = GnRH agonist plus high-dose conjugated estrogen/norethindrone.

interval at the beginning of a treatment cycle is unnecessary.[74]

Although not approved for use in the United States, gestrinone has been studied fairly extensively. Comparative trials show gestrinone to be roughly equivalent in pain relief to danazol[40] and GnRH agonists.[77] One study has even shown gestrinone to be slightly more efficacious than GnRH agonists for the relief of dysmenorrhea 6 months after discontinuation of medication.[77]

Given the above data, a number of conclusions can be reached regarding the medical treatment of endometriosis symptoms. It appears that most established medical therapies are effective for the primary treatment of endometriosis-associated pain, and all seem also to be roughly equivalent. Thus, for initial treatment the choice should probably be based on the cost and side-effect profile of the drug being considered. However, only GnRH agonists have been proved effective after the failure of a prior medical hormonal therapy.

MEDICAL TREATMENT OF ENDOMETRIOSIS-ASSOCIATED INFERTILITY

Most of the established medical therapies used to treat endometriosis have been applied to the problem of subfertility in women with the disease. These medications inhibit ovulation, and thus are used to treat the disease for a period of time prior to allowing an attempt at conception. Five randomized trials with six treatment arms have compared one of these medical treatments directed at endometriosis to placebo or no treatment, with fertility as the outcome measure.[78-82] Another eight RCT compared danazol to a second medication. These latter trials have been summarized by a meta-analysis by Hughes et al[83] (Table 14.3). Whether in individual trials or a meta-analysis, no increase in fertility can be demonstrated with these medications compared to expectant management; nor has any medication proved superior to danazol in this regard.

Table 14.3 Meta-analysis of medical therapy for endometriosis-associated infertility

Study	Medical treatment	Placebo or no treatment	Relative risk	95% Confidence limits
Bayer[78]	11/37	17/36	0.63	0.32–1.22
Fedele[81]	17/35	17/36	1.03	0.60–1.76
Telimaa[79]	13/35	6/14	0.87	0.41–2.25
Thomas[82]	5/20	4/17	1.06	0.28–4.29
Harrison[80]	0/50	3/50	0.00	0.00–2.18
Total	46/177	47/153	0.85	0.59–1.22

However, for some studies follow-up was begun at the conclusion of therapy; thus those receiving no treatment began attempting to conceive immediately after the diagnostic laparoscopy, whereas those placed on drug therapy were not allowed to attempt conception until after the medication course was completed (generally 6 months). These studies were analyzed as if the time had begun at the conclusion of 'treatment', but for the patient the clock begins ticking at the time of diagnostic laparoscopy. The real question is not who gets pregnant faster after therapy is completed, but rather who gets pregnant faster from the time of diagnosis?

If we reanalyze the above data, with follow-up proceeding from the time of diagnosis instead of conclusion of treatment, a different image emerges. Now, suppressive medical therapy proves significantly detrimental to fertility (Table 14.4)! In essence, the interval spent on medical therapy has been wasted time, merely serving to prolong the infertility in a number of couples. Thus, traditional medical therapy for endometriosis has not proved to be of value, and in fact to the subfertile patient may actually be counterproductive.

This is not to suggest that traditional medical therapy is incapable of playing a role in the treatment of the infertile couple with endometriosis. It is quite possible that a subgroup of infertile women exist who could be helped with drug therapy. However, this subgroup is thus far unidentified; advocates should focus future trials upon somehow stratifying endometriosis patients and then randomizing them to drug versus no treatment. Until that time, it is clear that these medications have no role in the treatment of endometriosis-associated infertility.

Table 14.4 Meta-analysis of medical therapy for endometriosis-associated infertility: adjustment for follow-up from time of diagnosis

Study	Medical treatment	Placebo or no treatment	Relative risk	95% Confidence limits
Bayer[78]	11/37	17/36	0.63	0.32–1.22
Fedele[81]	10/35	13/36	0.79	0.36–1.68
Telimaa[79]	4/35	5/14	0.32	0.08–1.24
Thomas[82]	4/20	4/17	0.85	0.20–3.69
Harrison[80]	0/50	3/50	0.00	0.00–2.18
Total	29/177	42/153	0.60	0.38–0.93

EXPERIMENTAL MEDICAL TREATMENTS

RU486 (MIFEPRISTONE) AND SELECTIVE PROGESTERONE RECEPTOR MODULATORS

Progesterone receptor modulators (PRM) are progesterone receptor ligands that can produce one of three effects.[84] Type I ligands prevent or attenuate PR binding to the progesterone response element;[85] in so doing they act as pure antagonists of progesterone action. Examples of such ligands include the 13α-configured steroids onapristone and ZK 135,695. Type II progesterone receptor ligands promote progesterone receptor binding to DNA response elements, but their ability to alter gene expression is highly variable and may be site specific.[86] A number of existing molecules can act in this manner: RU486, ZK 137,316, and the SPRM (J867, J956, J912, J1042; also known as mesoprogestins). Finally, type III ligands promote progesterone receptor binding to the progesterone response element, but transcription does not occur under any circumstances. Thus, in vivo type I or type III ligands act as pure antagonists, whereas type II ligands may act as agonists, partial agonists, or antagonists, depending upon the dose, presence, or absence of progesterone, and the site of action. To date only type II ligands have been used in the treatment of endometriosis.

Progesterone antagonists and agonist–antagonists have been shown in the non-human primate model to cause endometrial atrophy, similar to the effect of progesterone. However, the mechanism is completely different. It appears that the primarily antagonistic RU-486 causes a periarteriolar degeneration of endometrial spiral arteries. Partial agonists, such as the SPRM, also result in a decreased number and size of spiral arteries, but no periarteriolar degeneration is evident.[84] Thus, despite the potential proliferative effect upon endometrium via an antiprogestin effect, the inhibition of vascular supply results in endometrial atrophy.

RU-486 (mifepristone) was the first of this class of drugs to be used to treat endometriosis.

The drug is primarily a progesterone antagonist that can inhibit ovulation and disrupt endometrial integrity. Daily doses of this medication range from 50 to 100 mg daily, with side effects ranging from hot flashes to fatigue, nausea, and transient liver transaminase changes. No effects upon lipid profiles or bone mineral density have been reported.

The ability of mifepristone to produce a regression of endometriotic lesions has been variable and apparently dependent upon duration of treatment. Trials of 2 months in the rodent model[87] and 3 months in humans[88] failed to produce regression of disease. However, 6 months of therapy result in less visible disease in women.[89]

Uncontrolled trials suggest a possible efficacy for endometriosis-associated pain, although numbers are small.[88] No data have yet been collected regarding fertility enhancement.

The mesoprogestins are partial antagonists of progesterone, but also behave like progesterone in some tissues (Figure 14.2). This mixed agonist–antagonist effect may prove valuable if an SPRM can inhibit endometrial growth while not producing other systemic effects of progesterone, such as breast tenderness, depression, or fluid retention. The mesoprogestin J867 (asoprisnil) is currently in phase III clinical trials; early studies have suggested efficacy in pain relief with minimal side effects.

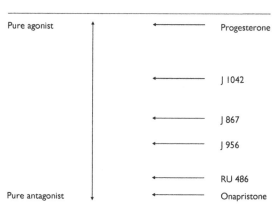

Figure 14.2 The relative agonist and antagonist activities of progesterone receptor modulators.

GnRH ANTAGONISTS

GnRH antagonists, like the long-utilized GnRH agonists, are a group of analogs of the native GnRH molecule (Figure 14.3). These drugs act by blocking the GnRH receptor directly and preventing it from activating. This results in a downregulation of the pituitary gland, a reduction of gonadotropin secretion, and suppression of ovarian steroid production. Thus, a hypoestrogenic state ensues, just as with GnRH agonists. Unlike GnRH agonists, however, these drugs do not cause an initial stimulation of gonadotropin and ovarian hormone release.

The GnRH antagonists have multiple changes compared to active GnRH. Substitutions in the first three amino acids result in binding to the GnRH receptor. Position six substitution creates a compound with a prolonged half-life, as this is the site generally attacked by degradation enzymes. Finally, early GnRH antagonists produced substantial histamine release, making their use problematic. Substitutions at positions eight and ten have eliminated this problem.

At the molecular level, the GnRH antagonist interrupts the basic activation process of the GnRH receptor. When GnRH binds to its receptor, the receptor dimerizes and initiates a cascade of events leading to synthesis and secretion of LH and FSH. With the antagonists, there is competition with the native molecule for the receptor. Given the high binding affinity, relative abundance, and long half-life of the antagonist, these molecules monopolize the GnRH receptors. Thus, dimerization of receptors is prevented (as GnRH cannot bind to them) and gonadotropes do not secrete LH or FSH.

Because of these characteristics the GnRH antagonists offer the theoretical advantage of working faster and more effectively than GnRH agonists, with better patient compliance owing to earlier amelioration of symptoms. Studies in animal models of endometriosis have been quite promising,[90] and preliminary clinical trials suggest the drug to be safe and efficacious.[91] A recent investigation demonstrated a GnRH antagonist to improve the health-related quality of life in women with endometriosis.[92] Phase III clinical trials are currently ongoing to further validate the use of this medication for endometriosis, as questions regarding relative efficacy and rate of side effects compared to GnRH agonists must be answered.

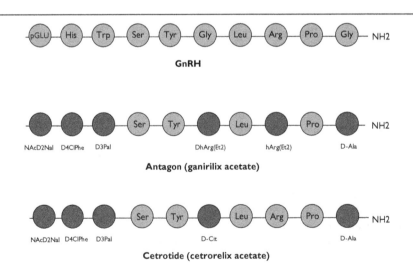

Figure 14.3 Structure of GnRH and GnRH antagonists.

AROMATASE INHIBITORS

It is well recognized that most if not all endometriosis is estrogen dependent, hence the effectiveness of medications that interfere with ovarian estrogen production. However, there are two other important sources of estrogen: peripheral tissue and endometriotic cells. Peripheral tissue sites such as adipose tissue and skin fibroblasts are capable of converting androgens to significant amounts of estrogen.[93] Furthermore, large quantities of estrogen can be produced locally within ectopically located endometrium via an intracrine mechanism (Figure 14.4).[94]

The mechanism by which endometriosis is able to produce its own estrogen is via the expression of the enzyme aromatase.[94] This enzyme, not expressed in normal endometrium, is stimulated by prostaglandin E_2 (PGE_2); the resulting estrogen production then stimulates PGE_2, further enhancing estrogen production. An obvious therapeutic target would thus be this aromatase enzyme. Aromatase inhibitors have now been tested in the rodent endometriosis model, with good success.[95] In addition, a case report of the use of anastrazole in a postmenopausal woman with severe endometriosis suggests the potential value of this treatment in women.[94] However, substantial bone loss in this woman highlights the need for caution with this class of medications, and reinforces the value of larger clinical trials to determine safety and efficacy.

TNF-α INHIBITORS

Tumor necrosis factor (TNF)-α is a cytokine that appears to be overproduced in endometriosis patients and may well be at least partially responsible for the influx of peritoneal macrophages known to occur in women with this disease. It has long been believed that this macrophage influx is at least partially responsible for many of the biochemical and symptomatic changes associated with endometriosis. In particular, it has been hypothesized that cytokine attraction of activated macrophages is one of the key initiators of growth

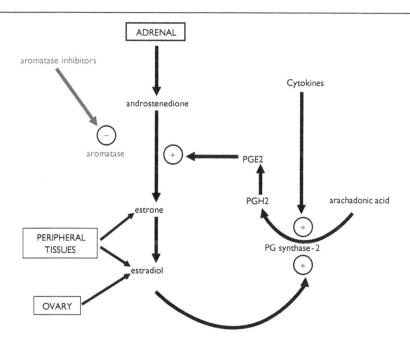

Figure 14.4 The intracellular pathway of aromatase action, and inhibition by aromatase inhibitors.

factor secretion in the peritoneal cavity, resulting in a favorable environment for endometriosis implantation, growth, and development.

One therapeutic approach that has been considered is some type of blockade of this cytokine. This has been attempted in the baboon, where recombinant human TNF binding protein-1 (TBP-1) was administered to menstrual endometrium prior to seeding the peritoneal cavity with the tissue.[96] In this scenario the development of endometriosis was inhibited. Additionally, baboons with endometriosis were treated with TBP-1, GnRH antagonist, or placebo; significantly less endometriosis was noted with TBP-1 and GnRH antagonist treatment. These studies suggest that TBP-1 is effective in treating the physical manifestations of endometriosis in the baboon, and may be of value in humans. Clinical trials, however, have not yet been conducted.

ANGIOGENESIS INHIBITORS

According to the transplantation theory of endometriosis, when shed endometrium is placed in the peritoneal cavity the establishment of a new blood supply is essential for the survival of the implant and the development of endometriosis. This process, termed angiogenesis, is a complex process involving a number of different but coordinated functions. These include proliferation, migration, and extension of endothelial cells, adherence of these cells to the extracellular matrix, remodeling of this matrix, and the formation of a lumen.[97]

Several angiogenic factors – that is, factors that aid in the development of new blood vessels – have been noted as being present in endometrium and endometriosis. The most prominently studied is vascular endothelial growth factor (VEGF), which is responsible for inducing early vascular growth. This molecule has been noted in endometriosis lesions,[98] endometriomas,[99] and the peritoneal fluid[100,101] of endometriosis patients, although in the latter case it is unclear whether levels are the same as or increased over controls. In any event, one logical therapeutic step would be to attempt inhibition of these new vas-

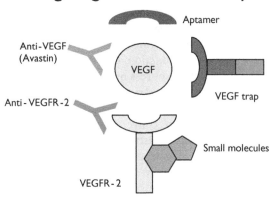

Figure 14.5 The chemical strategies for developing drugs to inhibit VEGF.

cular structures as a way of deterring the development of endometriosis (Figure 14.5). This has been attempted in the mouse model, where several angiogenic inhibitors (endostatin, TNP-470, celecoxib, and rosaglitazone) reduced the number and size of lesions.[102] The only human study thus far conducted with an angiogenesis inhibitor was the treatment of endometriosis-associated pain with thalidomide; pain relief was noted in these patients.[103]

MATRIX METALLOPROTEINASE INHIBITORS

Matrix metalloproteinases (MMP) are a family of endopeptidases which play a role in the degradation and turnover of extracellular matrix proteins. Their action is regulated by specific tissue inhibitors called tissue inhibitors of metalloproteinases (TIMP). The activity of these enzymes in the endometrium is generally regulated by steroid hormones: estrogen is known to increase endometrial MMP, and progesterone suppresses MMP activity.[104] The mechanism for these actions, as well as the many additional regulators of the system, are complex and are reviewed elsewhere.[104]

Increased matrix metalloproteinase activity has been described in endometriosis, and is believed to be integral in the ability of endometrium to invade tissue and implant successfully. Inhibition of these enzymes might be effective in inhibiting the development of endometriosis. Only one study has been conducted to date: the MMP inhibitor ONO-4817 was used in the mouse model to deter the development of experimental adenomyosis.[105] The value and practicality of this approach in endometriosis remains to be tested.

PENTOXIFYLLINE AND OTHER IMMUNOMODULATORS

Pentoxifylline is a multisite immunomodulating drug. It inhibits phagocytosis and the generation of toxic oxygen species and proteolytic enzymes by macrophages and granulocytes, stifles the production of TNF-α, and reduces the inflammatory action of TNF-α and interleukin (IL)-1 on granulocytes.[106,107] Thus, this medication influences both the production of inflammatory mediators and the responsiveness of immunocompetent cells to inflammatory stimuli. Given the many immunologic abnormalities described in endometriosis, this medication has some rationale in an attempt to correct immune dysfunction. As it is not an inhibitor of ovulation, pentoxifylline has an advantage over ovulation suppressors when attempting to treat endometriosis-associated infertility: it can be administered throughout the period of attempted conception. Doses have ranged from 400 to 1200 mg daily. The drug is extremely well tolerated, with the major adverse effects being gastric discomfort and dizziness; both are seen in few patients using the recommended dose, and neither has been shown to occur more often in treated patients than placebo controls when giving commercial preparations of the drug.[108]

Of the experimental treatments for endometriosis, only pentoxifylline has been investigated as a treatment for endometriosis-associated infertility. A single placebo-controlled RCT with 60 patients resulted in a 12-month pregnancy rate of 31% with pentoxifylline and 18.5% with placebo, a difference not statistically different but intriguing none the less.[109] Hopefully, additional larger trials will further investigate this approach to help clarify the value of this and similar drugs.

Two other immunomodulators have been used experimentally. In the rat model the administration of intraperitoneal loxoribine, an immunomodulator that enhances cytokine activity, resulted in regression of endometrial explants.[110] Interferon-α_{2b} has been shown to inhibit endometrioma cell growth in culture.[111] No primate studies have been conducted with either drug.

ESTROGEN RECEPTOR β AGONISTS

It is well established that endometriosis is an estrogen-dependent disease. However, recently it was discovered that estrogen has two receptors: ER-α and ER-β.[112] Whereas ER-α has clearly been related to the proliferation of endometrium, the function of ER-β is unclear. This receptor is expressed in a wide variety of tissues, including much of the immune system. However, it is expressed minimally if at all in reproductive tissues. ER-β mRNA has been seen in endometrial stroma, epithelium, and endometrioma,[113,114] but as yet the actual receptor protein has not been found in these tissues. Nevertheless, in animal models, ER-β agonist produces a regression of experimental endometriosis. Several possible mechanisms exist. One explanation could be that ER-β agonists are acting as mouse intraperitoneal immunomodulators, enhancing the immunologic response to the explants. A second possible explanation lies in the recognition of ER-β in endothelial cells of endometrial vasculature (D. Zhao, personal communication); an antiangiogenic effect might also explain the regression of endometrial tissue in the rodent model. Finally, it is still possible that improved assays will uncover the presence of ER-β in endometriosis, with the possibility that the receptor acts intracellularly as an ER-α inhibitor by dimerizing with the ER-α molecules to form a faulty product.[115] These possibilities will all be explored in future studies.

MEDICAL THERAPY IN CONJUNCTION WITH SURGERY

The use of medical therapy for the treatment of endometriosis is not restricted to standalone agents. Frequently, clinicians have used drugs in combination with surgery in an attempt to improve results compared to either modality alone. When this approach is utilized, the medications can be administered either prior to surgery, following surgery, or both. Understanding that surgical technique undoubtedly plays a role in the effectiveness of these approaches, it is still worth examining the available evidence regarding this rather aggressive attempt at treating endometriosis.

PREOPERATIVE MEDICAL THERAPY

The concept behind using medication to treat endometriosis prior to surgical elimination is that the surgery itself may be significantly easier. A possible disadvantage, however, is that medical suppression of the lesion may lead to incomplete surgical removal of the disease owing to lack of recognition. This may ultimately result in a greater risk of recurrence of disease and symptoms.

Only one randomized trial has attempted to examine the value of preoperative medical therapy versus surgery alone.[116] The study was able to demonstrate a significant reduction in the amount of visible disease at the time of laparoscopy, although this would have been expected. No assessment of efficacy in terms of pain relief or fertility enhancement was performed.

A single comparative study has randomized patients treated preoperatively to either GnRH-a or danazol.[117] Again, patients ware analyzed only for the amount of disease seen at laparoscopy (following the medical treatment); no difference was seen between the two groups.

POSTOPERATIVE MEDICAL THERAPY

The use of postoperative medical therapy is grounded in the concept that it is difficult if not impossible to remove all endometriosis at the time of surgery. Thus, surgical treatment should be looked upon as a debulking procedure, and medical therapy would be expected to enhance the improvement resulting from surgery alone. There is also the possibility that the period of medical treatment following surgery will serve to decrease the opportunity for the development of new lesions, resulting in a longer time until recurrence.

Numerous studies have tested these hypotheses. Four trials have compared medical treatment after surgery to surgery alone,[118–121] and another three have compared surgery followed by medical treatment to surgery followed by placebo.[122–124] Taken together, these studies fail to demonstrate any advantage to postoperative medical treatment in terms of pain or disease recurrence.[125] However, lumping all such studies together may be misleading, as they were heterogeneous in terms of length of drug administration. For example, danazol was found not to enhance the results of surgery when administered for only 3 months,[118] but 6 months of postoperative administration reduced pain versus placebo for at least 6 months after discontinuation of the drug.[124] Five studies have compared GnRH-a to either no treatment or placebo; two utilized medication for 3 months and found no effect,[119,123] but studies treating postoperatively for 6 months demonstrated a significant reduction in pain scores and delayed recurrence of pain (Figure 14.6).[120,122] Interestingly, the use of oral contraceptives for 6 months following surgery has been shown to be ineffective in improving upon the results of surgery alone.[121] Finally, a pilot RCT comparing the postoperative use of a levonorgestrel-containing IUD versus surgery alone found that all forms of pelvic pain were significantly reduced postoperatively by the addition of the IUD.[126]

Three trials have compared two different medications used after surgery.[124,127,128] Taken together, these studies suggest no difference in effect between GnRH-a, danazol, and high-dose progestogen.

One RCT has examined the use of a single postoperative medical therapy versus two sequential medical treatments following surgery.

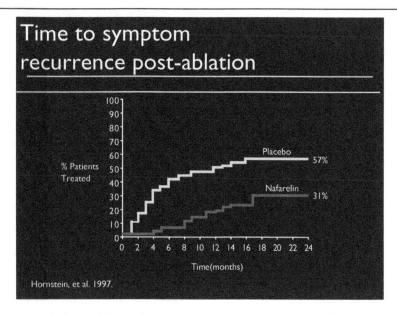

Figure 14.6 Rate of recurrence of pelvic pain following treatment with surgery alone versus surgery followed by GnRH agonist therapy.

Morgante and colleagues compared the use of 6 months of postoperative GnRH agonist therapy to 6 months of GnRH agonist followed by 6 months of danazol, 100 mg/day.[129] Twelve months after surgery (at the conclusion of danazol for one group, and after 6 months of no treatment for the other) there was significantly less pain in those treated with the two sequential medical treatments.

Three studies have investigated the use of postoperative medical therapy for fertility enhancement, utilizing GnRH agonists[121,122] and raloxifene,[130] a selective estrogen receptor modulator. None have demonstrated any enhancement of fertility in women with endometriosis utilizing this approach.

PREOPERATIVE COMPARED TO POSTOPERATIVE MEDICAL THERAPY

Only one study has compared the use of medical therapy preoperatively versus postoperatively. Audebert and colleagues randomized patients to GnRH-a for 6 months either before or after their operation; no differences were seen between groups in terms of either physician or patient perception of pain symptoms.[131]

SHOULD COMBINATION THERAPY BE USED?

Although these studies suggest that some postoperative medical therapies may be of value when used for 6 months or more, a word of caution must be interjected. As is the case with all surgical trials, the degree of surgical skill and the technique used may be critical in determining the results. At least one retrospective trial has indicated that excision of endometriosis results in greater pain relief than ablation of lesions (Winkel C, unpublished data), yet ablation is generally the treatment of choice with these studies. Furthermore, we have no way of ascertaining the degree of surgical skill that was applied in the treatment of these patients. Additional high-quality studies are needed in a variety of settings by a larger number of surgeons to further examine this issue and confirm the above results.

CONCLUSIONS

The use of medical therapy in the treatment of endometriosis has a long history, with a wide variety of medications having been utilized. For decades we had little in the way of scientific information to guide us, but today the proliferation of randomized clinical trials in the literature provides the discerning clinician with excellent clues as to how best to approach the treatment of symptomatic disease. One clear deficiency in the literature, however, is the lack of a direct comparison between medical and surgical therapy in the treatment of endometriosis-associated pain. Although several randomized trials have been attempted, none has ever been completed. Data from placebo and sham controlled studies suggest similar success rates, but these investigations have been carried out in different patient populations under differing conditions. Until an RCT comparing medicine and surgery is carried out, the relative merits of each are purely speculative.

None the less, what is clear from the above is that medical therapy can be of value in the treatment of endometriosis, particularly in regard to pain symptomatology. Furthermore, with a wide variety of investigational medications in the pipeline, it is likely that the role of medication for this disease will expand. As this occurs and our treatment options increase, we are likely to see an era of improved efficacy with fewer side effects for more patients, a situation clearly advantageous to the many women suffering from endometriosis.

REFERENCES

1. Goebel R, Rjosk HK. Laboratory and clinical studies with the new antigonadotropin, danazol. Acta Endocrinol 1977;85(Suppl 212):134 [Abstract].
2. Floyd WS. Danazol: endocrine and endometrial effects. Int J Fertil 1980;25:75–80.
3. Barbieri RL, Canick JA, Makris A et al. Danazol inhibits steroidogenesis. Fertil Steril 1977;28:809–13.
4. McGinley R, Casey JH. Analysis of progesterone in unextracted serum: a method using danazol [17α-pregn-4-en-20-yno(2,3-d)-osoxazol-17-ol] a blocker of steroid binding to proteins. Steroids 1979;33:127–38.
5. Buttram VC Jr, Belue JB, Reiter R. Interim report of a study of danazol for the treatment of endometriosis. Fertil Steril 1982;37:478–83.
6. Alvarado RG, Liu JY, Zwolak RM. Danazol and limb-threatening arterial thrombosis: two case reports. J Vasc Surg 2001;34:1123–6.
7. Vercellini P Tresid L, Panazza S et al. Very low dose danazol for relief of endometriosis-associated pelvic pain: a pilot study. Fertil Steril 1994;62:1136–42.
8. Janicki TI. Treatment of the pelvic pain associated with endometriosis using danazol vaginal suppositories. Two year followup. Fertil Steril 2002;77:S52.
9. Igarashi M, Iizuka M, Abe Y, Ibuki Y. Novel vaginal danazol ring therapy for pelvic endometriosis, in particular deeply infiltrating endometriosis. Hum Reprod 1998;13:1952–6.
10. Bruner KL, Eisenberg E, Gorstein F, Osteen KG. Progesterone and transforming growth factor-beta coordinately regulate suppression of endometrial matrix metalloproteinases in a model of experimental endometriosis. Steroids 1999;64:648–53.
11. Olive DL. Medical treatment: alternatives to danazol. In: Schenken RS, ed. Endometriosis: Contemporary Concepts in Clinical Management. Philadelphia: JB Lippincott, 1989; 189–211.
12. Muneyyirci-Delale O, Karacan M. Effect of norethindrone acetate in the treatment of symptomatic endometriosis. Int J Fertil Womens Med 1999;43:24–7.
13. Fedele L, Bianchi S, Zanconato G, Portuese A, Raffaelli R. Use of a levonorgestrel-releasing intrauterine device in the treatment of rectovaginal endometriosis. Fertil Steril 2001;75:485–8.
14. Lau TM, Affandi B, Rogers PAW. The effects of levonorgestrel implants on vascular endothelial growth factor expression in the endometrium. Mol Hum Reprod 1998;5:57–63.
15. Hamblen EC. Androgen treatment of women. South Med J 1957;50:743.
16. Hirvonen E, Malkonen M, Manninen V. Effects of different progestogens on lipoproteins during postmenopausal replacement therapy. N Engl J Med 1981;304:560.
17. Fahraeus L, Sydsjo A, Wallentin L. Lipoprotein changes during treatment of pelvic endometriosis with medroxyprogesterone acetate. Fertil Steril 1986;45:503.
18. Andrews MC, Andrews WC, Strauss AF. Effects of progestin-induced pseudopregnancy on endometriosis: clinical and microscopic studies. Am J Obstet Gynecol 1959;78:776.
19. Scott RB, Wharton LR Jr. The effect of estrone and progesterone on the growth of experimental endometriosis in rhesus monkeys. Am J Obstet Gynecol 1957;74:852.
20. Noble AD, Letchworth AT. Medical treatment of endometriosis: a comparative trial. Postgrad Med J 1979;55 (Suppl 5):37.
21. Meresman GF, Auge L, Barano RI et al. Oral contraceptive treatment suppresses proliferation and enhances apoptosis of eutopic endometrial tissue from patients with endometriosis. Fertil Steril 2001;76:S47–8.
22. Sharpe-Timms KL, Zimmer RL, Jolliff WJ et al. Gonadotropin-releasing hormone agonist (GnRH-a) therapy alters activity of plasminogen activators, matrix metalloproteinases and their inhibitors in rat models for adhesion formation and endometriosis: potential GnRH-a-regulated mechanisms reducing adhesion formation. Fertil Steril 1998;69:916–23.
23. Dmowski WP. The role of medical management in the treatment of endometriosis. In: Nezhat CR, Berger GS, Nezhat FR, Buttram VC Jr, Nezhat CH, eds. Endometriosis: Advanced Management and Surgical Techniques. New York: Springer-Verlag, 1995; 229–40.
24. Barbieri RL. Endometriosis and the estrogen threshold theory. Relation to surgical and medical treatment. J Reprod Med 1998;43:287–92.

25. Hurst BS, Gardner SC, Tucker KE, Awoniyi CA, Schlaff WD. Delayed oral estradiol combined with leuprolide increases endometriosis-related pain. JSLS 2000;4:97–101.

26. Cornillie FJ, Brosens IA, Vasquez G, Riphogen I. Histologic and ultrastructural changes in human endometriotic implants treated with the antiprogesterone steroid ethylnorgestienone (gestrinone) during 2 months. Int J Gynecol Pathol 1986;5:95.

27. Robyn C, Delogne-Desnoeck J, Bourdoux P, Copinschi G. Endocrine effects of gestrinone. In: Raynaud J-P, Ojasoot, Martini L, eds. Medical Management of Endometriosis. New York: Raven Press, 1984; 207.

28. Olive DL, Pritts EA, Morales AJ. Evidence-based medicine: study design for evaluation and treatment. J Am Assoc Gynecol Laparosc 1998;5:75–82.

29. Hughes EG. Systematic literature review and meta-analysis. Semin Reprod Endocrinol 1996;14:161–9.

30. Cooke ID, Thomas EJ. The medical treatment of mild endometriosis. Acta Obstet Gynecol Scand 1989;150(Suppl):27.

31. D'Hooghe TM, Bambra CS, Isahakia M, Koninckx PR. Evolution of spontaneous endometriosis in the baboon (*Papio anubis, Papio cynocephalus*) over a 12-month period. Fertil Steril 1992;58:409.

32. Jones G, Kennedy S, Barnard A, Wong J, Jenkinson C. Development of an endometriosis quality-of-life instrument: The Endometriosis Health Profile-30. Obstet Gynecol 2001;98:258–64.

33. Kauppila A, Puolakka J, Ylikorkala O. Prostaglandin biosynthesis inhibitors and endometriosis. Prostaglandins 1979;18:655.

34. Dmowski WP, Cohen MR. Treatment of endometriosis with an antigonadotropin, danazol: a laparoscopic and histologic evaluation. Obstet Gynecol 1975;46:147.

35. Barbieri RL, Evans S, Kistner RW. Danazol in the treatment of endometriosis: Analysis of 100 cases with a 4-year follow-up. Fertil Steril 1982;37:737.

36. Doberl A, Jeppsson S, Rannevik G. Effect of danazol on serum concentrations of pituitary gonadotropins in post-menopausal women. Acta Obstet Gynecol Scand 1984;123(Suppl):95.

37. Buttram VC Jr, Reiter RC, Ward S. Treatment of endometriosis with danazol: Report of a six-year prospective study. Fertil Steril 1985;318:485.

38. Henzl MR, Corson SL, Moghissi K et al. Administration of nasal nafarelin as compared with oral danazol for endometriosis. N Engl J Med 1988;318:485.

39. Telimaa S, Puolakka J, Ronnberg L, Kaupilla A. Placebo-controlled comparison of danazol and high-dose medroxyprogesterone acetate in the treatment of endometriosis. Gyecol Endocrinol 1987;1:13.

40. Fedele L, Bianchi S, Viezzoli T, Arcaini L, Cendiani GB. Gestrinone vs. danazol in the treatment of endometriosis. Fertil Steril 1989;51:781.

41. Worthington M, Irvine LM, Crook D et al. A randomized comparative study of the metabolic effects of two regimens of gestrinone in the treatment of endometriosis. Fertil Steril 1993;59:522.

42. Hornstein MD, Gleason RE, Barbieri RL. A randomized double-blind prospective trial of two doses of gestrinone in the treatment of endometriosis. Fertil Steril 1990;53:237.

43. Cedars MI, Lu JK, Meldrum DR, Judd HL. Treatment of endometriosis with a long-acting gonadotropin-releasing hormone agonist plus medroxyprogesterone acetate. Obstet Gynecol 1990;75:641–5.

44. Surrey ES, Gambone JC, Lu JK, Judd HL. Fertil Steril 1990;53:620–6.

45. Henzl MR, Corson SL, Moghissi K et al. Administration of nasal nafarelin as compared with oral danazol for endometriosis. A multicenter double-blind comparative clinical trial. N Eng J Med 1998;318:485–9.

46. Surrey ES, Voigt B, Fournet N, Judd HL. Prolonged gonadotropin-releasing hormone agonist treatment of symptomatic endometriosis: the role of cyclic sodium etidronate and low dose norethindrone 'add-back' therapy. Fertil Steril 1995;63:747–55.

47. Bayer SR, Seibel MM. Medical treatment: Danazol. In: Schenkel RS, ed. Endometriosis: Contemporary Concepts in Clinical Management. Philadelphia: JB Lippincott, 1989; 169–87.

48. Miller JD, Shaw RW, Casper RF et al. Historical prospective cohort study of the recurrence of pain after discontinuation of treatment with danazol or a gonadotropin-releasing hormone agonist. Fertil Steril 1998;70:293–6.

49. Regidor PA, Regidor M, Schmidt M et al. Prospective randomized study comparing the GnRH-agonist leuprorelin acetate and the gestagen lynestrenol in the treatment of severe endometriosis. Gynecol Endocrinol 2001;15:202–9.

50. Vercellini P, Trespidi L, Colombo A et al. A gonadotropin-releasing hormone agonist versus a low-dose oral contraceptive for pelvic pain associated with endometriosis. Fertil Steril 1993;60:75.

51. Frontino G, Vercellini P, De Giorgi O et al. Continuous use of oral contraceptive (OC) for endometriosis-associated recurrent dysmenorrhea not responding to cyclic pill regimen. Fertil Steril 2002;77:S23–4.

52. Dlugi AM, Miller JD, Knittle J. Lupron depot (leuprolide acetate for depot suspension) in the treatment of endometriosis: a randomized, placebo-controlled, double-blind study. Fertil Steril 1990;419–27.

53. Anonymous. Goserelin Depot versus danazol in the treatment of endometriosis. The Australian/New Zealand experience. Aus NZ J Obstet Gynaecol 1996;31:55–60.

54. Chang SP, Ng HT. A randomized comparative study of the effect of leuprorelin acetate depot and danazol in the treatment of endometriosis. Chinese Med J (Taipei) 1996;57:431–7.

55. Cirkel U, Oochs H, Schneider HPG. A randomized, comparative trial of triptorelin depot (D-Trp6-LHRH) and danazol in the treatment of endometriosis. Eur J Obstet Gynecol Reprod Biol 1995;59:61–9.

56. Crosignani PG, Gastaldi A, Lombardi PL et al. Leuprorelin acetate depot versus danazol in the treatment of endometriosis: results of an open multicentre trial. Clin Therapeutics 1992;14(Suppl A):29–36.

57. Dmowski WP, Radwanska E, Binor Z, Tummon I, Pepping P. Ovarian suppression induced with buserelin or danazol in the management of endometriosis: a randomized, comparative study. Fertil Steril 1989;51:395–400.

58. Fraser IS, Shearman RP, Jansen RP, Sutherland PD. A comparative treatment trial of endometriosis using the gonadotropin-releasing hormone agonist, nafarelin, and the synthetic steroid, danazol. Aus NZ J Obstet Gynaecol 1991;158–63.

59. Adamson GD, Kwei L, Edgren RA. Pain of endometriosis: effects of nafarelin and danazol therapy. Int J Fertil Med Stud 1994;39:215–17.

60. Wheeler JM, Knittle JD, Miller JD. Depot leuprolide versus danazol in treatment of women with symptomatic endometriosis. I. Efficacy results. Am J Obstet Gynecol 1992;167:1367–71.

61. Dawood MY, Ramos J, Khan-Dawood FS. Depot leuprolide acetate versus danazol for treatment of pelvic endometriosis: changes in vertebral bone mass and serum estradiol and calcitonin. Fertil Steril 1995;63:1177–83.

62. The Nafarelin European Endometriosis Trial Group (NEET). Nafarelin for endometriosis: a large-scale, danazol-controlled trial of efficacy and safety, with 1-year follow-up. Fertil Steril 1992;57:514–22.

63. Rolland R, van der Heijden PF. Nafarelin versus danazol in the treatment of endometriosis. Am J Obstet Gynecol 1990;162:586–8.

64. Kennedy SH, Williams IA, Brodribb J, Barlow DH, Shaw RW. A comparison of nafarelin acetate and danazol in the treatment of endometriosis. Fertil Steril 1990;53:998–1003.

65. Rock JA. A multicenter comparison of GnRH agonist (Zoladex) and danazol in the treatment of endometriosis. Fertil Steril 1991;56:S49.

66. Shaw RW. An open randomized comparative study of the effect of goserelin depot and danazol in the treatment of endometriosis. Zoladex Endometriosis Study Team. Fertil Steril 1992;58:265–72.

67. Prentice A, Deery A, Goldbeck-Wood S, Farquhar C, Smith S. Gonadotropin-releasing hormone analogues for pain associated with endometriosis (Cochrane Review). In: The Cochrane Library, Issue 3, 1999. Oxford: Update Software.

68. Ling FW. Randomized controlled trial of depot leuprolide in patients with chronic pelvic pain and clinically suspected endometriosis. Obstet Gynecol 1999;93:51–8.

69. Surrey E, Judd H. Reduction of vasomotor symptoms and bone mineral density loss with combined norethindrone and long-acting gonadotropin-releasing hormone agonist therapy of symptomatic endometriosis: a prospective randomized trial. J Clin Endocrinol Metab 1992;75:558–63.

70. Makarainen L, Ronneberg L, Kauppila A. Medroxyprogesterone acetate supplementation diminishes the hypoestrogenic side-effects of gonadotropins-releasing hormone agonists without changing its efficacy in endometriosis. Fertil Steril 1996;65:29–34.

71. Tabkin O, Yakinoghe AH, Kucuk S et al. Effectiveness of tibolone on hypoestrogenic symptoms induced by goserelin treatment in patients with endometriosis. Fertil Steril 1997;67:40–5.

72. Edmonds D, Howell R. Can hormone replacement therapy by used during medical therapy of endometriosis? Br J Obstet Gynaecol 1994;101:24–6.

73. Kiiholma P, Korhonen M, Tuimala R, Korhonen M, Hagman E. Comparison of the gonadotropin-releasing hormone agonist goserelin acetate alone versus goserelin combined with estrogen–progestogens add-back therapy in the treatment of endometriosis. Fertil Steril 1995;64:903–8.

74. Moghissi KS, Schlaff WD, Olive DL, Skinner MA, Yin H. Goserelin acetate (Zoladex) with or without hormone replacement therapy for the treatment of endometriosis. Fertil Steril 1998;69:1056–62.

75. Hornstein MD, Surrey ES, Weisberg GW, Casino LA and the Lupron Add-Back Study Group. Leuprolide acetate depot and hormonal add-back in endometriosis: a 12-month study. Obstet Gynecol 1998;91:16–24.

76. Lee PI, Yoon JB, Joo KY et al. Gonadotrophin releasing hormone agonist (GnRHa)-Zoladex (Goserelin) and hormonal add-back therapy in endometriosis: a 12 month study. Fertil Steril 2002;77:S23.

77. The Gestrinone Italian Study Group. Gestrinone versus a gonadotropin-releasing hormone agonist for the treatment of pelvic pain associated with endometriosis: a multicenter randomised, double-blind study. Fertil Steril 1996;66:911–19.

78. Bayer SR, Seibel MM, Saffan DS, Berger MJ, Taymor ML. Efficacy of danazol treatment for minimal endometriosis in infertile women: a prospective, randomized study. J Reprod Med 1988;33:179–83.

79. Telimaa S. Danazol and medroxyprogesterone acetate inefficacious in the treatment of infertility in endometriosis. Fertil Steril 1988;50:872–5.

80. Harrison RF, Barry-Kinsella C. Efficacy of medroxyprogesterone treatment in infertile women with endometriosis: a prospective, randomized, placebo-controlled study. Fertil Steril 2000;74:24–30.

81. Fedele L, Parazzini F, Radici E et al. Buserelin acetate versus expectant management in the treatment of infertility associated with minimal or mild endometriosis: A randomized clinical trial. Am J Obstet Gynecol 1992;166:1345–50.

82. Thomas E, Cooke I. Successful treatment of asymptomatic endometriosis: Does it benefit infertile women? Br Med J 1987;294:1117–19.

83. Hughes E, Ferorkow D, Collins J, Vandekerckhone P. Ovulation suppression for endometriosis (Cochrane review). In: The Cochrane Library, issue 1, 2000. Oxford: Update Software.

84. Chwalisz K, Brenner RM, Fuhrmann UU et al. Antiproliferative effects of progesterone antagonist and progesterone receptor modulators on the endometrium. Steroids 2000;65: 741–51.

85. Klein-Hitpass L, Cato ACB, Henderson K et al. Two types of antiprogestins identified by their differential action in transcriptionally active extracts from T47D cells. Nucleic Acids Res 1991;19:1227–33.

86. Elger W, Bartley J, Schneider B et al. Endocrine pharmacological characterization of progesterone antagonists and progesterone receptor modulators with respect to PR-agonist and antagonistic activity. Steroids 2000;65: 713–23.

87. Tjaden B, Galetto D, Woodruff JD, Rock JA. Time-related effects of RU486 treatment in experimentally induced endometriosis in the rat. Fertil Steril 1993;59:437.

88. Kettel LM, Murphy AA, Mortola JF et al. Endocrine responses to long-term administration of the antiprogesterone RU486 in patients with pelvic endometriosis. Fertil Steril 1991;56:402.

89. Kettel LM, Murphy AA, Morales AJ et al. Treatment of endometriosis with the antiprogesterone mifepristone (RU486). (Unpublished data).

90. Jones RC. The effect of a luteinizing hormone-releasing hormone antagonist on experimental endometriosis in the rat. Acta Endocrinol 1987;114:379–82.

91. Martha PM, Gray ME, Campion M, Kuca B, Garnick MB. Initial safety profile and hormonal dose response characteristics of the pure GnRH antagonist, Abarelix-depot, in women with endometriosis. (Unpublished data).

92. Woolley JM, De Paoli AM, Gray ME, Martha PM. Reductions in health related quality of life in women with endometriosis. (Abstract) Seventh Biennial World Congress of Endometriosis, London, 14–17 May 2000.

93. Bulin SE. Aromatase in aging women. Semin Reprod Endocrinol 1999;17:349–58.

94. Bulun SE, Zeitoun KM, Takayama K, Sasano H. Molecular basis for treating endometriosis with aromatase inhibitors. Hum Reprod Update 2000;6:413–18.

95. Yano S, Ikegami Y, Nakao K. Studies on the effect of the new non-steroidal aromatase inhibitor fadrozole hydrochloride in an endometriosis model in rats. Arzneimittelforschung 1996;46:192–5.

96. D'Hooghe TM, Cuneo S, Nugent N et al. Recombinant human TNF binding protein-1 (r-hTBP-1) inhibits the development of endometriosis in baboons: a prospective, randomized, placebo and drug controlled study. Fertil Steril 2001;76:S1.

97. Folkman J, Shing Y. Angiogenesis. J Biol Chem 1992;267: 10931–4.

98. Donnez J, Smoes P, Gillerot S, Casanas-Roux F, Nisolle M. Vascular endothelial growth factor (VEGF) in endometriosis. Hum Reprod 1998;13:1686–90.

99. Fasciani A, D'Ambrogio G, Bocci G et al. High concentrations of the vascular endothelial growth factor and interleukin-8 in ovarian endometriomata. Mol Hum Reprod 2000;6:50–4.

100. Mahnke JL, Dawood MY, Huang JC. Vascular endothelial growth factor and interleukin-6 in peritoneal fluid of women with endometriosis. Fertil Steril 2000;73:166–70.

101. Barcz E, Kaminski P, Marianowski L. VEGF concentration in peritoneal fluid in patients with endometriosis. Gynekol Pol 2001;72:442–8.

102. Levine Z, Efstathiou JA, Sampson DA et al. Angiogenesis inhibitors suppress endometriosis in a murine model. J Soc Gynecol Invest 2002;9:264a.

103. Scarpellini F, Sbracia M, Lecchini S, Scarpellini L. Anti-angiogenesis treatment with thalidomide in endometriosis: a pilot study. Fertil Steril 2002;78:S87.

104. Osteen KG, Yeaman GR, Bruner-Tran K. Matrix metalloproteinases and endometriosis. Semin Reprod Med 2003;21: 155–63.

105. Mori T, Yamasaki S, Masui F et al. Suppression of the development of experimentally induced uterine adenomyosis by a novel matrix metalloproteinase inhibitor, ONO-4817, in mice. Exp Biol Med 2001;226:429–33.

106. Steinleitner A, Lambert H, Roy S. Immunomodulation with pentoxifylline abrogates macrophage-mediated infertility in an in vivo model: a paradigm for a novel approach to the treatment of endometriosis-associated subfertility. Fertil Steril 1991;55:26–31.

107. Steinleitner A, Lambert H, Suarez M. Immunomodulation in the treatment of endometriosis-associated subfertility: use of pentoxifylline to reverse the inhibition of fertilization by surgically induced endometriosis in a rodent model. Fertil Steril 1991;56:975–9.

108. Physicians' Desk Reference. Montvale, NJ: Medical Economics Company Inc., 2002; 784.

109. Balasch J, Creus M, Fabregues F et al. Pentoxifylline versus placebo in the treatment of infertility associated with minimal or mild endometriosis: a pilot randomized clinical trial. Hum Reprod 1997;12: 2046–50.

110. Keenan J, Williams-Boyle P, Massey P et al. Regression of endometrial explants in a rat model of endometriosis treated with the immune modulators loxoribine and levamisole. Fertil Steril 1999;721:135–41.

111. Badawy S, Etman A, Cuenca V, Montante A, Kaufman L. Effect of interferon alpha 2b on endometrioma cells in vitro. Obstet Gynecol 2001;98: 417–20.

112. Kuiper GGJM, Enmark E, Pelto Huikko M, Nilsson S, Gustafsson JA. Cloning of a novel estrogen receptor expressed in rat prostate and ovary. Proc Natl Acad Sci USA 1996;93: 5925–30.

113. Lecce G, Meduri G, Ancelin M, Berferon C, Perrot-Applanat M. Presence of estrogen receptor beta in the human endometrium throughout the cycle: expression in glandular, stromal, and vascular cells. J Clin Endocrinol Metab 2001;86: 1379–86.

114. Fujimoto J, Hirose R, Sakaguchi H, Tamaya T. Expression of estrogen receptor alpha and beta in ovarian endometriomata. Mol Hum Reprod 1999;5:742–7.

115. Pavao M, Traish AM. Estrogen receptor antibodies: specificity and utility in detection, localization and analyses of estrogen receptor alpha and beta. Steroids 2001;66: 1–16.

116. Donnez J, Anaf V, Nisolle M et al. Ovarian endometrial cysts: the role of gonadotropin-releasing hormone agonist and/or drainage. Fertil Steril 1994;62:63–6.

117. Wright S, Valdes CT, Dunn RC, Franklin RR. Short-term Lupron or danazol therapy for pelvic endometriosis. Fertil Steril 1995;63:504–7.

118. Bianchi S, Busacca M, Agnoli B. Effects of three month therapy with Danazol after laparoscopic surgery for stage III–IV endometriosis: a randomized study. Hum Reprod 1999;14:1335–7.

119. Busacca M, Somigliana E, Bianchi S et al. Post-operative GnRH analogue treatment after conservative surgery for symptomatic endometriosis stage III–IV: a randomized controlled trial. Hum Reprod 2001;16:2399–402.

120. Vercellini P, Crosignani PG, Fedini R. A gonadotropin-releasing hormone agonist compared with expectant management after conservative surgery for symptomatic endometriosis. Br J Obstet Gynaecol 1999;106:672–7.

121. Muzii L, Marana R, Caruana P et al. Postoperative administration of monophasic combined oral contraceptives after laparoscopic treatment of ovarian endometriomas: a prospective, randomized trial. Am J Obstet Gynecol 2000;183:588–92.

122. Hornstein MD, Hemmings R, Yuzpe AA, Heinrichs WL. Use of nafarelin versus placebo after reductive laparoscopic surgery for endometriosis. Fertil Steril 1997;68:860–4.

123. Parazzini F, Fedele L, Busacca M et al. Postsurgical medical treatment of advanced endometriosis: results of a randomized clinical trial. Am J Obstet Gynecol 1994;171:1205–7.

124. Telimaa S, Ronnberg L, Kauppila A. Placebo-controlled comparison of danazol and high dose medroxyprogesterone acetate in the treatment of endometriosis after conservative surgery. Gynecol Endocrinol 1987;1:363–71.

125. Yap C, Furness S, Farquhar C. Pre and post operative medical therapy for endometriosis surgery. Cochrane Library, Update Software (in press).

126. Frontino G, Vercellini P, De Giorgi O et al. Levonorgestrel-releasing intrauterine device (Lng-IUD) versus expectant management after conservative surgery for symptomatic endometriosis. A pilot study. Fertil Steril 2002;77:S25–6.

127. Chang SP, Ng HT. A randomized comparative study of the effect of leuprorelin acetate depot and danazol in the treatment of endometriosis. Chin Med J 1996;57:431–7.

128. Regidor PA, Regidor M, Schmidt M et al. Prospective randomized study comparing the GnRH-agonist leuprorelin acetate and the gestagen lynestrenol in the treatment of severe endometriosis. Gynecol Endocrinol 2001;15:202–9.

129. Morgante G, Ditto A, La Marca A, De Leo V. Low dose Danazol after combined surgical and medical therapy reduces the incidence of pelvic pain in women with moderate and severe endometriosis. Hum Reprod 1999;14:2371–4.

130. Alvarez-Gil L, Fuentes V. Raloxifene and endometriosis. Fertil Steril 2002;77:S37.

131. Audebert A, Descampes P, Marret H. Pre or postoperative medical treatment with Nafarelin in stage III–IV endometriosis: a French multicentered study. Eur J Obstet Gynecol Reprod Biol 1998;79:145–8.

15. Surgical Treatment of Women with Endometriosis

John D. Buek and Craig A. Winkel

INTRODUCTION

The most appropriate method for the management of women with endometriosis remains a subject of considerable debate and one that is unlikely to be resolved scientifically in the near future. To a great extent, this debate continues because of lack of well designed, randomized controlled trials to assess comparative treatment paradigms based on outcomes that can be measured objectively. Thus, the proponents of surgical treatment and the proponents of medical therapy commonly argue their separate cases on the basis more of personal passion rather than of objective, scientific data.

A significant difficulty in the clinical management of women with endometriosis-related complaints or symptoms remains our lack of understanding of the pathophysiology of the disease. Described pathologically as the finding of tissue with histological characteristics consistent with endometrial glands and stroma in sites outside the uterus, endometriosis may or may not be associated with symptoms or complaints. Largely found in the dependent portions of the abdominopelvic cavity, endometriosis lesions may also be identified in unusual sites such as the urinary and alimentary tracts, the pleural cavity and the pulmonary system, the diaphragm, and even in the skin and lymphatic system. Despite growing recognition of the significance of endometriosis as a medical problem that affects large numbers of women, it is still not possible to state with certainty why women develop this disease. Whether is develops through coelomic metaplasia, hematologic or lymphatic spread from the endometrial cavity, or simplify via the dissemination of retrograde menstrual fluid cannot be identified at present. The problem is further obfuscated by the fact that a considerable number of women with endometriosis are completely asymptomatic and suffer no apparent consequence of the disease.[1]

As already mentioned, decisions regarding the best approach to the clinical management of women with endometriosis are often made on the basis of the clinician's level of comfort with surgical versus medical treatment options, past experiences, and perhaps scientifically unsound comparisons of the reported outcomes for various therapeutic approaches. Given the paucity of comparative randomized controlled trials, it is reasonable to conclude that the most effective basis upon which to make therapeutic decisions might be the wishes of the patient in the context of her current situation while considering the nature of the complaints believed to be associated with the endometriosis. Thus, appropriate treatment options should vary significantly given the woman's age, immediate versus future desire for pregnancy, and the nature of the complaints or symptoms. The decision whether to pursue surgical or medical treatments or a combination of both should rest on the patient's current and future situation, rather than the personal biases of the clinician. As an example, it would be difficult to conclude that the best treatment for an asymptomatic woman of reproductive age who is desirous of immediate pregnancy is medical, as there is little evidence in the literature supportive of a positive effect of medical therapy on fertility.

Given the belief that decisions regarding therapeutic options for the treatment of women with endometriosis should be based primarily on the context in which the woman finds herself at the time that therapy is believed indicated, this chapter is organized on the basis of the varied situations in which surgical treatment is considered appropriate. Every effort has been made to base recommendations on the highest quality of medical evidence available, and to make the reader aware of the quality of that evidence.

SURGERY FOR DIAGNOSIS

A discussion of surgical therapy for the management of women with endometriosis would not be complete without some discussion of the role of diagnostic laparoscopy as a surgical procedure. Our purpose in raising this topic lies not in a desire to provide a thorough and complete review of the means for making a diagnosis of endometriosis, but in the recognition that one of the significant problems with surgical therapy as an approach to such patients lies in the accuracy with which the disease can be identified. Inherent in the surgical approach is the assumption that the disease process or anatomical abnormality can be identified effectively at the time of the surgical procedure. It would be difficult to imagine that surgical management of colonic polyps, for example, could be effective if the surgeon were limited in ability to visualize the presence and the extent of the individual polyps.

Von Rokitansky, in 1860, first noted lesions in the pelvic cavity that he called 'adenomyoma', but it was Sampson, reporting in 1920, who provided the classic description of endometriosis as we know it today.[2] Whereas Sampson originally alluded to the varied appearances of endometriosis lesions, modern laparoscopists have defined the protean appearances of endometriosis as visualized through the laparoscope.[3] The difficulty that has recently become apparent, however, is the relatively low positive predictive value (PPV) of visualization as a means of identifying individual lesions. In two separate studies the authors found that the PPV of visualization of lesions for histologic confirmation of endometriosis was 43–45%.[4,5] Given the significant possibility that lesions are not accurately identifiable in significant number of women, the effectiveness of laparoscopic evaluation as a diagnostic tool must be called into question.

To further compound the problem, it must be recalled that endometriosis may be identified in women who have no related symptoms or complaints.[1,6] Endometriosis can also be identified microscopically when no lesions are identifiable visually.[7–10] Thus, the findings at laparoscopy do not correlate with clinical symptoms and may be associated with a significant incidence of false positive and false negative conclusions. On the basis of this information, it is reasonable to conclude that the value of laparoscopy as a means of diagnosing endometriosis is questionable.

OVERVIEW OF SURGICAL TREATMENTS

The surgical treatments for women with endometriosis may be classified generally as either conservative or radical. Conservative surgical procedures are most often accomplished today via a laparoscopic approach that aims to conserve the functional capacity of uterus, fallopian tubes, and ovaries. The radical approach is taken to mean total hysterectomy and bilateral salpingo-oophorectomy. The latter is often labeled 'definitive' surgery in spite of the fact that women who have undergone this type of procedure frequently experience recurrence of endometriosis and of symptoms.[11–15] In addition to recurrence of disease following radical surgical treatment, there is also a significant incidence of endometriosis-related complications following hysterectomy.[16,17] Finally, women have even reported continued vaginal bleeding following 'definitive' surgery for endometriosis.[18] Thus, it is probably unwise to continue to label hysterectomy and bilateral salpingo-oophorectomy as 'definitive' surgery, as to do so may lead to unreasonable expectations on the part of the patient.

LAPAROTOMY VERSUS LAPAROSCOPY

To address the issue of laparotomy versus laparoscopy as the better approach to the surgical management of endometriosis requires outcome data that currently do not exist. There are a few reports comparing the effectiveness of one approach to the other and no randomized, prospective controlled trials. In spite of this, many proponents of the laparoscopic approach are quite vocal in their claim that the laparotomy approach is no longer appropriate.[19]

In a retrospective, comparative study, Bateman et al compared outcomes of laparoscopy to results obtained by chart review in a similar number of women who had previously undergone laparotomy for surgical treatment of endometriosis.[20] During a 1-year follow-up period they found that 19% of women operated on via laparotomy experienced recurrence of an ovarian endometrioma, compared to 13.4% of women who had undergone laparoscopy. Women who underwent laparoscopy had shorter hospital stays and shorter recovery times, but the two groups were comparable in operating room times and blood loss.

In another study, the investigators compared the two surgical approaches employing a parallel, retrospective cohort design study. Crosignani et al operated on 155 women with moderate to severe pelvic pain who had AFS (American Fertility Society) Stage IV disease.[21] Laparoscopy was performed in 47 women and laparotomy in 108. A potential bias in this study was the fact that the choice of approach was determined by the surgeon. Patients completed pain surveys using a three-point scale before and after surgery. Both surgical approaches were found to be about equally effective during the 24-month follow-up period. Pain recurrence rates were statistically similar.

In addition, there are reports from two other parallel retrospective cohort studies concerning the issue of surgical approach. In one, the investigators compared laparoscopy to laparotomy in 81 women with all stages of endometriosis who required repeat surgery for endometriosis-related pain symptoms.[22] Similar rates of recurrence of acyclic pelvic pain (23% versus 34%), dyspareunia (25% versus 30%), and dysmenorrhea (23% versus 34%) were reported, respectively, for laparoscopy versus laparotomy.

The other study involved surgery by one surgeon in 132 women with ovarian endometriomas.[23] The surgery was accomplished either laparoscopically or via laparotomy using a microsurgical dissection technique. The investigators found similar results with the two surgical approaches, although length of stay and febrile morbidity were significantly lower for those women undergoing laparoscopy.

Based on these recent reports, it seems reasonable to conclude that both the laparoscopic approach and laparotomy are likely to yield similar results. For obvious reasons, laparoscopy might be favored because of the reduced hospitalization and shorter recovery time following surgery. At the same time, the experience of the surgeon is a critical issue, as not all surgeons are equally comfortable with laparoscopic operative techniques.

LAPAROSCOPIC SURGICAL TREATMENT

One of the difficulties in discussing the surgical treatment of endometriosis is the almost complete lack of prospective, randomized controlled trials (RCT). The studies reported in the literature, upon which it is possible to base this discussion, are commonly the observations of a surgeon who has performed the technical procedure that he or she believes most likely to address the clinical problem appropriately. Surgical skill and expertise vary between authors. Thus, it remains difficult to determine the extent to which skill of the surgeon affects the outcome, rather than surgical procedure itself. Finally, the literature on this topic is replete with variations in the outcomes measured, the length of follow-up before assessing outcome, and the applicability of the report to the general practice of gynecologic surgery. Moreover, assessment of the outcomes may be obfuscated by the combination of procedures employed, for example lesion ablation plus LUNA (laser uterosacral nerve ablation).

Having accepted the premise that the laparoscopic approach is associated with outcomes no different from those expected with laparotomy, it is important to recognize some difficulties inherent in attempting to determine the most effective technique for destruction or removal of endometriosis lesions. First, as has already been mentioned, the accuracy of visualization is less than perfect, but the technique can only be effective if lesions are identified before the technique is applied. Second, differences in surgical techniques have not been compared effectively in any well designed RCT. Thus, we are left to glean insights from non-comparative studies to determine the best surgical technique.

SURGICAL EXCISION

Koninckx et al reported that deeply infiltrating endometriosis lesions (labeled type III lesions) were associated most commonly with pain, whereas superficial lesions were commonly associated with no symptoms and were often found incidentally.[24] As a consequence, many experts argue that the most effective approach must be radical dissection and excision of the entire lesion. On the other hand, there are numerous experts who contend that destructive techniques involving fulguration, vaporization, or ablation are similarly effective.[25-29]

The techniques of surgical excision of endometriosis are varied, and most surgeons have their own particular instruments and energy sources to which they adhere. In general, the technique is based on a thorough knowledge of pelvic anatomy, patience, and attention to detail. The lesion to be removed is first visualized and examined. A significant issue when this is accomplished laparoscopically is to assess the lesions visually as well as through palpation, in an attempt to discern the actual size of the lesion, its depth of penetration, and its relationship to adjacent vital structures.

Once the lesion has been identified, initial dissection is aimed at delineating the adjacent structures. Thus, if the lesion involves the pelvic side wall, the ureter and the large vessels need to be identified and isolated from the lesion. This can often be accomplished by incising the peritoneum at a site away from the visible portion of the lesion. Once the peritoneum has been incised, the ureter, bowel, or vessels can be dissected. Care must be given to the areas in which the lesion may encroach upon these structures. At times, the lesion may actually penetrate structures such as bowel, bladder, or ureter. If such penetration is to sufficient depth, cyclic hematachezia or hematuria is common. Patients should be questioned

prior to surgery for these signs that might alter the evaluation and treatment approach.

Once the vital structures are isolated and good hemostasis achieved, the lesion itself can be resected. Because there is generally a fair amount of fibrosis surrounding endometriotic lesions, the surgeon should attempt to remove all associated fibrosis during the procedure. A hallmark of successful surgery is maintenance of excellent hemostasis. This will allow the surgeon to best visualize the endometriosis and afford the greatest opportunity to recognize encroachment on vital structures before they are injured.

Most of the data concerning the excision of endometriosis as a treatment approach have arisen from studies that focused primarily on the treatment of women with endometriosis-related pelvic pain. In one study, women were followed for up to 10 years after laparoscopic excision of endometriosis.[30] In this longitudinal, uncontrolled study the author reported the efficacy of surgical excision by determining the rate of recurrence of endometriosis at the time of reoperation. Unfortunately, the author did not evaluate the patients for recurrence of symptoms. Although the number of patients (359) was large, the total number of patient-years' follow-up over the 10-year study was only 67. In reality, the average length of follow-up was approximately 2 years. The cumulative rate of recurrence or persistence of disease was 19% at the fifth year, determined on the basis of finding lesions at the time of reoperation. Although it may be presumed that women who were subjected to repeat surgery were those who had experienced recurrence of pain symptoms, it is also likely that a large number of women who failed in follow-up also had recurrent symptoms but had simply chosen to go elsewhere for care. As there is no apparent correlation between extent of disease and the severity of pain,[31] or between clinical symptoms and clinical findings at the time of surgery,[32] it is difficult to interpret the meaning of these results. It is not possible to state whether excision may be better than ablative techniques. Likewise, it is not possible to define the situation(s) in which excision may be the better approach.

The effectiveness of excision compared to vaporization of endometriosis for the relief of pain has been reported based on a retrospective, longitudinal, uncontrolled trial of 240 women.[33] A significant difference was found in rates of recurrence of pelvic pain in women who had undergone excision compared to those who had undergone laser ablation (69% versus 23% at 24 months' follow-up, respectively). However, there are several problems with this study. First, the lack of randomization allows for potential bias in the selection of women with different stages of endometriosis in the treatment groups. Second, all women treated by ablation were treated during the first part of the study period, whereas all those treated by excision were treated in the latter portion of the study period. Interestingly, the recurrence of pain was similar among women treated by excision compared to those treated by ablation if postoperative therapy with a gonadotropin-releasing hormone agonist (GnRHa) was included as part of the treatment paradigm.

Given the general paucity of comparative trials, it remains difficult to recommend excision over ablative techniques on the basis of improved outcomes. On the other hand, there is information suggestive that excision may be associated with significantly increased risks of surgical complications. Implicit with the techniques for excision is the requirement for often difficult dissection in the pelvis in close approximation to vital structures such as the bowel, great vessels, and ureters. The true incidence of complications associated with excisional techniques is unknown. More likely than not, this is because most reports are submitted by truly expert surgeons. The average or inexperienced surgeon is unlikely to report small series, especially if they enumerate frequent complications.

Koninckx et al have reported complications associated with attempts to excise endometriotic lesions in their entirety.[34] In this series of women with pelvic pain and endometriosis, the authors found that in spite of an aggressive surgical approach, they could not remove the lesions in toto more than about 90% of the time. Perhaps this was because they found the lesions to be up to 20 mm deep. Importantly, in their attempt to remove lesions completely, they realized a high incidence (close to 25%) of serious complications. For example, enterotomy, at times requiring bowel resection, occurred in 13.6% of cases. Bowel injury recognized postoperatively with the onset of peritonitis occurred in 6%, and ureteral injury occurred in 3% of women in this study. Because of this experience, reported by a recognizably experienced surgeon, it would be difficult to recommend excision as the best approach to surgical treatment of women with endometriosis.

SURGICAL ABLATION

Surgical techniques that are not aimed at excision of lesions may be labeled by a variety of names, depending on the means by which the procedure is performed. The use of electrocautery involves dessication or fulguration of the lesion. The use of laser energy is often called vaporization. Distinctions between the different terminologies are germane to the physics involved, but there is little information to demonstrate that such distinctions are particularly relevant to the ultimate intent, that is, destruction of the lesion. For the purpose of this discussion we have chosen to use the term 'ablation'. The reader should not take this to imply an attempt to delineate the specific physics involved.

The actual procedure to be followed for destruction of endometriosis lesions varies somewhat depending on the energy source employed. The surgeon needs to be familiar with the instrumentation that is used, as the characteristics of the energy source determine parameters of use and safety issues. For example, bipolar cautery instruments typically apply current between the two poles of the grasping instrument. The surgeon needs to be aware that heat is created, and that closely adjacent tissues and structures may be injured.

Given the specifics of the instruments employed, the techniques for destruction involve visual identification of the lesion which, once identified, should be palpated with a probe to assess depth of penetration as well as actual volume of disease. Adjacent vital structures must be identified and their proximity to the lesion and intended area of destruction clearly identified, to avoid damage during the application of the destructive energy. Surgeons who favor CO_2 laser ablation frequently outline an area incorporating the lesion prior to applying laser energy to the entire area outlined. The depth of destruction is based upon visualization and the surgeon's impression of the depth of the lesion.

There is a large body of data regarding various investigators' results with a variety of techniques aimed at destruction of endometriotic lesions as opposed to excision. The studies are largely retrospective in nature and most are not comparative. In addition, they represent reports that involve a great number of different instruments and energy sources.

In 1990, Sutton and Hill[35] reported their results during a 5-year follow-up period of surgical treatment of women with endometriosis who suffered pelvic pain and/or infertility. All women underwent CO_2 laser vaporization of lesions. As no biopsies were taken, it is not possible to state that all women actually had endometriosis. Of the original 228 women, 216 were followed for intervals that ranged between 1 and 6 years. Seventy percent of the women who suffered pain were pain free or improved at the end of the first year of follow-up. The other 30% either experienced no pain relief or pain relief of less than 6 months' duration. No information was provided regarding techniques for pain assessment.

As mentioned, there are a number of reports of retrospective studies of surgical ablation for the management of pelvic pain believed related to endometriosis.[26,35,36] Based on these studies, it is possible to conclude that the failure rate (defined as recurrence of pain symptoms) appears to be about 40% within 2 years following ablative therapy. Because the means of assessing recurrent pain is not uniform among the studies, it is difficult to state how confident we are in the veracity of this statistic.

The highest quality of medical evidence is that derived from the results of a randomized, prospective placebo-controlled trial. There is only one such study of the effectiveness of surgical treatment for the management of pain-related symptoms reported in the literature. In 1994, Sutton et al reported the results of their evaluation, surgical treatment, and follow-up of 74 women identified clinically to have endometriosis.[37] The patients were asked to rate the severity of their pain prior to surgical intervention using a visual analog scale. Seventy-four women found to have AFS Stage I, II, or III endometriosis were assigned randomly to one of two treatment groups: one group underwent laser ablation of lesions and uterosacral nerve ablation. The other group underwent diagnostic laparoscopy only, with no further surgical procedure (sham surgery). Neither the patients nor the follow-up investigators were aware of which treatment had been performed. Follow-up was accomplished 3 and 6 months postoperatively.

Sixty-three of the original 74 women completed 6 months of follow-up. There was no significant difference in pain relief between the two groups at the time of the 3-month check. At the 6-months check 62.5% of the treated group had experienced an improvement in pain symptoms, whereas 22% of the sham treated group noted symptom improvement. This difference was statistically significant.

Although this study is the only one of its kind in the current medical literature, one must still be careful in drawing conclusions based on the results. First, the authors found that the best outcomes were noted in women with Stage III disease, whereas the worst outcomes were noted in those women with Stage I disease. This is interesting, as usually more women with Stage I disease have pain. This fact also implies that perhaps not all lesions were identified accurately in women with Stage I disease, and perhaps that is why the outcome was less improvement in this group. Finally, a very important fact is identified and proved by this study. That is, there is clearly a placebo effect of laparoscopic surgery. Nearly 50% of sham operated women noted improvement at 3 months following surgery. Moreover, at 6 months' follow-up nearly a quarter (22%) still had persistent placebo-related improvement.

Interpretation of these results is also confounded by the fact that the authors chose to treat women with endometriosis and pelvic pain not just by laser ablation of lesions, but also performed uterosacral nerve ablation on all women in whom lesions were ablated. Thus, it remains impossible to determine whether the outcome measured in pain relief was the result of lesion destruction, nerve destruction, or a combination of both.

This same group of women were studied for an additional 6 months in a follow-up study.[38] The 20 patients who had experienced pain improvement at 6 months in the original study were followed for an additional 6 months. Two developed recurrent pain symptoms and underwent further surgery. Of the 12 women in the surgical treatment group who had not reported pain improvement at 6 months, two reported an absence of symptoms at 1 year. The authors subjected the 24 women in the original sham treated group who had pain at 6 months to repeat laparoscopy. Laser ablation was performed in 23 of these women in whom endometriosis lesions were identified. These women were followed for an additional 6 months. Thirty-one percent reported no improvement at the end of the study period. Curiously, during the second laparoscopy procedure the authors apparently chose not to perform laser sacral nerve ablation. Thus, no additional information is elucidated regarding the impact of uterosacral nerve ablation.

An additional prospective, randomized trial designed to assess the efficacy of postoperative treatment with a GnRH agonist to prolong pain-free interval provides supporting data regarding the effectiveness of laparoscopic destruction of endometriotic lesions.[39] The study, conducted at several centers, involved 109 women who underwent laparoscopic ablation of endometriosis lesions followed by treatment with either a placebo or a GnRH agonist. The outcome measured was the length of time after surgery before medication for recurrent pain was required. Median time to the initiation of additional pain therapy for the placebo-treated women was 11.7 months, and 57% of this group required additional pain

therapy at the end of the 2-year follow-up period. Thus, at the end of a 24-month follow-up, about 60% of women experienced pain relief. This is a result very similar to that reported by Sutton.[37]

Based on published data, it appears that laparoscopic treatment of endometriosis for relief of pain symptoms can be expected to provide 2 years of pain relief for about 60% of women if ablative or excisional techniques are employed. Proponents of the latter continue to argue that the outcomes are better based on what is believed to be true regarding endometriosis lesions. That is, that deep lesions, assumed to be associated with pain, are better destroyed in their entirety if the surgeon makes a conscious effort to excise them, recognizing that ablative techniques often will fail to destroy the entire lesion. At the same time, excision requires additional skills and experience and is likely to be associated with surgical complications compared to ablative techniques.

ANCILLARY SURGICAL PROCEDURES

Many experienced surgeons perform either a presacral neurectomy or uterosacral nerve destruction in conjunction with the destruction or excision of endometriosis lesions. It seems logical to conclude that an impetus for the addition of one of these ancillary procedures rests on the basis of less than satisfactory results with the destruction or ablative procedure per se. The question that must be answered is whether these ancillary procedures actually contribute to the success of the procedure.

Presacral neurectomy was first described in 1899 by two separate authors, Jaboulay[40] and Ruggi,[41] and then reported in the United States in 1937.[42] The concept behind presacral neurectomy is the fact that the superior hypogastric plexus is the primary pathway for nociceptive (painful) stimuli that originate in the uterus and adjacent structures. Theoretically, destruction of the plexus would be expected to interrupt the nociceptive pathway and eliminate or ameliorate pain sensations.

The concept behind uterosacral nerve ablation is similar to that for presacral neurectomy. The sensory parasympathetic nerve fiber to the cervix and the sensory sympathetic fibers to the corpus of the uterus traverse the cervical division of the Lee–Frankenhauser plexus that lies in, under, and around the uterosacral ligaments. Transection of these fibers was proposed by Doyle to eradicate the transmission of pain sensation.

Although a number of reports have been published regarding the effectiveness of presacral neurectomy,[43–48] most are difficult to interpret because of inherent biases, flaws, and inconsistencies. Nezhat and Nezhat[49] reported that 49 of 52 women reported relief from dysmenorrhea up to 1 year following laparoscopic presacral neurectomy. In a longitudinal follow-up study of 25 women who underwent laparoscopic presacral neurectomy, Perez[50] reported that all women experienced a decrease in pain during the 12-month follow-up. In a study of 27 women at a community hospital, 22 experienced complete relief of midline pain but little or no effect on lateral pain.[51] A large longitudinal study followed women for up to 72 months using a structured pain questionnaire.[52] Although only two-thirds of the women returned the initial questionnaire, 74% experienced pain relief. No statistical analysis was undertaken.

A number of reports have been published regarding the effectiveness of uterosacral nerve ablation or transection via a laparoscopic approach. Similar to the difficulty encountered in interpreting the literature regarding presacral neurectomy, most of the reports regarding uterosacral nerve ablation involve longitudinal, uncontrolled series of patients. Daniell[53] reported that 72% of women with either endometriosis or dysmenorrhea experienced pain relief following uterosacral nerve ablation. Chaperon and Dubuisson[54] found that 84% of patients with dysmenorrhea experienced symptom relief for at least 1 year following surgery. Deep dyspareunia was relieved in 94% and chronic pelvic pain was relieved in 77%. No control group was studied. Symptom relief was assessed on history and direct questioning alone. A more extensive study was reported by the same authors in 1999.[55] One hundred and ten consecutive women were studied retrospectively as part of the Canadian Endometriosis Task Force. Improvement was reported in 82% of women with dysmenorrhea. Again, this was not a controlled study and the authors provided no information on length of follow-up.

There is one report of a comparative trial involving presacral neurectomy versus uterosacral nerve ablation,[56] in which the authors randomly assigned 33 women to presacral neurectomy and 35 to uterosacral nerve ablation, both via a laparoscopic approach. The women were followed at 3 months and 12 months after the surgical procedures. Pain was assessed at each time by employing a five-point linear scale. These women were found to have no pelvic pathology at the time of laparoscopy. At 3 months, 87.9% of the women who underwent presacral neurectomy and 82.9% of those who underwent uterosacral nerve ablation were improved. At 12 months, 81.8% of the women treated by presacral neurectomy were improved, compared to only 51.4% of those treated by uterosacral nerve ablation. This latter difference was statistically significant.

Based on the body of literature currently available, a number of conclusions can be drawn regarding the role of ancillary surgical procedures for the management of endometriosis-related pelvic pain. First, it is unclear whether either procedure contributes in any significant way to the relief of pain associated with the destruction or excision of endometriosis. Second, both presacral neurectomy and uterosacral nerve ablation are somewhat effective for the relief of midline pain, and perhaps dyspareunia. Finally, for the relief of midline pain it appears that presacral neurectomy may be the better procedure. There are no studies that provide reliable information regarding the length of time the effects of either procedure may last.

SURGICAL MANAGEMENT OF OVARIAN ENDOMETRIOMAS

The primary goal of preoperative evaluation of ovarian masses is to rule out malignancy. A variety of imaging techniques are useful for this purpose, but none is 100% accurate. Although ultrasound findings of homogeneous internal echoes, consistent with old blood, may be helpful in differentiating endometriomas from other ovarian neoplasms, the gold standard is histological evaluation. The goals of surgical therapy for the management of endometriomas include relief of associated symptoms, the prevention of recurrence, and preservation of fertility potential.

The formation of endometriomas is hypothesized to commence with the formation of endometrial implants on the surface of the cortex of the ovary. Endometriotic tissue leads to the formation of small cysts that repeatedly perforate and reseal. Each time this occurs blood accumulates anew within the cyst cavity until perforation again takes place.[57] Over time this results in the formation of adhesions around the ovary, with adherence to parietal peritoneum in the dependent portions of the pelvis, such as the cul de sac. The breakdown of the blood within the cyst cavity over time results in the formation of a structure commonly labeled a chocolate cyst. Other hemorrhagic cysts may fill with similar chocolate-colored material, but because such cysts are intrinsic to the ovary they do not usually become adherent to the parietal peritoneum as do endometriomas.

A variety of techniques have been suggested by which to manage ovarian endometriomas. Nisolle-Pochet et al[58] studied the effect of hormonal therapy on ovarian endometriomas and demonstrated that such therapies are associated with incomplete suppression. Thus, surgical options, including oophorectomy, excisional biopsy, removal of the cyst wall, drainage, and vaporization or fulguration are advocated by most experts for the management of these ovarian conditions.

The choice of surgical approach by laparotomy or by laparoscopy is probably less important than precise technique and adherence to good microsurgical principles. In one of the first such studies, Fayez et al compared different laparoscopic techniques for the treatment of endometriomas.[59] The women included in this study were patients with pain dysmenorrhea or dyspareunia for 1 year and an endometrioma 5 cm or larger. The women were randomly assigned to one of four treatment groups, which were similar in age and parity: 26 underwent excisional biopsy with removal of the overlying ovarian cortex; 24 had the cyst opened and lining removed; 30 had the cyst opened and the wall vaporized with a CO_2 laser; and 44 had the endometrioma opened and drained only. All patients received postoperative medical treatment with danazol and then underwent a second-look laparoscopy 8 weeks later. The authors reported no difference among groups in recurrence of the endometriomas or the associated pain. At second-look laparoscopy all of the women in the excision group, 37% in the group in whom the cyst wall was removed, 30% in the laser-treated group, and 27% in the drainage-only group had periadnexal adhesions. Only the excision group was statistically significantly different from the other three. Because of this report, most experts today do not recommend excisional biopsy as a treatment for endometriomas. Although this study was well designed, the patients were followed for only a short time postoperatively. Moreover, the addition of postoperative medical therapy also confounds the results and makes them difficult to interpret regarding the outcomes attributable to surgical therapy.

Vercellini et al compared coagulation or laser vaporization of the endometrioma cyst wall to excision of the pseudocapsule in an attempt to define the optimal surgical approach.[60] These authors reviewed four studies that compared surgical treatments for endometriomas,[59,61–63] only one of which was a prospective RCT,[62] one was a partially randomized trial,[59] and the other two were retrospective comparisons. The period of follow-up ranged from 1 to 3 years in the different studies. The data reported from the RCT indicated a mean follow-up of 24 months. Recurrence of an ovarian endometrioma, as determined by sonographic evaluation, was statistically different between the two treatment groups: 6/32 women who had vaporization, but only 2/32 who had excision. Recurrence of dysmenorrhea, deep dyspareunia, and non-menstrual pain after

24 months of follow-up were 53%, 75%, and 53%, respectively, for the women treated by ablation. For those treated by excision, the authors reported a much lower incidence of these three symptoms (16%, 20%, and 10%, respectively). When the data from all four studies were pooled, the authors calculated an odds ratio of recurrence of 3.09 (95% CI 1.78–5.36) that appears to favor excision of endometriomas over ablative procedures.

In the same review, however, there were conflicting data on postoperative fertility rates. Two of the studies addressed fertility directly.[61,62] Beretta et al reported pregnancy rates at 24 months of 24% in the 17 women in whom the endometrioma was coagulated, and of 67% in the nine women treated by excision.[62] In the other study, Hemming et al reported cumulative pregnancy rates at 36 months of 60% in 67 patients who had ablative treatment and 47% in 65 patients who had excision.[61] These differences are consistent with the previous suggestion that excision is more likely to be associated with postoperative adhesion formation.[59]

Given the limited data regarding comparative techniques, it is difficult to advocate one technique over another for the management of ovarian endometriomas regarding the preservation of fertility potential. It appears that excision is superior to drainage alone or ablation of the cyst wall when the outcome measured is recurrence of an endometrioma. Thus, when fertility is not an immediate concern, excision of the endometrioma appears to be the treatment option with the best expected outcome. The issue of adhesion formation as a result of excisional techniques remains open to debate, and further studies are needed to balance the issue of recurrence versus adhesion formation.

Another issue that has generated significant controversy is that of management of the ovary following removal, drainage, or ablation of an endometrioma. Many experts have argued in favor of primary surgical closure of the ovarian cortex after removal of the endometrioma, whereas others have argued in favor of allowing for spontaneous, secondary closure. There are insufficient reports in the literature to argue effectively in support of either approach. The best information to date is derived from animal models. Based on the report of Brumsted et al, allowing the ovarian cortex to heal spontaneously rather than closure by a suturing technique appears to result in less adhesion formation.[64]

SUMMARY

The most appropriate method for the management of women with endometriosis remains a subject of considerable controversy and serious debate. Given the difficulties with visualization of endometriosis lesions as a method for making the diagnosis, surgical therapy may be no more effective than medical therapy. Unfortunately, there is a lack of data from properly designed clinical trials to answer the question in a scientific manner.

Surgical treatment remains a very important approach, especially for the woman who is desirous of conception, as virtually all hormonal therapies are likely to result in impeded ovulation and conception. Laparoscopy has been shown to be as effective for the surgical management of women with endometriosis as the laparotomy approach, provided that the surgeon is sufficiently experienced and possesses the appropriate skills.

It is not clear that one surgical technique – i.e. either excision or ablation – is likely to result in better outcomes regarding pain relief or the recurrence of symptoms. From an evidence-based approach, however, there are ample data to support the concept that postoperative treatment with a GnRH agonist is likely to prolong the pain-free interval if pain management is the primary goal.

The addition of ancillary surgical procedures, such as uterosacral nerve ablation or presacral neurectomy, does not appear to enhance the outcomes that can be expected beyond what would be expected with destruction of the endometriosis lesions. However, both of these ancillary procedures have some effectiveness for the management of midline pain, and especially dyspareunia.

Surgical management is the method of choice for ovarian endometriomas, as hormonal suppressive treatments do not seem to result in a consistent response and reduction in the cysts or associated symptoms. Whether postoperative treatment can enhance the outcome of surgical management remains to be determined.

REFERENCES

1. Balasch J, Creus M, Fabregues F et al. Visible and non-visible endometriosis at laparoscopy in fertile and infertile women and in patients with chronic pelvic pain: a prospective study. Hum Reprod 1996;11:387–91.
2. Schenken RS. Pathogenesis. In: Schenken RS, ed. Endometriosis: Contemporary Concepts in Clinical Management. Philadelphia: JB Lippincott, 1989:1–48.
3. Martin DC, Hubert GD, Vander Zwaag R, el-Zeky FA. Laparoscopic appearances of peritoneal endometriosis. Fertil Steril 1989;51:63–7.
4. Walter AJ, Hentz JG, Magtibay PM, Cornella JL, Magrina JF. Endometriosis: correlation between histologic and visual findings at laparoscopy. Am J Obstet Gynecol 2001;184:1407–13.
5. Stratton P, Winkel CA, Sinaii N et al. Location, color, size, depth, and volume predict endometriosis in lesions resected at surgery. Fertil Steril 2002;78:743–9.
6. Rawson J. Prevalence of endometriosis in asymptomatic women. J Reprod Med 1991;7:513–15.
7. Murphy AA, Guzick DS, Rock JA. Microscopic peritoneal endometriosis. Fertil Steril 1989;51:1072–4.
8. Vasquez G, Cornillie F, Brosens IA. Peritoneal endometriosis: scanning electron microscopy and histology of minimal pelvic endometriosis lesions. Fertil Steril 1984;42:696–703.
9. Nisolle M, Paindaveine B, Bourdon A et al. Histologic study of peritoneal endometriosis in infertile women. Fertil Steril 1990;53:984–8.
10. Portuondo JA, Herran C, Echanojauregui AD, Riego AG. Peritoneal flushing and biopsy in laparoscopically diagnosed endometriosis. Int J Gynecol Obstet 1982;20:371–8.
11. Redwine DB. Endometriosis persisting after castration: clinical characteristics and results of surgical management. Obstet Gynecol 1994;83:405–13.
12. Dmowski WP, Radwanska E, Rana N. Recurrent endometriosis following hysterectomy and oophorectomy: the role of. Residual ovarian fragments. Int J Gynecol Obstet 1988;26:93–103.
13. Noller KL. Endometriosis persisting after castration: clinical characteristics and results of surgical management. Obstet Gynecol 1994;84:321–2.
14. Namnoum AB, Hickman TN, Goodman SB, Gehlbach DL, Rock JA. Incidence of symptom recurrence after hysterectomy for endometriosis. Fertil Steril 1995;64:898–902.
15. Clayton RD, Hawe JA, Love JC, Wilkinson N, Garry P. Recurrent pain after hysterectomy and bilateral salpingo-oophorectomy for endometriosis: Evaluation of laparoscopic excision of residual endometriosis. Br J Obstet Gynaecol 1999;106:740–4.
16. Sen SK, Treherne CA, Perry FA, Ashhurst JC. Endometriosis of the ureter in a post-hysterectomy patient. J Nat Med Assoc 1967;59:327–9.
17. Manyonda IT, Neale EJ, Flynn JT, Osborn DE. Obstructive uropathy from endometriosis after hysterectomy and oophorectomy. Eur J Obstet Gynecol Reprod Biol 1989;31:195–8.
18. Bouier A, Rohrenbach M. Menses due to endometriosis in a woman following hysterectomy. J Am Osteo Assoc 1990;90:259–63.
19. Crosignani PG, Vercellini P. Conservative surgery for severe endometriosis: Should laparotomy be abandoned? Hum Reprod 1995;10:259–63.
20. Bateman BG, Kolp LA, Mills S. Endoscopic versus laparotomy management of ovarian endometriomas. Fertil Steril 1994;62:690–5.
21. Crosignani PG, Vercellini P, Biffignandi F et al. Laparoscopy versus laparotomy in conservative surgical treatment for severe endometriosis. Fertil Steril 1996;66:706–11.
22. Busacca M, Fedele L, Bianchi S et al. Surgical treatment of recurrent endometriosis: laparotomy versus laparoscopy. Hum Reprod 1998;13:2271–4.
23. Catalano GF, Marana R, Caruana P, Muzii L, Mancuso S. Laparoscopy versus microsurgery by laparotomy for excision of ovarian cysts in patients with moderate or severe endometriosis. J Am Assoc Gynecol Laparosc 1996;3:267–70.
24. Koninckx PR, Meuleman C, Demeyere S, Lesaffre E, Cornillie FJ. Suggestive evidence that pelvic endometriosis is a progressive disease, whereas deeply infiltrating endometriosis is associated with pelvic pain. Fertil Steril 1991;55:759–65.
25. Lomano JM. Nd:YAG laser ablation of early pelvic endometriosis. A report of 61 cases. Lasers Surg Med 1987;55:759–65.
26. Keye WR Jr, Hansen LW, Astin M, Poulson AM Jr. Argon laser therapy of endometriosis: a review of 92 consecutive patients. Fert Steril 1987;47:208–12.
27. Martin DC, Vander Zwagg R. Excisional techniques for endometriosis with the CO2 laser laparoscope. J Reprod Med 1987;32:753–8.
28. Marrs RP. The use of the potassium–titanyl–phosphate laser for laparoscopic removal of ovarian endometriosis. Am J Obstet Gynecol 1991;164:1622–6.
29. Chang FH, Chou HH, Soong YK et al. Efficacy of isotopic 13CO2 laser laparoscopic evaporation in the treatment of endometriosis. J Am Assoc Gynecol Laparosc 1997;4:219–23.
30. Redwine DB. Conservative laparoscopic excision of endometriosis by sharp dissection: life table analysis of reoperation and persistent or recurrent disease. Fertil Steril 1991;56:628–34.
31. Fedele L, Parazzini F, Bianchi S, Arcaini L, Candiani G. Stage and localization of pelvic endometriosis and pain. Fertil Steril 1990;53:155–8.
32. Adamson GD, Nelson HP. Surgical treatment of endometriosis. Obstet Gynecol Clin North Am 1997;24:375–408.
33. Winkel CA, Bray M. Treatment of women with endometriosis using excision alone, ablation alone, or ablation in conjunction with leuprolide acetate (Abstract). In: Proceedings of the Fifth World Congress on Endometriosis. Yokohama, Japan, 1996; 55.
34. Koninckx PR, Timmermans B, Meuleman C, Penninckx F. Complications of CO2-laser endoscopic excision of deep endometriosis. Hum Reprod 1996;11:2263–8.
35. Sutton C, Hill D. Laser laparoscopy in the treatment of endometriosis. Br J Obstet Gynaecol 1990;97:181–5.
36. Howard FM. The role of laparoscopy in chronic pelvic pain: promise and pitfalls. Obstet Gynecol Surv 1993;48:357–87.
37. Sutton CJG, Ewen SP, Whitelaw N, Haines P. Prospective, randomized, double-blind, controlled trial of laser laparoscopy in the treatment of pelvic pain associated with minimal, mild, and moderate endometriosis. Fertil Steril 1994;62:696–700.
38. Sutton CJ, Pooley AS, Ewen SP, Haines P. Follow-up report on a randomized controlled trial of laser laparoscopy in the treatment of pelvic pain associated with minimal to moderate endometriosis. Fertil Steril 1997;68:1070–4.

39. Hornstein M, Hemmings R, Yuzpe A, Heinrichs W. Use of nafarelin versus placebo after reductive laparoscopic surgery for endometriosis. Fertil Steril 1997;68:860–4.

40. Jaboulay M. Le traitement de la neuralgie pelvienne par paralysie du sympathique sacré. Lyon Medicien 1899;90:102–8.

41. Ruggi C. La simpaticectomia addominale utero-ovarica come mezzo di cura di alcune lesioni interne degli organi genitali della donna. Bologna: Zanichelli, 1899.

42. Cotte G. Resection of the presacral nerves in the treatment of obstinate dysmenorrhea. Am J Obstet Gynecol 1937;33:1034–40.

43. Elaute L. Surgical anatomy of the so-called sacral nerve. Surg Gynecol Obstet 1933;57:581–9.

44. Labate JS. The surgical anatomy of the superior hypogastric plexus-'pre-sacral nerve.' Surg Gynecol Obstet 1936;67:199–211.

45. Black WT Jr. Use of presacral sympathectomy in the treatment of dysmenorrhea – a second look after 25 years. Am J Obstet Gynecol 1964;89:16–22.

46. Tjaden B, Schlaff WD, Kimball A, Rock JA. The efficacy of presacral neurectomy for the relief of midline dysmenorrhea. Obstet Gynecol 1990;76:89–91.

47. Soysal ME, Soysal S, Gurses E, Ozer S. Laparoscopic presacral neurolysis for endometriosis-related pelvic pain. Hum Reprod 2003;18:588–92.

48. Candiani GB, Fedele L, Vercellini P, Biachi S, DiNola G. Presacral neurectomy for the treatment of pelvic pain associated with endometriosis. Am J Obstet Gynecol 1992;167:100–3.

49. Nezhat C, Nezhat F. A simplified method of laparoscopic presacral neurectomy for the treatment of central pelvic pain due to endometriosis. Br J Obstet Gynaecol 1992;99:659–63.

50. Perez JJ. Laparoscopic presacral neurectomy. Results of the first 25 cases. J Reprod Med 1990;35:625–30.

51. Biggerswtaff ED 3rd, Foster SN. Laparoscopic presacral neurectomy for treatment of midline pelvic pain. J Am Assoc Gynecol Laparosc 1994;2:31–5.

52. Nezhat CH, Seidman DS, Nezhat FR, Nezhat CR. Long-term outcome of laparoscopic presacral neurectomy for the treatment of central pelvic pain attributed to endometriosis. Obstet Gynecol 1998;91:701–4.

53. Daniell JF. Fibreoptic laser laparoscopy. Baillières Clin Obstet Gynaecol 1989;3:545–62.

54. Chaperon C, Dubuisson JB. Laparoscopic treatment of deep endometriosis located on the uterosacral ligaments. Hum Reprod 1996;11:868–73.

55. Chaperon C, Dubuisson JB, Fritel X et al. Operative management of deep endometriosis infiltrating the uterosacral ligaments. J Am Assoc Gynecol Laparosc 1999;6:31–7.

56. Chen FP, Chang SD, Chu KK, Soong YK. Comparison of laparoscopic presacral neurectomy and laparoscopic uterine nerve. J Reprod Med Obstet Gynecol 1996;41:463–6.

57. Williams TJ. Endometriosis. In: Thompson JD, Rock JA, eds. TeLinde's operative gynecology. Philadelphia: JB Lippincott, 1992; 463–98.

58. Nisolle-Pochet M, Casanas-Roux F, Donnez J. Histologic study of ovarian endometriosis after hormonal therapy. Fertil Steril 1988;49:423–6.

59. Fayez JA, Vogel MF. Comparison of different treatment methods of endometriomas by laparoscopy. Obstet Gynecol 1991;78:660–5.

60. Vercellini P, Chaperon C, DeGiorgi O et al. Coagulation or excision of ovarian endometriomas? Am J Obstet Gynecol 2003;188:606–10.

61. Hemmings R, Bissonnette F, Bouzayen R. Results of laparoscopic treatments of ovarian endometriomas: laparoscopic ovarian fenestration and coagulation. Fertil Steril 1998;70:527–9.

62. Beretta P, Franchi M, Ghezzi F et al. Randomized clinical trial of two laparoscopic treatments of endometriomas: cystectomy versus drainage and coagulation. Fertil Steril 1998;70:1176–80.

63. Saleh A, Tulandi T. Reoperation after laparoscopic treatment of ovarian endometriomas by excision and by fenestration. Fertil Steril 1999;72:322–4.

64. Brumsted JR, Deaton J, Lavigne E, Riddick DH. Postoperative adhesion formation after ovarian wedge resection with and without ovarian reconstruction in the rabbit. Fertil Steril 1990;53:723–6.

16. Assisted Reproduction and Endometriosis

Eric S. Surrey

The mechanisms by which endometriosis may compromise fertility and the roles of surgical and medical therapy are discussed in detail in earlier chapters. Appropriate surgical technique should overcome the mechanical distortion induced by endometriosis, but would not be expected to have a significant impact on the alterations in angiogenesis, cytokine regulation, and other inflammatory processes associated with this disease state. Similarly, traditional medical therapies, which may be beneficial for patients with symptomatic endometriosis, have not been demonstrated to enhance fecundity.[1,2] In contrast, the assisted reproductive technologies (ART), which primarily include in vitro fertilization (IVF) and, to a lesser extent, gamete intrafallopian transfer (GIFT) and zygote intrafallopian transfer (ZIFT), should theoretically maximize the potential for conception by removing gametes and embryos in the early stages of development from an inhospitable peritoneal environment (Table 16.1). Similarly, abnormal pelvic anatomy, which may impede oocyte pickup and transport by the fallopian tube, can, in the case of IVF, be successfully bypassed.

In this chapter we shall critically review the relative success rates achieved with ART when performed in patients with various stages of endometriosis, as well as the benefits of adjunctive interventions that may serve to enhance outcomes.

DOES ENDOMETRIOSIS AFFECT ART OUTCOMES?

Pregnancy rates achieved with ART have increased progressively in recent years and, in endometriosis patients, achieve levels of success which are significantly higher than those obtained with alternative therapies.[1-4] Kodama et al[5] reported dramatically higher cumulative conception rates in endometriosis patients ≥32 years of age who underwent IVF after laparoscopy (59%) versus those who were managed expectantly postoperatively (29%).

A controversial issue is whether endometriosis per se exerts a deleterious effect on ART outcomes. Several early studies implied that IVF fertilization, implantation, and pregnancy rates in endometriosis patients were significantly compromised in comparison to controls,[6-9] but it is important to note that these rates were compromised in control groups as well. Guzick and colleagues[10] reported that delivery rates after GIFT were also significantly lower in 114 endometriosis cycles (35.5%) compared to 214 matched control cycles (47.2%). In contrast, other researchers demonstrate no impact. Olivennes and colleagues[11] reported a delivery rate per embryo transfer of 30% in 360 IVF cycles performed on 214 endometriosis patients, in contrast to a rate of 37.5% in 166 cycles performed on 111 tubal factor controls, a difference which was not statistically significant. Geber et al[12] confirmed these findings in a similar study design, reporting a 40% overall pregnancy rate in 140 endometriosis patients in

---

Table 16.1 Treatment of endometriosis-related infertility

Expectant management*

Medical suppression of endometriosis†

Surgical resection vs ablation

Controlled ovarian hyperstimulation ± intrauterine insemination (IUI)*

Assisted reproductive technologies
- In vitro fertilization (IVF)
- Gamete intrafallopian transfer (GIFT)*
- Zygote intrafallopian transfer (ZIFT)*
- Tubal embryo transfer (TET)*

*Requires normal tubal anatomy
†Enhanced fecundity from medical therapy alone has not been shown

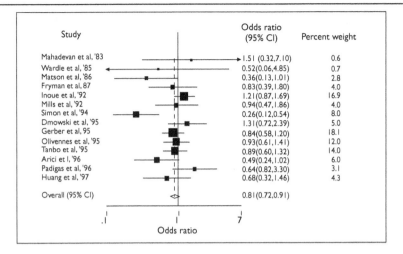

Figure 16.1 Unadjusted meta-analysis of odds of achieving pregnancy in endometriosis patients vs tubal factor controls. (Reprinted from Barnhart K, Duinsmoor-Su R, Coutifaris C. Effect of endometriosis on in vitro fertilization. Fertil Steril 2002;77:1148–55 with permission from the American Society for Reproductive Medicine.)

comparison to three control groups. Hickman[13] also reported no differences in pregnancy implantation rates in a retrospective cohort trial.

In an effort to resolve these issues, Barnhart and colleagues[14] published a meta-analysis that included 27 trials published between 1983 and 1998. After performing bivariate and multivariate logistic regression analyses, the authors concluded that the chance of conceiving from IVF was significantly lower for endometriosis patients than for tubal factor controls (odds ratio 0.56; 95% CI 0.44–0.70) (Figure 16.1). These authors also reported that endometriosis patients experienced significantly lower fertilization and implantation rates as well as number of oocytes obtained. Needless to say, these pregnancy rates still remain higher than those achieved with other forms of therapy.

The effect of disease severity on cycle outcome has also been evaluated. Several large investigations have demonstrated no relationship between disease severity and ongoing pregnancy or miscarriage rates.[11,12] Earlier trials had reported significantly lower pregnancy rates after IVF in patients with more advanced disease.[15,16] It is important to note that in these trials oocytes were obtained laparoscopically as opposed to by transvaginal ultrasound-guided techniques. Dense pelvic adhesions and ovarian disease may have significantly limited the ability to aspirate oocytes effectively with this technique, thus compromising outcome. More recently, Azem et al[17] noted reduced fertilization, pregnancy, and birth rates per cycle in 58 patients with Stages III and IV endometriosis compared to 60 controls with tubal factor infertility. No comparisons were made to patients with less extensive disease, however. Interestingly, delivery rates were low in both of the groups (6.7% vs 16.6%). Pal and colleagues[18] reported that although fertilization rates were significantly lower in patients with Stage III and IV in comparison to Stage I and II endometriosis, implantation, clinical pregnancy, and miscarriage rates were similar between the groups. Aboulghar et al[19] reported that Stage IV endometriosis patients who had undergone surgery prior to IVF had significantly higher cancellation rates owing to a poor response (29.7% vs

Table 16.2 Proposed mechanisms by which endometriosis could effect IVF outcome

- Reduced ovarian access with laparoscopic retrieval
- Embryotoxic effect of maternal serum
- Peritoneal cytokine expression
- Reduced oocyte developmental potential
- Reduced VEGF gene expression
- Increased follicular apoptosis
- Decreased endometrial αvβ3 integrin expression
- Decreased endometrial nitric oxide synthetase expression

1.1%) and lower clinical pregnancy rates (15.3% vs 52.5%) than an age-matched control group with tubal factor infertility who had been stimulated with a similar protocol.

As part of the aforementioned meta-analysis, Barnhart and co-workers[14] compared outcomes in patients previously diagnosed with Stage I–II endometriosis to those with Stage III–IV disease. Women with severe disease were noted to have significantly lower peak estradiol levels, number of oocytes retrieved, implantation and pregnancy rates than those with mild endometriosis.

Several possible explanations have been proposed as to why IVF pregnancy rates may be lower in endometriosis patients than in other infertility patients, if indeed this is the case (Table 16.2). As previously mentioned, outcomes in earlier studies may have been compromised by limited ovarian access in patients with dense pelvic adhesions undergoing laparoscopic oocyte retrieval. This problem should be obviated by transvaginal ultrasound-guided oocyte aspiration. Maternal serum from endometriosis patients has been shown to have a deleterious effect on murine fertilization and embryo development.[20–22] Interestingly, this effect appears to be partially reversed after combination therapy with conservative surgery and either danazol or a GnRH agonist.[22] Others have shown that this embryotoxic effect was decreased after glucocorticoid therapy.[23] Nevertheless, the elimination of the addition of maternal serum to culture media should obviate this effect.

The developmental potential of oocytes derived from women with endometriosis may also be a contributing factor. Norenstedt et al[24] reported that endometriosis patients undergoing IVF employing intracytoplasmic sperm injection techniques were noted to have significantly poorer follicular responses to controlled ovarian hyperstimulation and embryo cleavage rates than controls with male factor infertility. These findings were confirmed by Pal et al,[18] at least with regard to patients with moderate or severe endometriosis. Others have suggested that oocyte developmental capacity is not affected at all.[11,12] Gutierrez and co-workers have evaluated IVF outcome in oocyte donors with endometriosis using embryos transferred to recipients without endometriosis, and noted a significant decline in oocyte developmental capacity and fertilization rates in comparison to controls.[25] One possible explanation of this phenomenon is the suggestion that vascular endothelial growth factor (VEGF) gene expression from granulosa cells derived from patients undergoing controlled ovarian hyperstimulation for in vitro fertilization–embryo transfer is reduced in endometriosis patients.[26] A positive correlation between endometriosis severity, apoptotic bodies in follicular aspirates, and reproductive outcome has been reported.[27]

Others have suggested that endometrial receptivity may be compromised. Decreased expression of endometrial αvβ3 integrin and endometrial endothelial nitric oxide synthase has been described.[28,29] Nevertheless, Diaz and co-workers[30] essentially ruled out an implantation effect in these patients by employing an elegant case–control design. Oocytes derived from a single donor were shared between recipients who had been diagnosed laparoscopically with Stage III–IV endometriosis and infertile controls who were free of disease. Implantation, miscarriage, and livebirth rates were similar between the two groups. Similarly, these authors have also shown that endometrial receptivity, as reflected by pinopode expression – formations on the endometrial glandular cell surface which may be involved in blastocyst adhesion – was not altered in endometriosis patients.[31]

ALTERNATIVES TO IVF: CONTROLLED OVARIAN HYPERSTIMULATION

One group of researchers has reported that the fecundity of women with minimal or mild endometriosis is similar to that of women with unexplained infertility.[32] Several investigators have therefore attempted to treat these patients in a fashion similar to other patients with unexplained infertility by employing controlled ovarian hyperstimulation (COH), with or without intrauterine insemination (IUI), and have reported varying degrees of success. Clearly, one of the caveats for proceeding with this approach is that the endometriosis patient has either inherently normal pelvic anatomy or that anatomic relationships have been surgically restored to normal. In addition, male factor and decreased ovarian reserve should be ruled out.

Two studies addressed the use of clomiphene citrate. Simpson et al[33] completed a prospective non-randomized trial of clomiphene use and described an odds ratio for pregnancy in comparison to untreated controls of 2.9 (95% CI 1.2–7). Deaton and colleagues[34] published a prospective randomized crossover trial of clomiphene and IUI versus no treatment combining couples who had either unexplained infertility or surgically corrected endometriosis. Monthly fecundity rates in the treated group (0.095) were significantly higher than those in the untreated group (0.033) after the completion of life-table analysis. There were no differences in outcome between the 27 patients with endometriosis and the 24 with unexplained infertility.

Gonadotropin therapy has also been explored in two well-designed prospective randomized trials in this patient population. Fedele and coworkers[35] evaluated 49 patients with Stage I or II endometriosis randomized to receive human menopausal gonadotropins (hMG) and human chorionic gonadotropin (hCG) for three cycles versus expectant management for six cycles, and reported that cycle fecundity was significantly greater in the treated group (0.15% vs 0.045%; $P<0.05$). However, the cumulative pregnancy rates

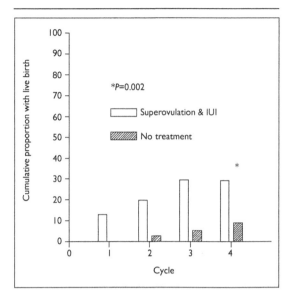

Figure 16.2 Cumulative proportion of livebirth rates in endometriosis patients after undergoing gonadotropin ovarian hyperstimulation and IUI versus expectant management. (Reprinted from Tummon IS, Asher LJ, Martin JSB, Tulandi T. Randomized controlled trial of superovulation and insemination for infertility associated with minimal or mild endometriosis. Fertil Steril 1997;68:8–12 with permission from the American Society for Reproductive Medicine.[36])

were not statistically different (37.4% vs 24%). Employing a somewhat similar study design, Tummon et al[36] randomized 103 couples to undergo gonadotropin therapy and IUI or expectant management for four cycles, and also reported a superior outcome with COH (odds ratio 5.6; 95% CI 1.8–17.4). Interestingly, all of the pregnancies during therapy occurred within the first three cycles (Figure 16.2). In contrast, other investigators have reported that the addition of COH had little additional impact over that achieved with IUI alone in a 3-month trial evaluating 50 patients with minimal endometriosis.[37] In a meta-analysis of 962 cycles of therapy with gonadotropin COH in conjunction with IUI performed in patients with a primary diagnosis of endometriosis, Peterson and coworkers[38] reported pregnancy rates per cycle of 15% in patients with Stage I and II disease, and 8% for those with Stage III and IV disease. These statistics are similar to those reported by Bérubé for untreated patients with minimal disease.[32]

Thus, the use of COH with or without IUI may be beneficial for a short (3-month) course of therapy in those endometriosis patients with normal pelvic anatomic relationships and in the absence of a significant male factor or a decrease in ovarian reserve, prior to considering more aggressive approaches. It is important to appreciate that pregnancy rates are relatively limited and the risks of high-order multiple pregnancy not insignificant with these approaches.

OVARIAN ENDOMETRIOTIC CYSTS AND ART

The presence of ovarian endometriotic cysts (endometriomas) should perhaps be addressed as an independent factor. However, for several reasons it is difficult to truly assess the effect of these lesions on ART outcome. First, the effect of endometrioma size has not been evaluated as an independent variable. Second, it is extremely difficult to evaluate the effect of the endometrioma per se on cycle outcome, given that the majority of patients with these lesions are likely to have concomitant peritoneal disease, which could have an independent effect.

Dlugi et al[39] reported uniformly poor outcomes in patients with endometriomas with regard to ovarian response, the number of embryos available for transfer, as well as fertilization and pregnancy rates in comparison to controls with hydrosalpinges. Yanushpolsky and colleagues[40] reported a higher incidence of pregnancy loss and an adverse effect on number of oocytes retrieved with transvaginal ultrasound-guided techniques as well as embryo quality in endometriosis patients.[40] Al-Azemi et al[41] described a decrease in ovarian response requiring the use of higher gonadotropin doses in patients with such lesions. However, cumulative pregnancy and livebirth rates were unaffected. In contrast, Olivennes et al[11] demonstrated no effect of persistent endometriomas on any outcome parameter of either controlled ovarian hyper-stimulation or IVF. It is interesting to note that at least one group of investigators would suggest that limited inadvertent exposure of oocytes to endometrioma fluid does not appear to have a significant impact on fertilization rates or early embryo development.[42] However, it is only logical to make every effort to avoid placing the aspirating needle through an endometrioma during oocyte retrieval procedures, to prevent rupture and inadvertent exposure if at all possible.

The effect of surgical resection of endometriomas prior to IVF has also been evaluated. Canis et al[43] reported the outcome of a series of 41 patients who had undergone precycle laparoscopic resection of large (>3 cm diameter) ovarian endometriotic cysts (unilateral in 30 patients and bilateral in 11) in comparison to 139 controls with endometriosis but without endometriomas, and 59 additional controls with tubal infertility. No differences were described regarding the resulting number of oocytes or embryos, despite extensive ovarian surgery. In contrast, Loh et al[44] reported reduced follicular response in natural and clomiphene-stimulated cycles, but no effect on ovarian response after gonadotropin stimulation in a retrospective report of 40 patients with ovarian endometriotic cysts of mean diameter 4.23 ± 2.2 cm who had undergone precycle resection. Donnez and colleagues[45] reported on 187 cycles in 85 patients who underwent laparoscopic cyst wall vaporization of ovarian endometriomas prior to IVF, and compared their responses to 633 cycles in 289 patients with tubal factor infertility. Response to stimulation and clinical pregnancy rates were similar between the groups.

Marconi and colleagues[46] also reported that there were no differences in ovarian response, oocytes retrieved, embryo quality, or clinical pregnancy rates in patients who had undergone laparoscopic resection of endometriomas compared to an age-matched control group with tubal factor infertility. These patients did require higher gonadotropin doses to achieve these endpoints, however.

The aforementioned studies do not address the question of whether resection of endometriomas is advantageous. In an interesting trial, Ho et al[47] compared ovarian response between the ovaries of patients who had undergone unilateral cystectomy for an endometrioma prior to IVF. The number of dominant follicles and oocytes retrieved was significantly lower in the ovaries that had been previously operated upon. This suggests that aggressive ovarian surgery could compromise ovarian blood supply or result in the destruction of normal ovarian tissue. In a retrospective series, Garcia-Velasco and co-workers[48] compared the outcomes of 50 patients who had at least one endometrioma >3 cm in mean diameter at the time of oocyte aspiration to those of 87 patients who had undergone laparoscopic resection of endometriomas within 3 months of an IVF cycle. Interestingly, there were no differences in ovarian response, fertilization rates, number of embryos available for transfer, or pregnancy rates between the groups. The authors concluded that although laparoscopic resection of ovarian endometriomas does not have a deleterious effect on IVF cycle outcome, it does not appear to offer any specific benefit. Resection of large lesions will clearly enhance access to follicles within underlying normal ovarian tissue and eliminate the potential for rupture during oocyte aspiration. However, meticulous surgical technique, with care taken to avoid compromising ovarian blood supply and destroying healthy ovarian tissue, is clearly mandatory.

SURGICAL OR MEDICAL THERAPY FOR ENDOMETRIOSIS AND ART OUTCOMES

The benefit of surgical management of endometriosis for achieving spontaneous conception has already been suggested.[1,4] The question of whether such intervention in the absence of ovarian endometriomas would enhance ART cycle outcome has also been addressed. One prospective randomized trial reported that although laparoscopic CO_2 laser ablation of endometriosis at the time of GIFT had no effect on cycle outcome, pregnancy rates in subsequent cycles of patients who failed to conceive from

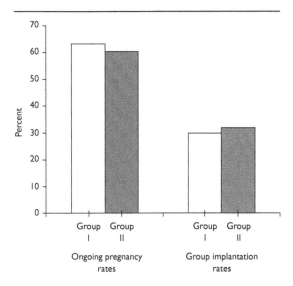

Figure 16.3 Ongoing pregnancy and implantation rates in endometriosis patients undergoing surgical resection for more than 6 months (Group I) or 6 months to 5 years (Group II) prior to oocyte aspiration. (Reprinted from Surrey ES, Schoolcraft WB. Does surgical management of endometriosis with 6 months of an in vitro fertilization/embryo transfer cycle improve outcome? J Assist Reprod Genet 2003;20:365–70 with permission from Kluwer Academic/Plenum Publishers.[50])

GIFT were significantly higher than in controls with endometriosis who underwent GIFT alone.[49] More recently, Surrey and Schoolcraft[50] reported that the cycle outcomes of COH and IVF were similar between two groups of endometriosis patients, one of which had undergone surgical resection within 6 months and the other had undergone surgical resection more than 6 months to 5 years prior to oocyte aspiration (ongoing pregnancy rates 63.6% vs 60.53%, respectively) (Figure 16.3). Regression analysis revealed no effect of the time interval between surgery and oocyte aspiration on implantation rates. Pagidas et al[51] have clearly shown that cumulative pregnancy rates from IVF were significantly higher than those achieved after reoperation for moderate–severe endometriosis. It would appear, therefore, that the aforementioned benefit derived from such surgery in enhancing spontaneous conception may be masked by the greater impact on implantation and pregnancy achieved with the assisted reproductive technologies.

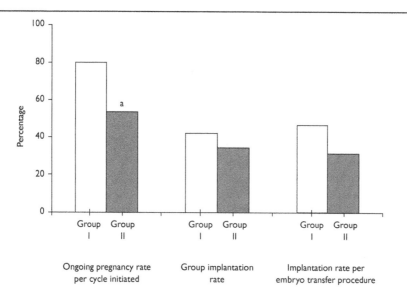

Figure 16.4 IVF cycle outcomes for endometriosis patients randomized to pretreatment with a GnRH agonist for 3 months (Group I) immediately prior to COH or undergoing standard COH (Group II). a: $P<0.05$ vs. Group I. (Reprinted from Surrey ES, Silverberg KM, Surrey MW, Schoolcraft WB. The effect of prolonged GnRH agonist therapy on in vitro fertilization-embryo transfer cycle outcome in endometriosis patients: a multicenter randomized trial. Fertil Steril 2002;78:699–704 with permission from the American Society for Reproductive Medicine.[52])

Interestingly, traditional medical therapy for endometriosis, such as progestins, danazol, and GnRH agonists, have been shown to have little impact on enhancing spontaneous pregnancy rates despite well described beneficial effects on symptomatic disease.[1,2] However, if the negative effect of this disease process on fertility returns rapidly after discontinuation of medication, then one could hypothesize that any benefits of medical suppression on enhancing fertility would be most evident if pregnancy could be achieved during a time of maximal suppression. This could only occur with the use of the assisted reproductive technologies.

In a recent prospective randomized multicenter trial, Surrey et al[52] evaluated the effect of a 3-month course of a GnRH agonist administered immediately prior to controlled ovarian hyperstimulation and IVF in patients with surgically confirmed endometriosis. Significantly higher ongoing pregnancy rates, with a trend towards higher implantation rates, were appreciated in this group of 25 patients compared to 26 controls with endometriosis treated with standard COH

techniques in the absence of prolonged GnRH agonist therapy (Figure 16.4). These findings have also been demonstrated by others. Seven previous studies of varying designs have assessed the effect of suppression with a GnRH agonist before IVF or GIFT.[53-59] The length of suppression varied from 6 weeks to 7 months. Some studies lacked control groups, but a beneficial effect of pretreatment was suggested by all.

Recently, Rickes et al[60] evaluated the effect of surgical treatment of endometriosis, either alone or in combination with a 6-month postoperative treatment course of a GnRH agonist, on IVF or COH–IUI outcome in a prospective randomized trial of 110 patients. The pregnancy rates were significantly higher for both forms of therapy in patients treated postoperatively with a prolonged course of GnRH agonists. However, when patients were stratified based on disease stage, a statistically significant difference was only appreciated among patients with Stages III and IV endometriosis who underwent IVF. There are no trials evaluating the relative benefit of duration of suppressive therapy, or whether this approach should be offered to specific subgroups of endometriosis patients, given the associated increased expense and time delay before pregnancy can occur.

The mechanism of action for this effect has not been established. It has been suggested that GnRH agonists may have been a positive input on natural killer cell activity, metalloproteinase tissue inhibitor concentrations, peritoneal cytokine levels, and endometrial cell apoptosis.[61–64] Alternatively, suppressive therapy with danazol and GnRH agonists has been suggested to have a beneficial effect on restoring aberrant expression of endometrial αvβ3 integrin, which may enhance implantation.[65,66]

SUMMARY

The management of infertility associated with endometriosis remains challenging. The clinician must rule out all other causes before creating a treatment plan, paying particular attention to an evaluation of ovarian reserve and sperm parameters. After surgical reconstruction, or in patients with less extensive disease, controlled ovarian hyperstimulation techniques, potentially in conjunction with intrauterine insemination, can be successful, although prolonged therapy is not beneficial. It is important to monitor patients carefully, given the risk of high-order multiple gestation reported with these techniques. In vitro fertilization represents an extremely effective means of bypassing the hostile peritoneal environment and anatomic distortion associated with this disease state. Surgical management of disease has little beneficial impact on IVF outcome, with the possible exception of resection of large ovarian endometriomas. Although medical suppression of endometriosis alone has virtually no benefit in the asymptomatic patient, there appears to be significant benefit of pretreatment with GnRH agonists immediately prior to IVF cycle initiation. However, whether only a specific subset or all patients with endometriosis would most benefit from this approach has not yet been determined. The use of endometrial implantation

markers may be helpful in this regard, although definitive data remain lacking.

REFERENCES

1. Adamson GD, Pasta D. Surgical treatment of endometriosis-associated infertility: meta-analysis compared with survival analysis. Am J Obstet Gynecol 1994;171:1488–505.
2. Hughes EG, Fedorkow DM, Collins JA. A quantitative overview of controlled trials in endometriosis-associated infertility. Fertil Steril 1993;59:963–70.
3. Center for Disease Control and Prevention, American Society for Reproductive Medicine, Society for Assisted Reproductive Technologies, et al. 2000 Assisted reproductive technologies success rates: national summary and fertility clinic reports. Department of Health and Human Services, Atlanta, GA, 2002.
4. Marcoux S, Maheux R, Berhle S et al. Laparoscopic surgery in infertile women with minimal or mild endometriosis. N Engl J Med 1998;377:217–22.
5. Kodama H, Fukuda J, Karube H et al. Benefit of in vitro fertilization treatment for endometriosis-associated infertility. Fertil Steril 1996;66:974–9.
6. Bergendal A, Naffah S, Nagy C et al. Outcome of IVF in patients with endometriosis in comparison with tubal-factor infertility. J Assist Reprod Genet 1998;15:530–4.
7. Simon C, Gutierez A, Vidal A et al. Outcome of patients with endometriosis in assisted reproduction: results from in-vitro fertilization and oocyte donation. Hum Reprod 1994;9:725–9.
8. Wardle PG, Mitchell JD, McLaughlin EA et al. Endometriosis and ovulatory disorder: reduced fertilization in vitro compared with tubal and unexplained infertility. Lancet 1985;2:236–9.
9. Arici A, Oral E, Bukulmez O et al. The effect of endometriosis on implantation: results from the Yale University in vitro fertilization and embryo transfer program. Fertil Steril 1996;65:603–7.
10. Guzick DS, Yao YAS, Berger SL et al. Endometriosis impairs the efficacy of gamete intrafallopian transfer: results of a case–control study. Fertil Steril 1994;62:1186–91.
11. Olivennes F, Feldberg D, Liu HC et al. Endometriosis: a stage by stage analysis in the role of in vitro fertilization. Fertil Steril 1995;64:392–8.
12. Geber S, Paraschos T, Atkinson G et al. Results of IVF in patients with endometriosis: the severity of the disease does not affect outcome, or the incidence of miscarriage. Hum Reprod 1995;10:1507–11.
13. Hickman T. Impact of endometriosis on implantation: data from the Wilford Hall Medical Center IVF-ET program. J Reprod Med 2002;47:801–8.
14. Barnhart K, Dunsmoor-Su R, Coutifaris C. Effect of endometriosis on in vitro fertilization. Fertil Steril 2002;77:1148–55.
15. Chillik CF, Acosta AA, Garcia JP et al. The role of in vitro fertilization in infertile patients with endometriosis. Fertil Steril 1985;44:56–61.
16. Matson PL, Yovich JL. The treatment of infertility associated with endometriosis by in vitro fertilization. Fertil Steril 1986;46:432–4.
17. Azem F, Lessing JB, Geva E et al. Patients with stages III and IV endometriosis have a poorer outcome of in vitro fertilization–embryo transfer than patients with tubal infertility. Fertil Steril 1999;72:1107–9.
18. Pal L, Shifren JL, Isaacson K et al. Impact of varying stages of endometriosis on the outcome of in vitro fertilization–embryo transfer. J Assist Reprod Genet 1998;15:27–31.

19. Aboulghar M, Mansour R, Serour G et al. The outcome of in vitro fertilization in advanced endometriosis with previous surgery: a case controlled study. Am J Obstet Gynecol 2003;188:371–5.

20. Damewood M, Hesla J, Schlaff W et al. Effect of serum from patients with minimal to mild endometriosis on mouse embryo development in vitro. Fertil Steril 1990;54:917–20.

21. Miller K, Pittaway D, Deaton J. The effect of serum from infertile women with endometriosis on fertilization and early embryonic development in a murine in vitro fertilization model. Fertil Steril 1995;64:623–6.

22. Abu-Masa A, Takahashi K, Kitao M. The effect of serum obtained before and after treatment for endometriosis on in vitro development of two-cell mouse embryos. Fertil Steril 1992;57:1098–102.

23. Simón C, Gómez E, Mir A et al. Glucocorticoid treatment decreases sera embryotoxicity in endometriosis patients. Fertil Steril 1992;58:284–9.

24. Norenstedt S, Linderoth-Nagy C, Bergendal A et al. Reduced developmental potential in oocytes from women with endometriosis. J Assist Reprod Genet 2001;18:644–9.

25. Gutiérrez A, Oliveira N, Cano F et al. In vitro fertilization in infertile patients with endometriosis. Assist Reprod Rev 1994;4:162–71.

26. Yamashita Y, Ueda M, Takehara M et al. Influence of severe endometriosis on gene-expression of vascular endothelial growth factor and interleukin-6 in granulosa cells from patients undergoing controlled ovarian hyperstimulation for in vitro fertilization–embryo transfer. Fertil Steril 2002;78:865–71.

27. Nakahara K, Saito H, Saito T et al. Ovarian fecundity in patients with endometriosis can be estimated by the incidence of apoptotic bodies. Fertil Steril 1998;69:931–5.

28. Khorram O, Lessey B. Alterations in expression of endometrial nitric oxide synthase and αvβ3 integrin in women with endometriosis. Fertil Steril 2002;78:860–4.

29. Lessey B, Castelbaum A, Sawin S et al. Aberrant integrin expression in the endometrium of women with endometriosis. J Clin Endocrinol Metab 1994;79:643–9.

30. Diaz I, Navarro J, Blasco L et al. Impact of Stage III–IV endometriosis on recipients of sibling oocytes: matched case–control study. Fertil Steril 2000;74:31–4.

31. Garcia-Velasco J, Nikas G, Remohi J et al. Endometrial receptivity in terms of pinopode expression is not impaired in women with endometriosis in artificially prepared cycles. Fertil Steril 2001;75:1231–3.

32. Bérubé S, Marcoux S, Langevin M et al. Fecundity of infertile women with minimal or mild endometriosis and women with unexplained infertility. Fertil Steril 1998;69:1034–41.

33. Simpson CW, Taylor PJ, Collins JA. A comparison of ovulation suppression and ovulation stimulation in the treatment of endometriosis-associated infertility. Int J Gynecol Obstet 1993;59:1239–44.

34. Deaton JL, Gibson M, Blackmer KM et al. A randomized, controlled trial of clomiphene citrate and intrauterine insemination in couples with unexplained infertility or surgically corrected endometriosis. Fertil Steril 1990;54:1083–8.

35. Fedele L, Bianchi S, Marchini M et al. Superovulation with human menopausal gonadotropins in the treatment of infertility associated with minimal or mild endometriosis: a controlled randomized study. Fertil Steril 1992;58:28–31.

36. Tummon IS, Asher LJ, Martin JSB et al. Randomized controlled trial of superovulation and insemination for infertility associated with minimal or mild endometriosis. Fertil Steril 1997;68:8–12.

37. Serta RT, Rufo S, Seibel MM. Minimal endometriosis and intrauterine insemination: does controlled ovarian hyperstimulation improve pregnancy rates? Obstet Gynecol 1992;80:37–40.

38. Peterson CM, Hatasaka HH, Jones KP et al. Ovulation induction with gonadotropins and intrauterine insemination compared with in vitro fertilization and no therapy: a prospective, non-randomized, cohort study and meta-analysis. Fertil Steril 1994;62:535–4.

39. Dlugi AM, Loy RA, Dieterle S et al. The effect of endometriomas on in vitro fertilization outcome. J In Vitro Fertil Embryo Transfer 1989;6:338–41.

40. Yanushpolsky E, Best C, Jackson K et al. Effects of endometriomas on oocyte quality and pregnancy rates in in vitro fertilization cycles; a prospective case-controlled study. J Assist Reprod Genet 1998;15:193–7.

41. Al-Azemi M, Lopez Bernal A, Steele J et al. Ovarian response to repeated controlled stimulation in in vitro cycles in patients with ovarian endometriosis. Hum Reprod 2000;15:72–5.

42. Khamsi F, Yavas Y, Lacanna IC et al. Exposure of human oocytes to endometrioma fluid does not alter fertilization or early embryo development. J Assist Reprod Genet 2001;18:106–9.

43. Canis M, Pouly JL, Tamburro S et al. Ovarian response during IVF–embryo transfer cycles after laparoscopic ovarian cystectomy for endometriotic cysts of >3 cm in diameter. Hum Reprod 2001;12:2583–6.

44. Loh FH, Tan AT, Kumar J et al. Ovarian response after laparoscopic ovarian cystectomy for endometriotic cysts in 132 monitored cycles. Fertil Steril 1999;72:316–21.

45. Donnez J, Wyns C, Nisolle M. Does ovarian surgery for endometriomas impair the ovarian response to gonadotropin? Fertil Steril 2001;76:662–5.

46. Marconi G, Vilela M, Quintana R et al. Laparoscopic ovarian cystectomy of endometriomas does not affect ovarian response to gonadotropin stimulation. Fertil Steril 2002;78:876–8.

47. Ho H-Y, Lee R, Hwu Y-M et al. Poor response of ovaries with endometrioma previously treated with cystectomy to controlled ovarian hyperstimulation. J Assist Reprod Genet 2002;19:507–11.

48. Garcia-Velasco J, Corona J, Requena A et al. Should we operate ovarian endometriomas prior to IVF? Fertil Steril 2002;78:S203.

49. Surrey MW, Hill DL. Treatment of endometriosis by carbon dioxide laser during gamete intrafallopian transfer. J Am Coll Surg 1994;79:440–2.

50. Surrey ES, Schoolcraft WB. Does surgical management of endometriosis within 6 months of an in vitro fertilization–embryo transfer cycle improve outcome? J Assist Reprod Genet 2003;20:365–70.

51. Pagidas K, Falcone T, Hemmings R, Miron P. Comparison of reoperation for moderate (stage III) and severe (stage IV) endometriosis-related infertility with in vitro fertilization–embryo transfer. Fertil Steril 1996;65:791–5.

52. Surrey ES, Silverberg KM, Surrey MW, Schoolcraft WB. The effect of prolonged GnRH agonist therapy on in vitro fertilization–embryo transfer cycle outcome in endometriosis patients: a multicenter randomized trial. Fertil Steril 2002;78:699–704.

53. Chedid S, Camus W, Smitz J et al. Comparison among different ovarian stimulation regimens for assisted procreation procedures in patients with endometriosis. Hum Reprod 1995;10:2406–11.

54. Wardle P, Foster P, Mitchel J et al. Endometriosis and IVF: effect of prior therapy. Lancet 1986;8475:276–7.

55. Dicker D, Goldman GA, Ashkenazi J et al. The value of pretreatment with long-term gonadotropin-releasing hormone (GnRH) analogue in IVF-ET therapy of severe endometriosis. Hum Reprod 1990;5:418–20.

56. Marcus SF, Edwards RG. High rates of pregnancy after long-term down-regulation of women with severe endometriosis. Am J Obstet Gynecol 1994;171:812–17.

57. Curtis P, Jackson A, Bernard A, Shaw RW. Pretreatment with gonadotrophin releasing hormone (GnRH) analogue prior to in vitro fertilization for patients with endometriosis. Eur J Obstet Gynecol Reprod Biol 1993;52:211–16.

58. Nakamura K, Oosawa M, Kondou I et al. Menotropin stimulation after prolonged gonadotropin releasing hormone agonist pretreatment for in vitro fertilization in patients with endometriosis. J Assist Reprod Genet 1992;9:113–17.

59. Remorgida V, Anserini P, Croce S et al. Comparison of different ovarian stimulation protocols for gamete intrafallopian transfer in patients with minimal and mild endometriosis. Fertil Steril 1990;53:1060–3.

60. Rickes D, Nichel I, Kropf S, Kleinstein J. Increased pregnancy rates after ultralong postoperative therapy with gonadotropin-releasing hormone analogs in patients with endometriosis. Fertil Steril 2002;78:757–62.

61. Garzetti GG, Ciavattini A, Provinciali M et al. Natural cytoxicity and GnRH agonist administration in advanced endometriosis: positive modulation on natural killer cell activity. Obstet Gynecol 1996;88:234–40.

62. Sharpe-Timms KL, Keisler LW, McIntush EW et al. Tissue inhibitors of metalloproteinase-I concentrations are attenuated in peritoneal fluid and sera of women with endometriosis and restored in sera by gonadotropin-releasing hormone agonist therapy. Fertil Steril 1998;69:1128–34.

63. Taketani Y, Kuo T-M, Mizuno M. Comparison of cytokine levels and embryo toxicity in peritoneal fluid in infertile women with untreated or treated endometriosis. Am J Obstet Gynecol 1992;167:265–70.

64. Imai A, Takagi A, Tamaya T. Gonadotropin-releasing hormone analog repairs reduced endometrial cell apoptosis in endometriosis in vitro. Am J Obstet Gynecol 2000;182:1142–6.

65. Tei C, Maruyama T, Kuji N et al. Reduced expression of αvβ3 integrin in the endometrium of unexplained infertility patients with recurrent IVF–ET failures: improvement by danazol treatment. J Assist Reprod Genet 2003;20:13–20.

66. Lessey BA. Medical management of endometriosis and infertility. Fertil Steril 2000;73:1089–96.

17. The Structure and Future of Endometriosis Research

Elizabeth A. Dille and David L. Olive

Endometriosis is a common disorder in the reproductive age woman, and as a result has been intensively studied over the last one hundred years. In the early 20th century, the disease was thought to be relatively straightforward in its etiology and treatment. However, as investigators have delved into understanding this disorder, the complexity of endometriosis has become apparent. Indeed, as we learn more about this challenging pathology, more and more questions become apparent.

This chapter will focus not upon what we know about endometriosis, but rather what we do not know. Despite major leaps in understanding over the past two decades, there are still a large number of investigative pathways available to the inquisitive and persistent scientist. This chapter will help identify those areas, while hopefully illuminating future pathways to discern the answers to remaining issues.

WHAT IS ENDOMETRIOSIS?

Traditionally, endometriosis has been defined as the presence of endometrial stroma and epithelium in an ectopic location. However, is this the definition we need to make further advances in endometriosis research? This definition was created by pathologists, and clearly represents diagnostic criteria for their convenience. Yet Koninckx and colleagues raise an important issue: what if the occasional ectopic implant is a normal, physiologic process? What if progression to a definite level of invasiveness actually defines the abnormal process?[1] Such a scenario has been suggested by studies in the baboon, in whom endometriotic implants are often seen to be transient phenomena.[2] Studies utilizing repeat laparoscopy in women also suggest that in some cases the implants spontaneously resolve.[3] It remains a challenge for the endometriosis research community to better determine which ectopic implants represent pathology and which are indicative of a normal and reversible physiologic process.

While we puzzle over the relative importance of various implants, it is also worth considering exactly what defines an ectopic implant. The requirement for both glands and stroma was practical but arbitrary. As we are better able to identify cell types by means other than hematoxylin and eosin staining, as we progress with monoclonal antibodies directed at a wide variety of cell-specific markers, it is becoming increasingly clear that the capacity exists to clearly identify stroma in the absence of epithelia, and vice versa. In fact, we now have the ability to identify specific subtypes of endometrial cells. New work identifying and characterizing endometrial stem cells is demonstrating the utility of this concept.[4] It remains a challenge for researchers to determine which cells, in which combinations, represent endometriosis as a disease process.

It is worth considering the possibility that endometriosis is in fact not a single disease, but rather a group of pathologically distinct disorders with a common clinical manifestation. Such a scenario would not be unprecedented: polycystic ovarian disease very likely represents a number of primary abnormalities whose only common thread is a chronic anovulatory state without a deficiency of any required component.

If endometriosis is similarly a complex of diseases, it becomes imperative that we develop the means to identify and separate these existing subtypes.

EPIDEMIOLOGY OF ENDOMETRIOSIS

Few good epidemiologic studies of endometriosis have been conducted; the reasons for this are detailed elsewhere in this book. As diagnosis is costly and invasive, only a subset of women in many investigations are properly diagnosed. Case-control studies frequently use biased controls, only eligible due to a prior laparoscopic evaluation but not necessarily matched for significant confounders. This requires statistical correction for a large number of covariates that may have impact beyond that imagined. Population studies suffer from incomplete or imperfect diagnostic criteria, thus making their conclusions fraught with error.

The most important potential advance in the epidemiologic study of endometriosis would be a non-invasive mechanism for diagnosis. However, an alternative approach would be to define the clinical disease not by visualization of ectopic implants at surgery but rather by a clinical symptom or syndrome, perhaps that responds in a predictable way to a specific intervention. Perhaps the ability to sort out these subtypes of endometriosis will allow us to better characterize each and, by summation, the disease as a whole.

PATHOGENESIS OF ENDOMETRIOSIS

It appears highly likely that transplantation, generally via retrograde menstruation, is central to the development of ectopic endometrial lesions. However, given the near universality of retrograde menstruation, it is also likely that additional factors are involved in the development and maintenance of this disease. To date, deficiencies in immunologic function,[5] abnormalities of matrix metalloproteinase function,[6] as well as excesses of growth factors and chemokines[7] have been identified as probable promoters of endometriosis.

Immunologic function has been frequently examined, but still has little definitive information resulting from investigation. Peritoneal macrophages are known to be found in greater number and in a more highly activated state in the woman with this disease.[8,9] In addition, growth factors secreted by these cells are found to be at increased concentration in the patient with endometriosis.[10] These facts would suggest an overactive inflammatory response as a key ingredient in the recipe for endometriosis development. However, this does not jive with a failure to demonstrate higher rates of endometriosis in women with chronic inflammation of the pelvis (and patent tubes) due to infectious disease; surely, the same immunologic status would be expected in such subjects. Furthermore, macrophages act as the scavengers of the peritoneal cavity, removing damaged or inappropriate invaders or debris. Would not a highly charged immune response be more likely to remove retrograde menstruation, decreasing the chances of endometriosis? One could possibly envision a disconnect between phagocytic capacity and growth factor secretion among the monocytic cells of the peritoneal cavity.[11] This possibility has yet to be investigated.

Matrix metalloproteinases have been the beginning of a story for actual cell implantation into an ectopic locale. However, there is undoubtedly much more to this tale. Serious recent investigation into the ability of endometrial cells to bind, intercalate, and eventually submerge within peritoneum provides important clues to the mechanism of endometriosis initiation. However, the requirements for cell binding and further immersion within the peritoneum have yet to be elucidated. Furthermore, the qualities of this process that may differ in those with endometriosis versus those without are uninvestigated and of critical importance to understanding the disease process.

Many factors have been suggested as necessary once implantation occurs and growth or maintenance is required. Estrogen and a variety of growth factors are most commonly mentioned, yet articulation of the minimum necessary requirements as well as the environment most likely to promote growth of implants is thin. Further investigation into this arena will likely prove productive.

One particularly inviting area of investigation is the presence of aromatase in the endometriosis lesion. Noble et al first demonstrated that aromatase mRNA was found in ectopic and eutopic endometrium from women with endometriosis but was undetectable in disease free women.[12] However, Fazleabas et al recently demonstrated that induced endometriotic implants in baboons did not express aromatase until later in the disease process.[13] Future research in this area should focus on how and why this aberrant expression of aromatase occurs. It may well be that characteristics of aromatase expression are related to invasiveness or aggressiveness of the disease process.

A problem with much disease research is the development of reliable and accurate models for experimentation. All models have limitations, and often an investigator must choose a specific, flawed model for one type of study and another for a related but different experiment. Endometriosis presents a challenge in that it is often difficult to select a model that is reliable, efficient, and affordable. Cell culture is widely used and has allowed tremendous insight into a number of aberrant events at the cellular and subcellular level. While this approach allows us to study very precise perturbations of the endometrial cell, it fails to provide us with information about the behavior of this tissue as part of a complex system in situ. The rodent model has been used extensively in the endometriosis world, yet the lack of a menstrual cycle or spontaneous development of disease limit applicability for many avenues of investigation. Non-human primates are close to ideal, but have not been utilized to the necessary extent due to high cost and access difficulties. A major thrust in future endometriosis investigation will be to learn to more effectively integrate the results from these disparate systems into a holistic model of the disease.

PATHOPHYSIOLOGY

The two chief symptoms of endometriosis are pain and infertility. Many questions regarding the relationship between the disease and these symptoms have yet to be adequately addressed.

Infertility and its relationship to endometriosis remains an unsolved puzzle even after many years of investigation. While it is clear that extensive pelvic anatomic distortion can lead to decreased fecundity, it is unclear why early stage endometriosis decreases fertility. Suggestions have been proposed for abnormalities of oocyte development,[14] endometrial receptivity,[15] early embryo function,[16] and even post-implantation development.[17] Yet current studies are hampered by small numbers, failure of verification, and questionable selection of model systems. Careful basic research into each of these areas using each of the available model systems would seem fruitful to identifying the cause and effect mechanism (if it exists) between endometriosis implants and decreased fertility.

Investigation into pain carries similar uncertainties. Model systems have been slow to develop, with outcome measures in rodents and non-human primates difficult to construct. Even human investigation has suffered from poor quality instruments for pain quantitation. Validation is in short supply, and analysis of scales as linear rather than nonlinear scores is rampant. Furthermore, the outcome of choice is often some subset of pain or sum of pain scores, while quality of life measurement is likely to be more meaningful and productive. Attention to these facets of endometriosis pain research will help advance this area in the future.

DIAGNOSIS

The diagnosis of endometriosis is currently surgical, with the gold standard being visualization of the lesion (generally at laparoscopy). However, recent studies of excision of so-called lesions reveal those identified as endometriosis are pathologically confirmed less than half the time.[18,19] Excision of disease, however desirable, is impractical. Thus, we are left with a comparator for other diagnostic methods that is itself often incorrect.

Those other methods that have been developed include history and physical examination, serum markers, radiologic tests, endometrial biopsy analysis, and combinations of these techniques. To date, all have proven to be unacceptably inaccurate.[20] However, the basic flaw may lie not in the tests but rather in their comparison to the gold standard. It may not be optimal to determine by non-invasive test whether or not an ectopic lesion of endometrium exists, but rather if the test can predict response to symptom interventions. Thus, a serum test would be quite valuable if a high level indicated a very high likelihood of response of the patient's pain to medical therapy, while a low level suggested a lesser chance of response. This symptom directed validation is sorely needed for diagnostic methods, and should be the next generation of investigations in this area.

CLASSIFICATION OF ENDOMETRIOSIS

Over the previous decades of clinical interest in endometriosis, physicians have been intent upon developing a classification system for the disease. Numerous schemes have been developed, but most have been based upon anatomic presentation rather than prognosis. For a classification system to be meaningful, it must clearly relate to the ability of one or more interventions to relieve the symptom of concern to the patient. Past staging systems have attempted this with fertility and pain as the outcome of interest, but none have truly staged the disease based upon response to medical or surgical treatment.

What is needed is a classification scheme indicating what will respond when. This would suggest classifying the disease differently for different treatment choices and different symptoms. For instance, once the anatomic location and type of disease is described it might be calculated that the presentation is severe for medical therapy (poor prognosis for relief of pain) while moderate for surgical excision (modest prognosis for relief of pain). The same patient with the same disease presentation might also have minimal disease for assisted reproduction (excellent prognosis) if fertility is the issue.

The above type of dynamic classification is virtually impossible to construct by a single researcher or center. It would require a large cooperative effort for data collection of the disease characteristics, demographic data, and outcome based upon type of intervention. Once models are developed, validation in subsequent independent populations will be required. Currently, no large organizations are moving in such a direction for disease classification; it is likely that future classification methods will be of limited value at best.

TREATMENT OF ENDOMETRIOSIS

The last two decades have provided a tremendous amount of information regarding the treatment of endometriosis, due to a number of well-constructed randomized trials. However, we still have a number of therapeutic questions that have not been adequately addressed. Attention to these issues in upcoming years will greatly benefit the care of women suffering from this disease.

It is clear that endometriosis-associated pain can be effectively treated with medical therapies. However, not all have been adequately tested, and few have been tested as part of a sequential algorithm. Thus, if a patient fails to respond to a first-line therapy, it would be advantageous to know to what they might best respond as a second line drug. In addition, continuous oral contraceptives have not been adequately explored; nor have combinations of medications. Comparative studies in these areas will help clarify an optimal treatment approach.

The surgical treatment of endometriosis-associated pain now has also been shown to be efficacious, yet the two primary modes of treatment – excision and ablation – have never been directly compared. An RCT examining these two approaches in total as well as for specific types and locations of endometriosis would seem indicated.

Finally, controversy lingers regarding the use of combination medical/surgical therapy for endometriosis-associated pain. Preoperative medical therapy is thus far essentially unevaluated. Postoperative medication seems to be of value, but clarification is needed to assess its role following both ablation and excision. The optimal length of time to treat with postoperative drugs, as well as which might be best, is in need of investigation. It would also be of interest to investigate the need for adjunctive medical therapy based upon the skill or experience of the surgeon.

Endometriosis-associated infertility has yet to be shown to be responsive to any type of medical therapy directed at the disease. However, surgical intervention has been suggested to be of value in early-stage disease. No studies have examined late-stage endometriosis and its response to surgical treatment, when compared to any other effective therapy, such as controlled ovarian hyperstimulation and insemination or in vitro fertilization. In fact, IVF is in dire need of comparison to surgery as a primary treatment option, with outcomes of pregnancy and cost-effectiveness in need of examination. Lastly, the desirability of pre-IVF medical treatment for 3 months to suppress the disease has been suggested to be of value in a small study;[21] confirmation by a large, multi-center randomized trial would provide needed assurance of the correctness of this approach.

The greatest issue in the treatment of endometriosis-associated infertility continues to revolve around the best approach to ovarian endometriomas. Surgery is an expensive and time-consuming option, particularly for the patient known to be undergoing IVF. Yet superior IVF success rates might justify this action. Is it worth risking the adverse effect upon oocyte development by an endometrioma to avoid surgical excision? Might surgery damage the ovary sufficiently such that it is actually more disadvantageous than expectant management? Could aspiration be superior to excision in the future IVF patient, or might the reverse be true? And finally, might some patients (older patients, women with decreased ovarian reserve) benefit specifically from one of these approaches versus the others? These are issues being asked on a daily basis and in dire need of scientific answers.

CONCLUSIONS

The history of endometriosis research has been littered with supposition, false claims, incorrect interpretation, near religious philosophical attacks, and ultimately a diffuse effort by the scientific community to build a complete and complex story. In this way it has not differed from most other areas of medicine. However, the story is not yet complete. We continue to have huge gaps in our knowledge regarding this fascinating disorder, and this chapter (indeed, this text) has attempted to outline some of the future directions we need to pursue to unravel more of the mysteries of endometriosis.

As a research community, we can make this task difficult or streamlined. Our failure to work cooperatively, our need to take ownership of specific lines of investigation, and our inability to freely share ideas and techniques continues to hamper efforts. Furthermore, our reasonably slow adoption of more modern investigative techniques, both in the basic and clinical arenas, has proven damaging. It is hoped that we as a cohort of interested and knowledgable investigators will, in the future, learn to be more effusive with our ideas, techniques, and findings. Cooperation of individuals, centers, and ultimately organizations will be the key to maximizing future productivity in research and seducing a new generation of eager minds into taking on the challenge we call endometriosis.

REFERENCES

1. Koninckx PR. Barlow D. Kennedy S. Implantation versus infiltration: the Sampson versus the endometriotic disease theory. Gynecol Obstet Invest 1999;47 Suppl1:3–9.
2. D'Hooghe TM, Bambra CS, Suleman Ma et al. Development of a model of retrograde menstruation in baboons (*Papio anubis*). Fertil Steril 1994;62:635–8.
3. Cooke ID, Thomas EJ. The medical treatment of mild endometriosis. Acta Obstet Gynecol Scand 1989;150 (Suppl):27–30.
4. Cho NH, Park YK, Kim YT, Yang H, Kim SK. Lifetime expression of stem cell markers in the uterine endometrium. Fertil Steril 2004;81:403–7.
5. Dmowski WP, Steele RW, Baker GF. Deficient cellular immunity in endometriosis. Am J Obstet Gynecol 1981;141:377–83.
6. Osteen KG, Yeaman GR, Bruner-Tran K. Matrix metalloproteinases and endometriosis. Sem Reprod Med 2003;21:155–63.
7. Oral E, Arici A. Pathogenesis of endometriosis. Obstet Gynecol Clin North Am 1997;24:219–33.
8. Haney AF, Muscato JJ, Weinberg JB. Peritoneal fluid cell populations in infertility patients. Fertil Steril 1981;35:696–8.
9. Halme J, Becker S, Hammond M, Raj MH, Raj S. Increased activation of pelvic macrophages in infertile women with mild endometriosis. Am J Obstet Gynecol 1983;145:333–7.
10. Halme J, White C, Kauma S, Estes J, Haskill S. Peritoneal macrophages from patients with endometriosis release growth factor activity in vitro. J Clin Endocrinol Metab 1988;66:1044–9.
11. Hastings JM, Fazleabas AT. Future directions in endometriosis research. Sem Reprod Med 2003;21:255–62.
12. Noble LS, Simpson ER, Johns A, Bulun SE. Aromatase expression in endometriosis. J Clin Endocrinol Metab 1996;811:174–9.
13. Fazleabas AT, Brudney A, Chai D, Langoi D, Bulun SE. Steroid receptor and aromatase expression in baboon endometriotic lesions. Fertil Steril 2003;80 Suppl:2820–7.
14. Simon C, Gutierrez A, Vidal A et al. Outcome of patients with endometriosis in assisted reproduction: results from in-vitro fertilization and oocyte donation. Human Reproduction 1994;9:725–9.
15. Lessey BA, Castelbaum AJ, Sawin SJ et al. Aberrant integrin expression in the endometrium of women with endometriosis. J Clin Endocrinol Metab 1994;79:643–9.
16. Garrido N, Navarro J, Garcia-Velasco J et al. The endometrium versus embryonic quality in endometriosis-related infertility. Hum Reprod Update 2002;81:95–103.
17. Pellicer A, Navarro J, Bosch E et al. Endometrial quality in infertile women with endometriosis. Ann NY Acad Sci 2001;943:122–30.
18. Stratton P, Winkel C, Premkumar A et al. Diagnostic accuracy of laparoscopy, magnetic resonance imaging, and histopathologic examination for the detection of endometriosis. Fertil Steril 2003;79:1078–85.
19. Walter AJ, Hentz JG, Magtibay PM, Cornella JL, Magrina JF. Endometriosis: correlation between histologic and visual findings at laparoscopy. Am J Obstet Gynecol 2001;184:1407–11.
20. Gagne D, Rivard M, Page M et al. Development of a nonsurgical diagnostic tool for endometriosis based on the detection of endometrial leukocyte subsets and serum CA-125 levels. Fertil Steril 2003;80:876–85.
21. Surrey ES, Silverberg KM, Surrey MW, Schoolcraft WB. Effect of prolonged gonadotropin-releasing hormone agonist therapy on the outcome of in vitro fertilization-embryo transfer in patients with endometriosis. Fertil Steril 2002 78:699–704.

Index